Chiropractic Standards of Practice and Quality of Care

Edited by
Herbert J. Vear, DC, FCCS, LLD
President
Council on Chiropractic Education (Canada)
Pickering, Ontario, Canada
and
President Emeritus
Western States Chiropractic College
Portland, Oregon

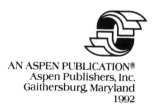

AN ASPEN PUBLICATION®
Aspen Publishers, Inc.
Gaithersburg, Maryland
1992

Library of Congress Cataloging-in-Publication Data

Chiropractic standards of practice and quality of care /
edited by Herbert J. Vear.
p. cm.
"An Aspen publication."
ISBN: 0-8342-0242-5
1. Chiropractic—Standards. I. Vear, Herbert J.
[DNLM: 1. Chiropractic—standards. 2. Quality of Health Care.
WB 905 C544]
RZ236.C48 1992
615.5'34—dc20
DNLM/DLC
for Library of Congress
91-22234
CIP

The authors have made every effort to ensure the accuracy of the information
herein, particularly with regard to drug selection and dose. However, appropriate
information sources should be consulted, especially for new or unfamiliar drugs or
procedures. It is the responsibility of every practitioner to evaluate the appropriateness of a particular opinion in the context of actual clinical situations and with
due consideration to new developments. Authors, editors, and the publisher cannot
be held responsible for any typographical or other errors found in this book.

Editorial Services: Ruth Bloom

Library of Congress Catalog Card Number: 91-22234
ISBN: 0-8342-0242-5

Printed in the United States of America

1 2 3 4 5

To Joyce

For her patience
and understanding

Table of Contents

Contributors

Robert Anderson, MD, PhD, DC
Director of Manual Medicine
San Francisco Spine Institute at Seton Medical
  Center
Professor of Anthropology
Mills College
Oakland, California

Lee E. Arnold, DC
Professor
Chiropractic Clinical Procedures and Diagnosis
National College of Chiropractic
Canadian Memorial Chiropractic College
Northwestern College of Chiropractic
St. Petersburg, Florida

Robert Boal, PhD
Professor of Biochemistry
Chair of Basic Sciences
Western States Chiropractic College
Portland, Oregon

Meridel I. Gatterman, MA, DC
Director, Division of Chiropractic Sciences
Associate Professor
Canadian Memorial Chiropractic College
Toronto, Ontario, Canada

Richard G. Gillette, MS
Assistant Professor of Physiology
Associate Director of Research
Western States Chiropractic College
Portland, Oregon

Daniel T. Hansen, DC
Board Certified Chiropractic Orthopedist
Fellow, International Collge of Chiropractors
Olympia, Washington

**Donald J. Henderson, BSc, DC,
  FCCS (C), DACBR, FCCR, FICC**
Chairman, Standards of Practice Committee
Canadian Chiropractic Association
Chairman, Chiropractic Advisory Committee
Healing Arts Radiation Protection Commission
Ministry of Health
Toronto, Ontario, Canada

Robert L. Hirtle, Jr., BSS, JD
Rogin, Nassau, Caplan, Lassman, & Hirtle
Hartford, Connecticut

Mark Kaminski, MS
Associate Professor of Physiology
Western States Chiropractic College
Portland, Oregon

Joseph C. Keating, Jr., PhD
Professor
Palmer College of Chiropractic-West
Sunnyvale, California

William C. Meeker, DC, MPH
Dean of Research
Palmer College of Chiropractic-West
Sunnyvale, California

Cynthia Peterson, RN, DC, DACBR
Anglo-European College of Chiropractic
Bournemouth, England
Former Chairperson, Department of Radiology
Western States Chiropractic College
Portland, Oregon

David H. Peterson, DC
Associate Professor of Chiropractic and Clinical
    Sciences
Chair of Chiropractic Sciences
Western States Chiropractic College
Portland, Oregon

Charles A. Simpson, DC, DABCO
Private Practice
Cornelius, Oregon

Richard H. Tilden, DC
Private Practice
Cornelius, Oregon

Susan L. Vlasuk, DC, DACBR
Charter President
American Chiropractic College of Thermology
Diagnostic Imaging Consultant
Bellevue, Washington

Walter J. Wardwell, PhD
Professor of Sociology Emeritus
University of Connecticut
Storrs, Connecticut

Foreword

As third-party reimbursements for chiropractors' services became more common, chiropractors evolved from what Freidson called "client dependent" to "colleague dependent,"[1] from needing only to attract and satisfy patients to having to meet practice standards generally accepted by the profession as a whole. The medical profession went through the same process earlier as it evolved from a simple group of isolated general practitioners to the complex system of interrelated hospital-based specialists that exists today. Because chiropractors have practiced mainly in ambulatory settings, they have not had the opportunity to develop the kind of peer review that hospitals (the prime promoters of health care quality) make possible. Consequently, the advantages of peer review for the maintenance and improvement of the quality of chiropractic care have been largely absent.

This book is about standards of practice established by colleagues. The questions of which colleagues should establish the standards and who is to enforce them are central for any profession. Because chiropractic is burdened with rival "schools," philosophies, and associations, these problems are especially difficult to resolve in chiropractic. The different definitions of the scope of practice enshrined in state licensing laws (something that medicine never had to confront) further complicate the issue and have delayed the process of achieving consensus.

Which colleagues should chiropractors depend on to establish practice standards? As Keating and Meeker emphasize in Chapter 2, they must be chiropractors, not members of other professions. Chiropractic practice is sufficiently different from medicine (concerned mostly with pharmacotherapy and surgical procedures) that only chiropractors can set the standards for chiropractic diagnosis, prognosis, and therapy. The public's interest will continue to be represented on licensing boards and college boards of trustees. Of course, it will be chiropractors who disseminate and interpret the standards—in colleges, in licensing examinations, and in regulating practice.

Besides chiropractors, malpractice attorneys, whether they represent plaintiffs or defendants, and third-party payers who review claims for chiropractic services will use these standards. Third-party payers, almost exclusively for financial reasons, insist on close scrutiny of both the *quality* of chiropractic care and its *quantity* (ie, the number of treatments). Whether their emphasis on costs serves to increase or decrease quality remains a matter for dispute. The administration of the standards should profit from medical and osteopathic experience whenever possible.

The establishment of appropriate standards of chiropractic care should improve quality by facilitating peer review and providing better ways to regulate practice. At the same time, it should encourage third-party payers to function more rationally and fairly. As we move toward a national health care system of a not-yet-determined type, these standards become ever more necessary. This book is a giant step toward that goal.

NOTE

1. Freidson E. *Profession of Medicine: A Study of the Sociology of Applied Knowledge.* New York: Dodd, Mead; 1970.

Walter J. Wardwell PhD
Professor of Sociology Emeritus
University of Connecticut
Storrs, Connecticut

Preface

As primary contact health care providers and a portal of entry to the health care delivery system, there is a responsibility for the chiropractic profession to adopt and practice a standard of quality care commensurate with that mandate. At the present time there is no collected work which provides documentation of standards and quality of care for use by educators, students, practitioners and special interest groups within the public and private sectors.

The purpose of this book is to provide documentation on how practice standards affect chiropractic education and clinical research, scope and standards of practice, quality and efficiency of care, contra-indications to chiropractic care, jurisprudence and malpractice, relationships with third-party payers and other health care professionals.

In Chapter 1, Vear provides a framework for the objectives of the book by examining the incongruity in chiropractic practice acts for definitions of key words and scope of practice. He reviews the development of educational standards and how restrictive basic science laws were slowly replaced by a professional commitment to formal accreditation of chiropractic education. This was followed by the Council on Chiropractic Education reaching consensus on adopting measurable clinical competency outcomes, which may have been the beginning of practice standards for the profession.

Keating and Meeker set the tone for the intent and purpose of the succeeding chapters in Chapter 2. They identify succinctly the conundrum created by chiropractic's mosaic structure, as demonstrated by philosophy (science vs. fundamentalism), dogma (cultist methods vs scientific rationale in clinical care), the lack of predictive values, and, most important, the traditional anecdotal/empirical constructs used for untested clinical procedures. They present a number of experimental and statistical strategies that may be used to establish consensual standards of practice based on extensive quantitative and experimental evaluations. Although they recognize the need for qualified chiropractic scientists in performing these evaluations, they also recognize the importance of the motivated individual practitioner to the process. They suggest that practitioners must read, evaluate, and use the findings of science. In addition, they advocate research in practice "in proposing diagnostic and treatment hypotheses, in reporting clinical observations, and in field testing the results of large scale, college- and university-based clinical trials."

In Chapter 3, Vear proposes a generic approach to a chiropractic scope-of-practice definition, as there is a serious vacuum in defining what chiropractic physicians agree on and what they do in clinical practice. Vear recognizes that states, provinces, and countries retain the sovereign right to define the parameters of practice for all health care disciplines and that it will be some time before a consensus on the scope of chiropractic practice will become a reality. There should be optimism, however, that chiropractic educational institutions, worldwide, can reach agreement on this important topic and other parallel issues by using consensus strategies.[1] It does not seem possible for the chiropractic profession to resolve the problems of standards of care, quality of care, and outcome measurements without first reaching agreement on the scope of chiropractic practice.

Vear presents a scope of practice model for chiropractic education in Chapter 4, along with definitions of key words. The model includes a primary chiropractic practice core for the minimum scope of practice in all jurisdictions. This is followed by a discussion of additional areas of clinical activity (eg, adjunctive procedures, nutrition) where statute allows for these activities. Chapter 4 also provides a generic approach to standards of practice, which can be construed to be a "patient's chiropractic bill of rights." A distinction is made between the process of chiropractic education, with its attendant standards, and the practice of clinical chiropractic, with its attendant standards mandated by statute, ethics, morality, and other measurements of quality practice assigned to health care providers. In some respects, Chapter 4 provides what Donabedian defined as "process."

> By asserting that the quality of medical care is an attribute that care may have to a greater or a lesser degree, I have implied that the primary object of study is a set of activities that go on within and between practioners and patients. A judgment concerning the quality of that process may be made either by direct observation or by review of recorded information, which allows a more or less accurate reconstruction of what goes on.[2(p41)]

The remainder of this book builds on Donabedian's concept of process and enters into what he defined as "outcomes," meaning a change in a patient's current and future health status that can be attributed to antecedent health care. By postulating a rather broad definition of health, I shall include improvement of social and psychological function in addition to the more usual emphasis on the physical and physiological aspects of performance.[2(p83)]

Chapter 5 emphasizes the importance of quality assurance and standards of care to chiropractic practice. In fact, the main thrust is a discussion of what constitutes reasonable and necessary services for reimbursement. The author, Hansen, concludes that public and private third-party agencies are influencing quality assurance and standards of care in an effort to control the escalating costs of health care, now at 12% of the gross national income.[3] The question of unnecessary and inappropriate care is reviewed as a component of rising health care costs. The essence of Chapter 5 is best expressed in Hansen's description.

This chapter follows the chiropractic profession through its struggle to decide what ethically comprises "chiropractic necessity" and how it might address standardization as it relates to utilization and quality assurance. Identification of the historical "false standards" and their impact on utilization of chiropractic services by the consumer public is put in context with current trends toward managed care, purchaser-generated utilization guidelines and development of problem-oriented clinical algorithms.

A major impact of Chapter 5 is the emphasis that Hansen places on defining the terminology used in the managed health care system, which places a responsibility upon the chiropractic profession to use such terminology in its proper accepted context. The glossary includes all terminology that Hansen recommends. Of particular importance to the reader are the figures that accompany the text and provide clarification.

Patients consult chiropractors for a great variety of physical complaints. Most problems are benign in origin, and treatment is without incident. These problems require the usual and expected standard of care and skill necessary in ensuring that there are no contraindications to treatment, however. In Chapter 6, Henderson emphasizes that one particular area, the upper cervical spine, demands that the chiropractor take extraordinary care and caution. In recent malpractice claims, it has been proved that cervical manipulation can lead to a cerebrovascular accident. Henderson provides a comprehensive approach to the cervical spine, emphasizing the importance of patient screening when upper cervical manipulative adjustments are contemplated. He sets forth the best current evaluative procedure in determining risk. He provides the chiropractic physician with an algorithm, but cautions that it cannot substitute for the conscientious and seasoned skill of a primary care practitioner. Material in the chapter that will be of daily value to the physician is a patient questionnaire to help identify vertebrobasilar insufficiency and a table listing radiographic findings with clinical concerns identified.

In Chapter 7, Boal, Kaminski, Peterson, and Gillette examine a practical model for determining the validity of clinical procedures used in chiropractic practice. They recognize that the issue of standards for the diagnostic and therapeutic methods used in chiropractic practice is a difficult, controversial, and often emotional issue. However, they ask the simple question, How does a profession determine standards for the methods used in practice? They proceed to review the procedures available to investigators and present the details of the model of assessment for clinical validation that they have developed. It is their opinion that, although the model does not address ways to develop consensus, it does focus on the important questions that must be asked for diagnostic and treatment validation.

Chapters 8, 9, and 10 examine in considerable detail relationships with patients and other health care professionals where clinical investigation is concerned. Anderson begins this discussion with a description of protocols that should be adopted by chiropractic physicians when making referrals to other health care providers, including hospitals, and the importance of communication skills when addressing the public and other professionals. In his conclusion for Chapter 8, Anderson writes, "no clinician knows enough to take complete responsibility for every patient. . . . health care has become so complex that we must all work in a context of specialization and subspecialization." This statement supports the growing recognition of chiropractic as a limited profession in health care, a designation that the profession should embrace by defining the objectives of chiropractic health care within the totality of health care.

Peterson, the author of Chapter 9, and Vlasuk, the author of Chapter 10, examine standards and procedures for evaluating the patient's clinical condition. They set forth protocols to assist the clinician in arriving at a defensible diagnosis and treatment plan based on orthodox procedures and technology. Because clinical procedures and technology will be under constant review for validity and appropriateness in the future, standards must be fluid.

Chapters 11, 12, and 13 focus on the relationship of the chiropractic profession to the courts and third-party payers. In Chapter 11, Gatterman recognizes that the use of spinal manipulation, the primary therapeutic modality of the chiropractic profession, requires consideration of contraindications or nonindications, where manipulation may be life-threatening. Her analysis of this question reinforces what has been written in previous chapters, particularly in Chapter 6.

The literature is replete with unfortunate outcomes of the use of spinal manipulative therapy, even when great caution has been exercised.[4-6] The chiropractor's failure to exercise the prudence expected of a reasonable chiropractic physician is the primary cause of malpractice claims. Hirtle, in Chapter 12 examines this issue and the tort system or negligence system of tort lawsuits, which provides the basis for a patient's claim of malpractice. His emphasis on the responsibilities of the reasonable physician is amplified by this statement: "The chiropractic physician is bound to use toward his or her patients reasonable care, skill, and diligence. By that is meant the care, skill, and diligence that chiropractors in the same line of practice ordinarily have and exercise in like cases."

Simpson and Tilden, the authors of Chapter 13, cover in detail the responsibilities of physicians and the behavior that is expected and required of them in relationships with third-party payer organizations, which range from government-sponsored health insurance plans to small self-insured companies. Each is concerned with the standards and quality of care provided by health care providers to the insured patient. The process for insuring and providing health care in the United States is likely to lead to a universal coverage national health care insurance plan, as is already in place in Canada and other countries. If the experience of other countries is any indication, such a plan could radically change the role of chiropractic practice. This change will focus on standards of practice and care, quality assurance, and treatment outcomes. Thus, it is imperative for the profession as a whole to address the issue of communication and cooperation with the third-party system, and Simpson and Tilden have provided important guidelines for the profession in this area.

This book is not the first attempt to address the question of standards for chiropractic practice. The profession has come full circle from establishing its standards based on the wisdom of private interests, state and provincial practice acts, local and national associations, accredited colleges, and insurance and government organizations, and it must once again accept the responsibility for establishing its own standards. The danger rests with procrastination and disinterest by the average practitioner, who is not always exposed to the pressures of other health care professions.

It is the editor's hope and expectation that this book will provide a platform for the first step toward a more responsible profession. Responsibility must include consensus on definitions for scope of practice, chiropractic terminology, and standards of practice before any progress in establishing standards of care, quality assurance, and treatment outcomes can be realized.

REFERENCES

1. Fink A, et al. Consensus methods: characteristics and guidelines for use. *Am J Pub Health.* 1984;74:971–983.

2. Donabedian A. *Explorations in Quality Assessment and Monitoring,* vol. I. The definition of quality and approaches to its assessment. Ann Arbor, Mich: Health Administration Press, 1980:80–84.

3. Vital signs. *J Am Chiro Assoc.* 1990;27(11):12.

4. Livingston CP. Spinal manipulation causing injury: a three year study. *Clin Orthop.* 1971;81:82–86.

5. Ladermann JP. Accidents of spinal manipulation. *Annals Swiss Chir Assoc.* 1981;7:162–208.

6. Terrett AB. It is more important to know when not to adjust. *Chiropractic Technique.* 1990;2:1–8.

1

Introduction

Herbert J. Vear

> Don't attempt to maintain self respect by maintaining self deception. Chiropractic facts must not be buried by the embellishment of philosophy.
>
> —*Joseph J. Janse, DC*

In the past, standards for chiropractic practice were commonly based on the opinion and empirical experience of an author/entrepreneur and whatever biases that person brought to the work. In addition, the work focused on a single subject or topic within the broad base of chiropractic practice, such as chiropractic diagnosis, spinal adjustive technique, extremity adjusting, and spinal x-ray marking,[1-8] with few if any scientific references. The standards or guidelines emphasized the specifics of application for a particular system or procedure rather than patients' complaints and/or clinical outcomes. Although such specificity should continue, all such works must also include criteria firmly based in the scientific evaluation of clinical procedures and consensus by experts within the profession. Of course, not all clinical procedures can be "scientifically validated." In fact, it is unlikely that more than a small percentage will be so validated in the foreseeable future. Regardless, the principles underlying the clinical procedure should not be at variance with scientific knowledge as interpreted by a consensus of experts.

As the chiropractic profession prepares to celebrate its centennial, it faces unique challenges. First, the profession has a duty to create standards of practice that will advance the extent and quality of chiropractic health care, protect patient rights, and ensure the independence of chiropractic physicians in the health care marketplace; second, the profession must reach a consensus on standards of care through the assessment of outcomes, an analysis of the effectiveness of care, and quality assurance necessary for that care. The profession is currently pursuing standards of practice and care in a dynamic fashion that is exemplary for a patient-oriented health care profes-

1

sion. For example, the Consensus Conference on the Validation of Chiropractic Methods (Seattle, Washington, March 1989[9]), the International Conference on Spinal Manipulation (Washington, DC, May 1990), and the Consortia (Pacific) for Chiropractic Research Consensus Conference on Chiropractic Technique (Monterey, California, June 1991) are part of the profession's efforts to address a complex subject. In addition, numerous colleges and associations are beginning to emphasize practice standards in continuing education programs. The external forces that impeded chiropractic progress in the past still remain in many quarters, however.

After more than 95 years of providing effective conservative health care to millions of patients, the chiropractic profession is able to demonstrate scientifically the clinical efficacy of that care in only a few conditions. This unacceptable record stands in stark contrast to the exorbitant claims made for chiropractic spinal adjustments since 1895. In the beginning, anecdotal testimony by patients and practitioners provided all that was necessary to "stake out" the chiropractic therapeutic territory, a territorial imperative followed by all health care professions of that time.

In contrast, recent decades have witnessed a growing public clamor for greater accountability by all health care professions and for improved quality of care and clinical outcomes. For the chiropractic profession, this requires (1) reaching consensus on standards for today's professional practice, (2) conducting controlled clinical research studies in areas where there is no consensus, (3) reporting of clinical trials and/or single patient studies, and (4) reaching consensus for a scope of practice based on scientific criteria rather than relying on anecdotal data. Chiropractic is not the only profession in which there have been problems in documenting clinical efficacy in a scientific manner.[10] Rachlis and Kushner (1989) wrote, "As many as 80% of all treatments, including surgeries, have never been scientifically tested to prove their worth. Medical history is littered with abandoned therapies that were once common practice but are now utterly discredited."[11]

One of the major reasons that those in the chiropractic profession and colleges have not pursued clinical research with more vigor has been the isolated position in which the medical and higher education communities placed chiropractic practice and education prior to the acceptance of the Council on Chiropractic Education as the official accrediting body by the US Department of Education in 1974 and the Council on Postsecondary Accreditation in 1976. The financial loss to the profession attributed to the denial of research funds because of this involuntary isolation will never be known. No doubt, it could be measured in the billions. The "continental divide" between the anecdotal era and the scientific era of chiropractic practice followed the 1974 accreditation of chiropractic education and the February, 1975 National Institute of Neurological and Communicative Disorders and

Stroke (NINCDS) conference held in Bethesda, Maryland,[12] which examined the research status of spinal manipulative therapy.

CHIROPRACTIC PRACTICE ACTS

The majority of chiropractic practice acts in the United States and Canada were passed between 1913 and 1940. All jurisdictions in the United States and five provinces in Canada had chiropractic practice acts by 1975. Now, there are chiropractic practice acts that define the practice of chiropractic and establish regulations for licensure, discipline, and scope of practice in all 60 jurisdictions of the United States and Canada.

Chiropractic Definitions

The diversity of definitions for the chiropractic lexicon found in chiropractic practice acts exemplifies the problems that face the profession as negotiations for agreement on basic definitions begin. Regardless of the vehicle used to achieve consensus for definition and purpose of the profession, progress will be painfully slow. This is demonstrated by a recent news release in which the International Chiropractic Association announced policies on diagnosis, immunization, fluoridation, and scope of practice in isolation from other organized segments of the profession.[13]

An examination of the 52 chiropractic practice acts of the United States adds to the confusion of the definition problem facing the profession.[14,15(p10)] Reaching agreement on the definitions of subluxation and adjustment—two terms fundamental to all chiropractic physicians—and manipulation may prove to be a monumental task in itself. For example, subluxation, the most respected biological concept in chiropractic science, does not receive much respect in the 52 practice acts.

- Only four acts use the word *subluxation* alone, without definition or modifiers.
- Only four acts include a definition of the word *subluxation,* and there is no uniformity in definition from one act to another.
- Nine practice acts include modifiers to describe the word *subluxation* (eg, malposition, nerve transmission and expression, misalignment, imbalance with distortion).
- Six practice acts make no reference to the word *subluxation.*
- Twenty-eight practice acts use other terms, alone or in combination,

without the word *subluxation* (eg, anatomical displacements, abnormal functioning articulations, interference of transmission and expression of nerve energy, science of palpating articulations, treatment of human ailments, any misplaced tissues, malposition of articulations, realignment of the spine to release pressure on nerves).

• One practice act has no reference to any of these terms.

Adjustment, probably the most revered and defended word in chiropractic practice, identifies the preferred treatment modality. It fares better in the 52 practice acts.

• Twenty-three practice acts use the word *adjust* without any modifiers or definition.
• Three practice acts use the word *adjust* with a definition or modifier.
• Nineteen practice acts use the words *adjust* and *manipulation* equally and complementary to each other.
• Three practice acts use terms other than *adjust* or *manipulation* without reference to either (eg, externally applied mechanical pressures; correction, manual or mechanical).

Manipulation, a word very prominent in practice acts, is rejected by many chiropractors who adhere to a more fundamental philosophical focus. It is their position that manipulation is not chiropractic.

• Two practice acts use the word *manipulation* alone and without modifiers or definition.
• One practice act uses the word *manipulation* with a modifier (eg, preparatory procedure).

Those in the chiropractic profession would be wise to use the terminology that they adopt from the lexicon of the scientific community (eg, manual therapy, manipulation) according to the accepted definitions. The terminology that originates within chiropractic science (eg, adjustment, subluxation/fixation) must be defined on a consensus basis, however, and used uniformly as such by the profession and its educational institutions.

Scope of Chiropractic Practice

The same 52 practice acts only confuse the question further when they address the scope of chiropractic practice. The diversity of interpretation is bewildering at best. Definitive analysis of all 52 statutes' scope statements is unproductive, but three states, Pennsylvania, Illinois, and Alaska, have recently enacted new or amended practice acts with varying scope-of-practice descriptions.

Pennsylvania

In 1986, the Pennsylvania state legislature defined the scope of chiropractic practice under the heading Chiropractic.

> Chiropractic. A branch of the healing arts dealing with the relationship between the articulations of the vertebral column, as well as other articulations, and the neuro-musculo-skeletal system and the role of these relationships on the restoration and maintenance of health. The term shall include systems of locating misaligned or displaced vertebrae of the human spine and other articulations; the examination preparatory to the adjustment or manipulation of such misaligned or displaced vertebrae and other articulations; the adjustment or manipulation of such misaligned or displaced vertebrae and other articulations; the furnishing of necessary patient care for the restoration and maintenance of health; and the use of board approved scientific instruments of analysis including X-ray. The term shall also include diagnosis, provided that such diagnosis is necessary to determine the nature and appropriateness of chiropractic treatment; the use of adjunctive procedures in treating misaligned or dislocated vertebrae or other articulations and related conditions of the nervous system, provided that, after January 1, 1988, the licensee must be certified in accordance with this act to use adjunctive procedures; and nutritional counseling, provided that nothing herein shall be construed to require licensure as a chiropractor in order to engage in nutritional counseling. The term shall not include the practice of obstetrics or gynecology, the reduction of fractures or major dislocations, or the use of drugs or surgery.[16]

Although the Pennsylvania act does not define the terms *subluxation, adjustment,* or *manipulation,* the regulations and rules adopted by the State Board of Chiropractic may have such definitions.

Illinois

The Illinois Medical Practice Act of May, 1987, which regulates and licenses chiropractors, was amended in 1989 to include definitions for *chiropractic, subluxation, spinal adjustment,* and *spinal analysis.*

> "Chiropractic" means a limited primary health care profession that contributes to health through the analysis and adjustment of subluxations in the spinal column.
>
> "Subluxation" means a slight mal-articulation of a spinal column segment which occurs in such a way as to disturb nerve function and interfere with the ability of the human body to regain or maintain health.
>
> "Spinal adjustment" means a specific, localized force introduced to tissue overlaying a segment of the spinal column for the singular purpose of correcting subluxations within the spinal column.
>
> "Spinal analysis" means determining the presence and character of subluxations within the spinal column, and the appropriateness of chiropractic care, through the use of spinal radiographs, accepted non-surgical and non-medical examining and non-invasive instrumentation techniques. [17]

Prior to its amendment, the Illinois act did not define chiropractic by statute, but did provide a scope of practice: "the practice of any system or method of treating human ailments without the use of drugs or medicines and without operative surgery.[15(p82)] This may be the first time that chiropractic is defined by statute as "a limited health care profession," although the American Public Health Association (APHA) had earlier adopted a similar position.[18] Classifying chiropractic as a limited health care profession does not detract from the responsibilities and duties of a primary contact physician.

Alaska

The Alaska Chiropractic Act of May, 1988 is the most definitive and descriptive of current chiropractic practice acts.[19] Trevor V. Ireland of Anchorage (written communication, June 23, 1988) provided an excellent summary, from which the following is excerpted.

> The new law separates "Chiropractic Core Methodology" from "Ancillary Methodology." Ancillary methodology is viewed as common domain with the understanding that x-rays and physical therapy machines and devices, stethoscopes, thermometers, etc., are "tools of science" and therefore do not belong to any singular profession. It addresses "functional integrity of skeletal joint structures," "physiological efficiency of the nervous system," "subluxation complex," "chiropractic diagnostic impression," "biomechanical analysis," "ramifications of health and disease," "inher-

ent recuperative powers," "chiropractic adjustment," "interference with normal nerve transmission and expression," [and it] focuses on the detection, correction, and prevention of the subluxation complex.

The definition for *chiropractic adjustment* incorporates the phrase "angular movement." In *Dorland's Illustrated Medical Dictionary,* angular movement is defined as "a movement which changes the angle between two bones."[20]

> "Chiropractic adjustment" means the application of a precisely controlled force applied by hand or by mechanical device to a specific focal point of the anatomy for the express purpose of creating a desired angular movement in skeletal joint structures in order to eliminate or decrease interference with neural transmission and correct or attempt to correct subluxation complex; chiropractic adjustment utilizes, as appropriate, short lever force, high velocity force, short amplitude force, or specific line-of-correction force to achieve the desired angular movement, as well as low force neuro-muscular, neuro-cranial, or neuro-lymphatic reflex technique procedures.
>
> "Manipulation" means an application of a resistive movement by applying a nonspecific force without the use of a thrust, that is directed into a region and not into a focal point of the anatomy for the general purpose of restoring movement and reducing fixations.[20]

The definition for adjustment is lengthy, but it introduces the bioengineering concept of "angular movement." The added emphasis on types of "force" and the recognition of nonforce adjustments amplifies the importance of this singular treatment modality to the chiropractic profession. Rather than looking for short definitions for key words and phrases, such as adjustment, the profession may be advised to do a definitive description of all such words.

If there is a problem of definition, scope, and standards of practice in contemporary practice acts, that same problem is compounded when "old" statutes and regulations are examined. As Kusserow succinctly stated, "The State's practice act definitions of what a chiropractor may and may not do differ substantially across the nation. This variability seriously undermines the desire of many chiropractors to be regarded as a unified profession with clearly established standards for practice and treatment."[21] Lamm, who conducted a survey of North American practice acts concluded that

the results of the survey, while revealing a broad scope of chiropractic practices, also demonstrated a lack of consensus within the
chiropractic profession. It is not unexpected that this not only
causes confusion in the minds of those within the chiropractic
profession but also in the minds of those who access services from
or conduct business with chiropractors.[22]

As important as consensus is for defining chiropractic as a health discipline with an appropriate scope of practice, including agreement on definitions for subluxation, adjustment, and manipulation, there are even larger
problems facing the profession during this decade. Beyond the growing
public concern about excessive health care costs (largely due to overservicing
patients, unnecessary diagnostic and treatment procedures, and duplication
of costly resources), it is necessary to develop quality assurance parameters
for standards of care, quality of care, and outcome of care measurements.
This will not be an easy task. In fact, the resources required, not to mention
the costs, are astronomical for a small profession like chiropractic. Although
allopathic medicine may appear to be better placed and prepared for the task
than chiropractic, based on financial, physical, and professional resources,
the comprehensive scope of medical practice (medicine and surgery) makes
the task equally difficult in that profession.[23-25]

CLINICAL EDUCATION STANDARDS FOR CHIROPRACTIC COLLEGES

It is a widely held opinion that chiropractic practice acts in the United
States and Canada helped to establish the criteria for curriculum development
in chiropractic colleges.[26] Actually, the *Flexner Report on Medical Education in the United States and Canada,* published in 1910, established a
standard medical curriculum that became the model for chiropractic practice
acts and, inevitably, for curriculum planning and development in chiropractic
colleges.[27]

In the beginning, chiropractic educational standards were proprietary, with
no form of control other than competition between schools. Chiropractic
colleges had little in common for course offerings, length of the course of
study, curriculum design, educational facilities, admission standards, or faculty qualifications.[28] Chiropractic education ranged from short correspondence courses, to short apprenticeship experiences, to short residence courses.
(It was not until the 1930s that some colleges became independent, not-for-
profit institutions.) Furthermore, from the very beginning (circa 1910), colleges were separated by philosophical differences in regard to the scope of

practice and treatment modalities. These differences contributed to the potpourri of educational offerings.

In 1925, Connecticut and Wisconsin introduced the first basic science laws.[29] By 1970, there were basic science laws in 22 states. These laws required all health care graduates who applied for state licensure to pass a basic science examination administered by a state-appointed Basic Science Board. The majority of state basic science examinations covered anatomy, bacteriology, physiology, chemistry, hygiene, sanitation, and pathology.[30] Aspiring chiropractors were required to pass the basic science examination before writing chiropractic board examinations.[30] In some states, the failure rate was such that few, if any, chiropractors were licensed for a decade or more (personal communication with R. W. Gibbons, April 1988).

Although basic science laws were a serious deterrent to the free movement of chiropractors within the United States and received severe criticism from most chiropractic leaders, there were a few chiropractic academics who not only supported such laws, but also advocated them for the good of the profession. As Gatterman wrote on the significant contributions of W.A. Budden, DC to chiropractic education during his tenure as president of the Western States Chiropractic College (1929–1954):

> Dr. Budden was of the opinion that requirements of the basic science exams were not prejudicial to those wanting chiropractic to become one of the learned professions, with educational institutions of equivalent rating. He felt that those opposing these laws were willing to let the profession degenerate into a trade with their teaching institutions equivalent to trade schools.[31]

Soon after the introduction of basic science laws, most chiropractic colleges did indeed upgrade basic science faculty, facilities, and teaching. There can be no doubt, however, that the medical profession invented basic science laws as a legal weapon to control the proliferation of chiropractors.

Professional concern for the quality of chiropractic education dates back to 1935 when the first voluntary efforts were made to improve the situation. The National Chiropractic Association, later the American Chiropractic Association, formed a Committee on Educational Standards, which developed the first educational standards for chiropractic colleges. In 1941, the committee released its first list of 12 status institutions following an evaluation of compliance with the new standards by chiropractic colleges. During this time, the first standard basic curriculum was developed and approved by all the US chiropractic colleges and National Chiropractic Association and the International Chiropractors Associations.

In 1969, the Council on State Chiropractic Examining Boards, later the Federation of Chiropractic Licensing Boards, published a standard basic curriculum as its official position.[30] This action encouraged all colleges to meet this basic educational standard. Haynes stated, "In general the chiropractic licensing laws reflect the present knowledge explosion and academic norms. These laws have been amended so as to increase the educational requirements for chiropractic licensure, both as to quality and quantity."[30(p9)] Although written in 1970, the same statement applies today.

In 1971, the Council on Chiropractic Education (CCE) became an autonomous, national organization advocating high standards for chiropractic education. On December 11, 1975, the CCE became the official chiropractic accrediting agency under the US Department of Education, with funding support from the American Chiropractic Association, the International Chiropractic Association, the Federation of Chiropractic Licensing Boards, and the member CCE chiropractic colleges. Since then, the CCE has prescribed all educational standards, including admissions and curriculum, in the *Educational Standards for Chiropractic Colleges.*[32] These standards are intended as qualitative, not quantitative, guidelines for chiropractic institutions. The CCE wants colleges to be as educationally varied as possible within the standards. Moreover, after the CCE became the approved accrediting agency for chiropractic education, most basic science laws were rescinded.

On February 12, 1977, the Federation of Chiropractic Licensing Boards adopted a resolution by unanimous vote, stating

> that the purpose of a basic curriculum in the education of the chiropractic practitioner is to provide a thorough understanding of the structure and function of the human organism in health and disease.
>
> The curriculum should provide a means for identifying deviations from normal structure and function, while providing the essential facts required for diagnosis, prognosis, and treatment of disease. The curriculum shall encompass and shall be presented over a period of time as prescribed by the Council on Chiropractic Education or its equivalent as the official accrediting agency for the chiropractic profession approved by the United States Office of education.
>
> Current Educational Standards of the Council on Chiropractic Education require all candidates to furnish proof of having acquired at least two years or 60 acceptable semester hours, leading to a Baccalaureate Degree in the Arts and Sciences, including laboratory courses in biology and chemistry.

> The curriculum shall be presented over a minimum period of eight semesters or the equivalent, for a total of not less than 4,200 hours.[15(p82)]

The resolution ends with a list of the required curriculum offerings.

Once again, the Federation of Chiropractic Licensing Boards adopted the CCE standards for education and then translated these standards into state administrative rules. The early versions of a basic standard curriculum specified not only the subjects, but also the topics to be taught in each subject and the subject hour requirements.[30] Fortunately, the prescriptive nature of the standard curriculum no longer applies.

The CCE 1985 *Annual Report* provided a good description of the concern that CCE has for the licensing needs of the Federation of Chiropractic Licensing Boards and its state members.

> Due to the quality standards exhibited by the CCE, the Federation of Chiropractic Licensing Boards recommended to the various state licensing boards that applicants for licensure should be graduates from chiropractic colleges having status with the CCE's Commission on Accreditation or a college meeting equivalent standards. The licensing jurisdictions of the 50 states recognized the wisdom of this recommendation.
>
> As a responsible accrediting body, the CCE standards had to provide for the educational needs of all licensing jurisdictions in the United States. In some states, chiropractors are licensed to utilize treatment procedures that exclude only prescription drugs and major surgery. In other states, however, treatment procedures are more limited by definition. CCE does not interfere with institutional philosophy. If an institution chooses not to prepare students for practice in all states by limiting its teaching of treatment methods, it may do so provided it properly informs the student consumer of the practice limitations of that education as well as the current states in which he or she will not qualify for licensure. If, on the other hand, an institution does in fact undertake to prepare students for practice in liberal statutes by offering courses in a broad range of treatment procedures, it must then also provide adequate clinical experience in those treatment procedures.[28(p11)]

The advancement and progress of chiropractic education has been driven by societal demand for responsible chiropractic health care through chiropractic practice acts. Initially, in view of the abysmal level of chiropractic education at that time, the passage of chiropractic practice acts was not an unfavorable development. In fact, chiropractors had been demanding that legislatures pass practice acts to enforce the standards of education and practice that were being developed by the profession itself. Sutherland wrote, "How may a suitable standard of professional practice be maintained if there are no provincial statutes under which such a standard may be enforced? The answer is, of course, that it cannot be done."[33] As time passed and the chiropractic educational establishment matured, however, statutory prescriptions for curriculum became a deterrent to education growth in the colleges. All chiropractic acts specify subjects that candidates must pass for registration. In 1988, nearly all jurisdictions required graduation from a CCE-accredited college, a national examining board license, and successful completion of specified state or provincial examinations.

STANDARDS OF CARE AND CLINICAL COMPETENCY

In the references available, the term *clinical competency* is not defined separately, but rather is included with the descriptions of quality of care. For example, Campbell, Ladenheim, Sherman, and Sportelli examined compliance with the legal standard of care in some detail and classified quality care as a duty to provide all patients "with competent clinical services."[34] They went on to argue that competence and quality are not carved in stone, that changes occur for a number of reasons, and that the prudent chiropractic physician attempts to keep up-to-date on changes of statute, judicial edicts, new technology, college training, practice specialization, and advertising. Rutstein and associates stated, "Quality is the effect of care on the health of the individual and of the population. Improvement in the quality of care should be reflected in better health."[35(p582)] Vear noted that "Standards of Quality of Care [are] concerned with outcome which can be verified by the direct measurement of the improved health of the individual or population served."[36(p34)] Donabedian defined quality assurance as two components:

> The first is system design, which includes all the measures that a particular organization, and also society at large, use to safeguard and promote the quality of health care. The second component is monitoring, which is the process by which performance is periodically or continuously reviewed and, when found deficient, first modified and then monitored once again. System design and monitoring should be an inseparable, mutually supportive pair.[37(p83)]

Webster's definition of competence is "having the necessary quality and skills, showing adequate skill, having legal capacity or qualification."[38(p200)]

Burg, Lloyd, and Templeton provided the following as measures of competency:

> A definition of competence is usually a set of statements which describe the abilities needed by a person to perform adequately his or her role in a variety of specified situations. The statements—the "components of competence"—ideally describe:
> 1. The specific abilities manifested by the competent individual.
> 2. The conditions under which each ability will be manifested.
> 3. The standards of ability at or above which competence will be declared.[39]

Role of the National Board of Chiropractic Examiners

The first national organization to evaluate the academic and clinical qualifications of candidates for chiropractic licensure was the National Board of Chiropractic Examiners, which administered its first examination in 1965. The National Board "has committed itself to the development and administration of quality examinations, the results of which may be used by state licensing boards in their determination of a candidate's academic and clinical competency."[40]

In 1987, the National Board of Chiropractic Examiners administered its first Written Clinical Competency Examination (WCCE) in an attempt to assist the states in the assessment of clinical competency skills. The Federation of Chiropractic Licensing Boards had requested such an examination. The *WCCE Guide* states,

> The questions assess competency and skills that are nationally accepted as necessary in light of common practice requirements. Additionally the WCCE test questions are not dependent on particular chiropractic philosophies or techniques, but rather are based on an objective assessment of necessary practice skills.[41]

At the present time, the National Board of Chiropractic Examiners academic/clinical science and clinical competency examinations are the final assessment of the practice preparedness of graduates of accredited colleges before licensure by state boards. Canada has a similar system, which is administered by the Canadian Chiropractic Examining Board. It is clear that the chiropractic profession, through its own initiative and funding has developed unique procedures to assess the basic clinical competency of licensure candidates.

Role of the CCE

In the United States, the CCE has played a continuous and important role in developing standards of practice and clinical competency. The Mission Statement of the CCE includes the following:

> The functions of the Council on Chiropractic Education are:
> 1. to determine chiropractic institutional effectiveness for purposes of accreditation. In accomplishing this, the CCE:
>   a. establishes educational standards of program quality and effectiveness for chiropractic institutions.
>   b. assures CCE's publics that chiropractic institutions meet minimal levels of program quality and effectiveness.[42(p1)]

In addition to meeting this CCE requirement, "an institution must provide evidence that its instructional program includes a statement on Clinical Competencies which incorporates the intent of the Clinical Competency document dated October 1, 1984 or as it is amended."[42(p48)]

CCE Clinical Competency Document

The realization by the CCE that there was considerable variance among the clinical skills and competencies provided by the CCE colleges resulted in the formation of a Clinical Quality Assurance Panel in 1981. The following is an excerpt from the introduction of that document:

> In July, 1981, the Council on Chiropractic Education initiated an effort to identify those minimal clinical competencies requisite to entrance into the profession of chiropractic. Consistent with the mandate to ensure frank discussion of the various positions regarding the educational component of clinical competency, an ad hoc task force representing all concerned constituencies was appointed to complete this project. Following consultation with authorities in the area of professional education, the task force conducted an intraprofessional dialogue through a polling process and a series of meetings which resulted in this document. The document reflects the consensus of the separate representatives; the task force has approved each competency by unanimous decision.
> The clinical competencies delineated herein address the minimal acceptable clinical criteria necessary to the conduct of a competent practice of chiropractic. They are not intended to limit the skill level attained through the resident clinical experience; rather, they identify the various cognitive, affective and psychomotor skills

expected of the non-specialist, primary contact Doctor of Chiropractic that are implicit in the first professional degree awarded by a college holding status with the Council on Chiropractic Education. These competencies do not reflect the mastery of clinical skills acquired through extensive practice experience; rather, they represent those minimal skills a candidate should demonstrate when presenting for licensure after completing the educational program with resident clinical experience in a status-holding institution.

The clinical competencies delineated herein are not intended to establish a universal standard of chiropractic care. . . .

It is generally held that the development of competency cannot be accomplished within the resident clinical experience alone. The integration of those preclinical sciences basic to chiropractic practice with courses in the clinical disciplines is necessarily prerequisite to a clinical experience in which these competencies may be appropriately demonstrated. The nature of the cognitive, affective and psychomotor domains in which they are delineated may require assessment methods unique to their particular domains; cognitive competencies might best be assessed with written instruments, affective competencies possibly evaluated by repeated observation during the clinical experience and technical skills evaluated by practical demonstration. The document serves only to delineate those competencies expected of the graduate; it is not intended to prescribe a curriculum or specify the manner in which these competencies may be addressed and evaluated. That function, quite properly, remains within the purview of the college itself.[43]

The document goes on for 45 pages to define those clinical competencies necessary for a new practitioner. Fourteen sections are indexed.

1. history
2. physical examination
3. neuromusculoskeletal examination
4. roentgenologic examination
5. clinical laboratory examination
6. "special studies" examinations
7. diagnosis or clinical impression
8. referral
9. treatment plan
10. spinal adjusting competencies
11. extraspinal adjusting competencies

12. nonadjustive competencies
13. case follow-up and review
14. record keeping

The format used to delineate the competencies in all sections is

1. cognitive competencies
    a. knowledge and understanding
    b. clinical judgment
2. affective competencies
    a. attitudes and habits
    b. interpersonal skills
3. psychomotor competencies: technical skills

The Clinical Competency Document is a landmark in the development of academic and clinical skills of the chiropractic profession.

CCE Standards of Care Document

An interesting document prepared by the CCE Task Force on Standards of Care in 1987 did not receive wide distribution, but it appears to be the first CCE document to address standards of practice in a chiropractic college clinic.[44] It contains definitions of the terms *quality assurance, criteria, accountability, utilization, evaluating care, and chiropractic mission.* Although the definitions are useful, they are not widely accepted, nor are they supported by a literature search. This may be the reason that the document was not widely distributed. Regardless, with literature support, it could have formed the basis for a commentary or editorial in a chiropractic journal and added support to the standards movement.

The list of criteria for quality care in chiropractic college clinics is little more than an outline for a college clinic manual. It provides no descriptive analyses and does not define the terms listed as criteria for quality care.

CONCLUSION

Clinical competency procedures have been adopted by the majority of chiropractic colleges beyond what is required by the CCE. Because the chiropractic graduate is a primary contact physician, it is imperative that the educational environment provide competency evaluation for this comprehensive practice role. Several college documents suggest that this is being done. Two colleges—School of Chiropractic, Phillips Institute, Australia, and the Canadian Memorial Chiropractic College—have published the procedures that they follow.[45,46]

REFERENCES

1. Langworthy SM, Smith O, Paxson MC. *Modernized Chiropractic.* Cedar Rapids, IA: American School of Chiropractic; 1906.

2. Beatty HG. *Anatomical Adjustive Technique.* 2nd ed. Denver, CO: authors; 1939.

3. Carver W. *Chiropractic Analysis 4th ed.* Oklahoma City: Carver Chiropractic College; 1912.

4. Gillet H. *Belgium Chiropractic Research Notes.* 8th ed. Brussels; 1970.

5. Illi F. *The Vertebral Column-Life Line of the Body.* Chicago: National College of Chiropractic; 1951.

6. Loban J. *Technic and Practice of Chiropractic.* Denver: Bun-Loban; 1928.

7. Logan HB. *Logan Basic Methods.* St. Louis: Logan College of Chiropractic; 1950.

8. Janse J., Wells R., Houser B. *Chiropractic Principles and Practice.* Chicago: National College of Chiropractic; 1947.

9. Bergmann T, ed. Proceedings: Consensus conference on chiropractic methods, March 2-3, 1990. *Chiropractic Technique.* 1990;2:75–161.

10. Epstein AM. The outcomes movement-will it get us were we want to go? *N Engl J Med.* 1990;323:266–269.

11. Rachlis M, Kushner C. *Second Opinion.* Toronto: Collins Publishers; 1989:10.

12. Goldstein M, ed. The research status of spinal manipulative therapy. Bethesda. MD: *US Department of Health, Education and Welfare,* 1975. NINCDS Monograph No. 15.

13. ICA Board adopts major new policies and resolutions for the 90s. Arlington, VA; International Chiropractors Association; 1990, news release, April 18.

14. Scope of chiropractic practice by statute, board rule/regulation. *ACA Legal Handbook.* American Chiropractic Association; 1985;2:1–76.

15. *Official Directory of Chiropractic Examining Boards with Licensure and Practice Statistics.* Glendale, Calif: Federation of Chiropractic Licensing Boards; 1988:4–62.

16. House Bill No. 1362, An Act for the Licensing of Chiropractors and the Regulation of the Practice of Chiropractic. ch18, § 2. Pennsylvania House of Representatives and Senate, November 25, 1986.

17. Medical practice act of 1987, ch111, § 2, amended 1989. Illinois General Assembly; 1989 and 1990.

18. Joint Policy Committee, American Public Health Association. Revised Chiropractic Health Care Resolution 8331, November 23, 1983.

19. An Act Relating to the Practice of Chiropractic. AS08.20.055, ch. 20, Legislature of the State of Alaska, Fifteenth Legislature—Second Session: S.B. 264;26 May, 1988.

20. Friel JP, ed. *Dorland's Illustrated Medical Dictionary.* 25th ed. Philadelphia: W.B. Saunders; 1974:984.

21. Kusserow RP. *State Licensure and Discipline of Chiropractors.* Office of Inspector General; 1989:10. US Dept of Health and Human Services publication OAI-01-88-00581.

22. Lamm LC. Chiropractic scope of practice: what the laws say. *Am J Chiropractic Medicine.* December 1989:159.

23. Kanouse DE, et al. *Changing Medical Practice through Technology Assessment—A Rand Corporation Study.* Ann Arbor: Mich: Association for Health Services Research and Health Administration Press: 1989.

24. Chassin MR, et al. *The Appropriateness of Selected Medical and Surgical Procedures, A Rand Corporation Study.* Ann Arbor, Mich: Association for Health Services Research and Health Administration, 1989.

25. Young ALC., ed. Quality of care. *Health Care Financing Review.* Baltimore, Md: Health Care Financing Administration; 1987 (suppl).

26. Vear. HJ Impressions concerning chiropractic education. *J Canadian Chiro Assoc.* March 1971:12–14.

27. Flexner A. *The Flexner Report on Medical Education in the United States and Canada, 1910.* Carnegie Foundation for the Advancement of Teaching.

28. *Council on Chiropractic Education Annual Report.* Des Moines, Iowa:CCE;1985:7.

29. Evans HW. *Historical Chiropractic Data.* Stockton, Calif: World-Wide Report; 1978.

30. Haynes GA. Analysis and evaluation of chiropractic education in the United States, Part 2. *Chirogram.* 1971;38:11.

31. Gatterman M. WA Budden: The transition through proprietary education, 1924–1954. *Chiropractic History.* 1982;2:22.

32. *Educational Standards for Chiropractic Colleges.* Des Moines, Iowa: Council on Chiropractic Education; 1988.

33. Sutherland DC. Chiropractic in Canada. *J Canada Chiro Assoc.* December 1974:7.

34. Campbell JK, Ladenheim CJ, Sherman RP, Sportelli L. *Risk Management in Chiropractic.* Fincastle, Va: Health Services Publications;1991:23.

35. Rutstein DD, Berenberg W, Chalmers TC, Child CG. Measuring the quality of medical care—a clinical method. *N Engl J Med.* 1976;294(11):582–588.

36. Vear HJ. Standards of chiropractic practice. *Journ Manipul Physio Thera.* 1985;1:34.

37. Donabedian A. Commentary on some studies of the quality of care. *Health Care Financing Review.* Baltimore, Md: Health Care Financing Administration; 1987(Suppl).

38. *New Lexicon Dictionary.* New York: Lexicon Publications; 1987:200.

39. Burg FD, Lloyd JS, Templeton B. Competence in medicine. *Medical Teacher.* 1982;4:60.

40. *Candidates Guide.* 5th ed. Greeley, Colo: National Board of Chiropractic Examiners; 1989.

41. *Written Clinical Competency Examination Candidate's Guide.* Greenley, Colo: National Board of Chiropractic Examiners; 1988.

42. *Standards for Chiropractic Institutions.* West Des Moines, Iowa: Council on Chiropractic Education; 1991.

43. *Clinical Competency Delineations Document.* West Des Moines, Iowa: Clinical Quality Assurance Panel, Council on Chiropractic Education; 1984:50.

44. Savage LJ, Canterbury R, Dallas W, Pedigo M, Poole P, Sawyer C. *Criteria for Quality Standards of Patient Care for Chiropractic College Clinics.* West Des Moines, Iowa: Council on Chiropractic Education; 1987.

45. Kobrossi T, Shut B. The use of objective structured clinical examination (OSCE) at the Canadian Memorial Chiropractic College outpatient clinic. *Canada Chiro Assoc.* 1987;31:21–25.

46. Jamison JR. Clinical competence: The use of simulators/models in diagnosis of visceral conditions. *J Manip Physio Ther.* 1989;12:10–14.

2

Philosophy, Research Methods, and Chiropractic Standards

Joseph C. Keating, Jr., and William C. Meeker

The call for standards of practice in chiropractic has grown louder of late. No longer is the issue of what a chiropractor does and does not do a matter for internal dispute alone. In this age of increasing accountability, the role of healers and the methods that they employ are no longer left to individual whims. Although physicians continue to be licensed to exercise their best judgments in meeting the idiosyncratic needs of the patient, scrutiny from government, third-party payers, and society is increasing. The question seems not to be whether there will be chiropractic standards, but rather the extent to which chiropractors will participate in establishing these criteria.

PROFESSIONAL STANDARDS

Traditionally, the closest thing to standards in the chiropractic profession has been found in the various licensing statutes and the curricula of the chiropractic colleges and the technique organizations. The former vary widely,[1,2] and they are often too general in terminology to specify methods and techniques. This generality is probably for the best, as the legal system ordinarily does not provide the flexibility that clinical standards may require. On the other hand, chiropractic curricula are often very specific, but they vary so widely that they are anything but standard. Chiropractic methods of assessment and intervention have been a focus of contention rather than consensus, a point not lost on many patients who change chiropractic doctors.

The existence of a standard implies the authoritative establishment of a criterion or rule. As already suggested, the authority for chiropractic standards may come from society, government, third parties (eg, insurers), and/or from the members of the profession. These interested parties may each establish criteria by which the profession and its individual members will be judged. The more widely accepted (or imposed) a rule becomes, the more "standardized" (and less ambiguous) it becomes. The focus of this chapter is primarily on standards developed by the discipline itself.

Standards developed by professionals themselves are consensual standards. Although professional associations may impose penalties upon members who violate standards, compliance is essentially voluntary; the most severe penalty that a professional association can impose is loss of membership. The authority of these standards derives primarily from agreement among members on the criteria of practice. The establishment of standards by a profession may, however, significantly influence the standard-setting activities of other interested parties and provides opportunities for the discipline to exercise moral leadership among all standard setters. For example, the establishment of educational standards by the Council on Chiropractic Education has averted or obviated the basic science laws that challenged the profession 50 years ago (see Chapter 1).

Consensual standards are published statements about appropriate and preferred strategies of interaction with patients. Standards provide guidelines by which individual doctors may govern themselves and by which others may judge the doctors' professional behavior. These criteria may be very broad (eg, to maintain optimal neural function or to reduce "nerve interference") or very specific (eg, to adjust only the atlas, using a toggle-recoil procedure, or to delay irradiation of low back pain patients until 2 weeks of spinal manipulation have proved unsuccessful). Some standards specify purpose and ethics in professional life and are generally stable principles that are independent of research findings (eg, doctors should evaluate before they intervene, doctors should not abandon their patients). Others, especially standards related to clinical technique, should be based on rigorous clinical research.

Ideally, consensual standards of practice in a clinical science are based on extensive quantitative and experimental evaluations. In reality, however, only a fraction of the practices in general use today by all health care disciplines have been substantiated by adequate data, and the delivery of such services is even less well studied.[3-5] These deficiencies are especially severe in chiropractic, where rigorous clinical quantification and experimentation are still in their infancy. For all professions, scientific standards of practice are necessarily supplemented by judgments of what is "usual and customary" and/or "rational." Such judgments are usually based on less than direct, controlled tests of the clinical methods or health problem in question and are therefore less than ideal. Some of the designations that may be and/or have been assigned to clinical procedures are suggested in Table 2-1.

The rationality of a therapeutic method refers to judgments made by those knowledgeable in the basic sciences about the clinical procedure's logical consistency with accepted biological knowledge. Such a judgment about the

Table 2-1 Classification of Treatment Procedures

Dimension and Classification	Meaning	Other Classifications
Basic Science Rationale		
Rational	Use of the procedure for a particular health problem is consistent with the known facts of the basic sciences.	"Provisional acceptance"[6]
Without logical (basic science) foundation	Use of the procedure for a particular health problem is not consistent with the known facts of the basic sciences or based on knowledge outside the basic sciences.	"Unsubstantiated"[6]
Clinical/Experimental Status		
Proved/substantiated	Effectiveness for a particular health problem has been established by multiple replications in controlled outcome trials.	"Full acceptance"[6]
Experimental	Effectiveness for a particular health problem is under investigation by means of controlled outcome trials.	"Unsubstantiated"[6] "experimental" or "tentative"[7]
Pre-experimental	Effectiveness for a particular health problem has not yet been tested by controlled outcome trials.	"Empirical"
Quantitative	Effectiveness for a particular health problem has not yet been tested by controlled outcome trials, but quasi-experimental and/or quantitative, uncontrolled outcome reports (eg, case studies, uncontrolled clinical series) are available.	"Unsubstantiated"[6]
Private empiricism	Effectiveness for a particular health problem has not been reported in critically reviewed science journals; effectiveness is supported only by clinical legends, anecdotes, and/or testimonials.	"Unsubstantiated"[6]; "anecdotal"[7]
Clinical use/Acceptance		
Usual and customary	Widespread use for a particular health problem has been documented, or the legitimacy of widespread use has been affirmed by a sizable portion of the profession; pervasiveness of the procedure may be regional rather than national or international.	"Accepted by consensus"; "empirically proven"; "private empiricism"
Limited use	Use of the procedure for a particular health problem has found some small acceptance in the profession.	
Novel	Use of the procedure for a particular health problem is new and has been tried by only a few in the profession.	

merits of a clinical method is a sensible first step in technique evaluation, but it is not essential for determining the "full acceptance" of a procedure.[6] A method that initially appears unsound (ie, inconsistent with basic scientific knowledge) may be found effective if and when submitted to rigorous clinical tests.

The clinical/experimental status of an intervention strategy refers to the level of confirmation or disconfirmation (uncertainty) that may be derived from controlled clinical trials of the procedure. This is the strongest type of authority available in the development of clinical standards, because it is based on rigorous tests of the natural world. Even standards based on clinical experimentation are not carved in stone, however, because future investigations may provide new information that casts doubt on earlier findings or demonstrates superior health care procedures to replace those previously accepted. Relatively few health care practices in any discipline have received this level of endorsement, but some disciplines have outpaced others in systematic efforts to evaluate their practices by controlled tests.

Usual and customary standards of practice are rules of patient/doctor interaction that draw on the best available sources of clinical information and depend for their authority on the perceived (or sampled) normative clinical strategies in use at a given time in a given region. Practice methods that are justified by appeal to the principle of usual and customary are less firm than are those established by research, however, for they are based on inadequately tested data rather than established scientific facts. Usual and customary standards may vary greatly from one geographical region to another, based on differences of habit and opinion among groups of practitioners. Obviously, practice criteria that vary regionally are less "standard" than are those more universally accepted. Consensus concerning current normative practices may be reached by actually surveying the doctors who constitute the norm group or by "guestimation" of what is normative. Occasionally, groups of clinicians attempt to impose a standard by fiat.

BARRIERS TO THE DEVELOPMENT OF CLINICAL STANDARDS

Like many other health care disciplines, chiropractic has been sluggish in establishing rules by which it can be more accountable. Not only have chiropractors lacked the usual and customary guidelines by which interim standards have been set in some other health care disciplines, but also we have failed to develop a critical, quantitative data base that would facilitate the establishment of more authoritative consensual standards.[8,9] Furthermore, chiropractors have disagreed profoundly on fundamental philosophical questions and about the ways in which scientific knowledge is developed and disseminated. Whereas those in disciplines such as psychology, dentistry, and medicine generally acknowledge the value of clinical research in shaping standards of clinical practice, chiropractors have long disputed epistemological issues and still do not agree on principles of knowledge production in the profession.[10] Yet, as Watkins noted,

> The future of our profession depends more upon the manner by which we choose our methods of patient care than upon any other consideration. Four possible basic methods of choosing practice methods in chiropractic are as follows:
> 1. The Cultist Method:
>   It requires the chiropractor to use methods based upon a preconceived practice dogma set forth by established authority. . . .
> 2. The Empiric Method:
>   This system permits the chiropractor to choose his methods of patient care on the basis of his own experience or that of other chiropractors. . . .
> 3. Theoretical Practice Method:
>   This system would allow the chiropractor to choose his methods of practice from theories which have their roots in the basic sciences.
> 4. The Clinical Science Method:
>   Under this system the chiropractor selects his methods of patient care from methods which have been tested for demonstrable worth by clinical research.[11]

Fixed and Dogmatic Authority

In chiropractic, the philosophy of science has competed rather unsuccessfully with other epistemological strategies. Some (fundamentalist) chiropractors have argued that inflexible standards, often based on untestable theoretical constructs (eg, innate intelligence), largely untested theories (eg, of subluxation), or the personal authority of individuals (eg, the Palmers, technique gurus, "red-hot" philosophers), require chiropractors to practice by certain unchangeable rules (eg, use hands only, adjust only the atlas, ignore symptoms, use only brand name technique X). Clinical research has little purpose (other than public relations) in this perspective, as practice methods are held dogmatically to be correct and are not subject to change on the basis of new information about the natural world.

This strategy of standard setting can be successful only so long as all parties agree to submit to a particular authority. Obviously, this has not occurred in chiropractic. Although there has been no shortage of would-be "authorities" in chiropractic philosophy, theory, and technique, there is no logical means of differentiating among the many claimants to the throne. The result has been the unchecked proliferation of clinical systems.

Chiropractic Rationalism

Perhaps a majority of doctors adhere to an epistemology that combines rationalism and private empiricism in order to substantiate particular chiropractic methods. The rational chiropractic tradition holds that practice methods are scientific and/or justified *because* biological rationales can be formulated to "explain" their supposed effects.[12-15] Some rationalist chiropractors deny that clinical research can provide any useful basis for practice, or even that there can be a meaningful clinical science of chiropractic, because patients are so idiosyncratic in their responses to care.

Rationalists see chiropractic as an art based on science, but not per se as a science.[16] Like the fundamentalist philosopher, the rationalist perceives no need or benefit in subjecting chiropractic methods to rigorous evaluation. Untested strategies deduced from basic knowledge are not necessarily safe and effective, however. Health care methods ought not to be presumed to "work" merely because they seem sensible.

Private and Casual Empiricism

Many fundamentalist and most "rational" philosophers of chiropractic seem also to adhere to a private, uncritical empiricism in which anecdotal, uncontrolled, unreviewed, and frequently unpublished clinical observations are taken as "proof" that chiropractic works. Examples of this epistemological rationale are abundant; they range from the panacealike (eg, "it works, and that's what counts") to the specific (eg, "proved cure for psoriasis"— undocumented, of course). So long as someone opines that "sick people get well," the technique is considered valid. When combined with the "rational" chiropractic perspective, private empiricism provides seemingly incontrovertible "scientific" justification for chiropractic practices: techniques that are logically/rationally deduced from the "immutable laws of biology"[13] and proved everyday in doctors' offices for nearly a century.

Private and uncontrolled observations do not, however, meet the stringent requirements of data-based standards of care. The private empiricism of chiropractic ignores the undependability of casual, uncritical, and private clinical observation. Although some groups in the profession have acknowledged the importance of experimentation, testing, and publication in critical journals,[6,17] many doctors who agree that clinical research data are needed are motivated to "prove what we already know is true." This uncritical approach to clinical knowledge and technique development stands at odds with the scientific method.

Technique Marketing and Chiropractic Communications

The three antiscientific epistemologies of chiropractic (dogma, rationalism, and private empiricism) have encouraged and sustained the proliferation of clinical theories and techniques in chiropractic. Technical innovation in many cases has been patterned after the strategies of Old Dad Chiro himself: a doctor who discovers an apparent breakthrough in health care proceeds to offer the new service to patients and to teach the new method to clinicians and students. These clinical and educational offerings are all too often accompanied by sensational and untested claims, and justified by one or more of the antiscientific philosophies. Although the profit motive is not always incompatible with the scientific attitude and methods, the lucrative nature of private seminars and workshops has probably encouraged the proliferation of scientifically unsubstantiated techniques and claims. It is a hopeful sign, however, that a small number of technique leaders and organizations have recently begun to participate in and financially support at least some research.

Nonetheless, much of chiropractic education today is plagued by claims for the experimentally unproved value of various clinical theories and methods. Although the technical content of such instruction may be quite legitimate (there's nothing inherently wrong with teaching or using an unproved method), the unsubstantiated status of the clinical methods being taught frequently goes unmentioned. Indeed, clinical instructors often sensationalize the supposed merits of their methods. The resulting philosophical/intellectual climate is inimical to clinical research and quantitative standards, and pointed questions about effectiveness are deflected as pseudo-intellectual semantics or "treason." Such an attitude is a barrier to research-based standards of the chiropractic art, because it denies the need for a research base and the alternative authority that such data could provide. Although most doctors acknowledge a need for research, many seem to believe that the primary purpose of research is to determine how and why (but not whether) chiropractic methods may be effective.

There are several legitimate and perhaps obligatory types of public education and communications that do not violate the public trust by promoting unsubstantiated claims about the chiropractic profession. Some topics are appropriate for chiropractors' communications with the public; others, for intraprofessional dialogue; and some, for both kinds of public relations:

- current scientific status of spinal manipulation/adjustment for particular health problems
- potential merits of spinal manipulation (labeled as "potential" or experimental)
- conservative, holistic orientation to patient care and health maintenance
- patient self-care skills and responsibilities
- counseling in diet, nutrition, exercise, hygiene, stress reduction, life style
- history of the chiropractic profession
- education of chiropractic physicians
- public health issues, such as drug abuse, disease prevention, pollution, poverty

Clinical standard setting in a health care profession should be accompanied by communications standards that are clearly understood by all in the discipline and are guided by the same commitment to honest, critical information acquisition and dissemination.

Standards of Reimbursement vs. Standards of Quality

Although the need for research-based standards of quality for chiropractic care has long been recognized,[7,18] there has been no impetus within the profession to develop the necessary data base. Fueled by the nationwide surge in health care costs and the consequently more critical policies and review procedures of the insurers, however, a growing segment of the profession is now acknowledging that technique anarchy cannot persist and that chiropractors must either determine their own standards or have them set by others. Furthermore, a few in the profession have recognized that hard data are the best defense against arbitrary limits on chiropractic services (eg, 12 visits for Medicare, 20 visits for Blue Cross/Blue Shield of Minnesota).

Yet there are dangers inherent in meeting these growing demands for fiscal accountability. Vear pointed out the distinction between "standards of efficiency" (eg, cost-effectiveness criteria) and standards of quality of care.[7] The former often relate to the processes of providing care (eg, types of interventions, numbers of visits, total cost of care for patients with a particular disorder) and provide a basis for reimbursement policies. These reimbursement standards do not necessarily focus on patient outcome, however. Moreover, existing reimbursement schemes, which are increasingly based on the diagnosis-related groups (DRGs) that have been introduced in hospitals over the past decade, threaten to lock chiropractors into allopathically derived categories of health problems. Such classifications may not be the most useful clinical groupings for chiropractic patients and doctors. Given the current dearth of information concerning which patients with which problems will respond to which chiropractic interventions, it seems extremely presumptuous to assume that chiropractors will find medically-derived classifications ideal.

Doctors of chiropractic must take the initiative, through research, discussion, and consensus, if quality chiropractic standards are to evolve. Third-party payers can be expected to eventually call for standards of quality (eg, controlled outcome studies as a basis for reimbursement for a procedure) merely as a cost-cutting strategy. Recognition by insurers that the current status of all uniquely chiropractic methods of care (especially the adjustment) is at best investigational or experimental may well encourage them to reject doctors' and patients' claims on the grounds that the methods employed have not been properly validated. Despite the usual and customary designation that many chiropractic methods seem to deserve after decades of use, the profession can expect that a lack of initiative in establishing standards of quality will have a high price in the future.

BASING STANDARDS ON CLINICAL RESEARCH

Data obtained through clinical research provide a basis for evaluating the clinician's two major functions: assessment and intervention. Chiropractors are obliged to evaluate components of their patients' physiological condition as a basis for intervening. They may obtain information through an interview, physical examination, monitoring, and laboratory tests. The findings from these assessment methods provide the patient information base from which doctors decide how to try to help their patients.

Evaluation of Clinical Assessment

Clinical observations and measurements may or may not be useful. The mere act of examining or measuring patient characteristics does not guarantee that the resulting information is accurate, nor does it ensure that the information is meaningfully or strategically related to the patient's health problem. Several research designs, however, permit critical judgments of the reliability and validity of clinical assessment strategies.

- intra-observer reliability (test-retest reliability, stability)
- interobserver reliability (interexaminer and interrater reliability)
- concurrent validity
- sensitivity and specificity
- predictive validity
- trial validity
- social validity

These various research designs address different issues in the credibility of a measurement system. Methods useful in answering one type of question may not be useful in addressing other qualities of the same measurement procedure.

Intra-Observer Reliability

Designs to determine intra-observer reliability provide a means of judging the reproducibility and temporal stability of observations over specific, but variable, time periods. For example, in judging the reliability of passive motion palpation of the lumbosacral joint, an examiner may repeat the palpation of 50 low back pain patients over very short (eg, immediate repalpation) or longer (eg, minutes, hours, even weeks or months) time periods, depending on the examiner's theory of joint fixation. The investigator then compares the preliminary findings in these 50 patients with retest findings in the same subjects by means of concordance or correlational statistics.[19,20] No intervening health care is permitted between test and retest, and the specified delay between these measures must be constant across all subjects. Examples of intra-observer reliability data in the chiropractic literature include studies of the test-retest reliability of passive spinal motion palpation[21,22] and roentgenographic determinations of atlas laterality.[23-25]

Clinical measurements that fail to demonstrate temporal stability are not necessarily inaccurate, but may instead correctly reflect spontaneous change (or concurrent change agents) during the test-retest interval. In some cases, it may not be possible to conduct the measurement with an adequately brief test-retest interval (eg, when the duration of the measurement process is greater than the interval over which change is spontaneously occurring). In such cases, concurrent measurement by multiple examiners (ie, interobserver reliability evaluation) may provide an alternative basis for evaluating the accuracy of measurement.

Interobserver Reliability

Some evaluations of clinical assessments are based on interobserver reliability—the logic that an accurate measurement system ought to permit two or more observers who examine the same phenomenon at the same time to find the same result. Several chiropractic studies have examined the extent to which two or more examiners can agree on (or predict) one another's assessments of spinal motion palpation.[21,22,26,27] Agreement or correlation between or among examiners is evaluated by the same or similar statistical methods used to evaluate test-retest reliability. Positive interobserver findings do not guarantee valid measurement, as multiple examiners may err in a similar fashion and thereby agree. Repeated negative findings suggest a lack of measurement validity, however.

Concurrent Validity

Designs for the study of concurrent validity provide strategies for judging the extent to which an observation system actually measures what it is intended to measure. The basis for this research paradigm is the assumption that some previously developed measurement method is valid. Subjects are measured concurrently (or at very nearly the same time) by means of the accepted, "standard" procedure and the new system under study. Correlational or concordance statistics are then applied to determine whether covariation between the results of the two assessment procedures exceed the concordance or predictability that could be expected by chance alone. For example, Zachman and associates compared measurements of cervical ranges of motion made with a straight-arm goniometer (the standard) to those made with an inclinometer (pendulum goniometer).[28] The resulting correlation coefficients lend credibility to the meaningfulness of measuring head motion with the inclinometer.

Predictive Validity

Research focused on predictive validity seeks to determine how well a measurement tool can forecast future performance or clinical outcome. For example, radiographic findings in young adults may be compared to survey information obtained in their middle years (eg, spinal surgeries, work days lost to back pain, spinal health care costs incurred) in order to evaluate how well radiologic data predict subsequent back problems. Predictive paradigms provide a rather direct test of the clinical usefulness of some kinds of measurements.

Sensitivity and Specificity

Evaluations for sensitivity and specificity are alternative means of expressing concurrent and predictive validity data. These constructs are important in determining the diagnostic performance of a test and, thus, when and how a test or procedure should be used.

Testing for sensitivity and specificity requires a "gold standard," that is, an independent means of establishing the true presence or absence of the disease or other clinical target. The results of the new or unestablished test are then compared to the results of the gold standard, as indicated in the 2×2 table in Figure 2-1. Ideally, bias in the study is minimized by having the unestablished test interpreted by someone who is unaware of the results of the gold standard test. For example, in order to determine the sensitivity of a subluxation detection procedure to predict subsequent dysfunction or disease, it is necessary to establish an unambiguous standard for determining that the patient does or does not develop the condition. The presence of subluxation is then evaluated by an individual who is unaware of the disease findings.

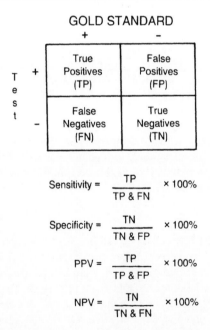

Figure 2-1 2×2 contingency table for computation of sensitivity, specificity, positive predictive value (PPV), and negative predictive value (NPV).

Sensitivity, specificity, and predictive values are mathematical concepts calculated from the 2×2 table. These concepts express the performance of the unestablished diagnostic test or procedure and suggest standards of clinical behavior in specific clinical situations. Sensitivity is expressed as the proportion of correct positive results in a group of patients who actually have the disease in question. Specificity is expressed as the proportion of correct negative results in a comparison group who do not have the target disease or condition. Positive and negative predictive values are calculated as the proportion of true positive or true negative results to the total number of positive or negative results.

Sensitivity and specificity are both considered in the decision to use a diagnostic test. Predictive values are important for interpreting the result. Generally speaking, highly sensitive tests are used to exclude or *rule out* disease; they are useful as screening procedures. Highly specific tests are used to confirm or *rule in* the presence of disease (or other target) as suggested by other examination procedures. Ideal observation systems have 100% sensitivity and 100% specificity; in the real world of clinical practice, however, few measurement systems are perfectly valid. Most tests and measures are skewed toward one or the other characteristic (ie, sensitivity or specificity).

Only a handful of chiropractic procedures have been evaluated for sensitivity and specificity,[29,30] and much remains to be done. Perhaps the most challenging task in this area of chiropractic is to develop highly sensitive and specific indicators of spinal subluxation in the absence of a universally accepted gold standard of subluxation.

Trial Validity

Trial validity investigations evaluate whether clinical observations and measurements dependably change as a function of interventions that are expected to influence the target clinical phenomena. For instance, if a method designed to detect subluxation were employed in a patient sample prior to adjustive intervention, it may be expected that fewer (or less pronounced, reduced) indicators of subluxation would subsequently be recorded in those patients who have received adjustments than in those patients in a waiting list control group. Nansel and associates[31] provide a chiropractic example of this paradigm. They found that cervical lateral flexion measured by a pendulum goniometer improved when subjects were adjusted on the side of greatest fixation, but not when they were adjusted on the side of least restriction nor when they were not adjusted.[31] Their data support the contention that the inclinometer can validly measure cervical motion.

The trial validity of measurement can be confounded with the validity (effectiveness) of clinical interventions. If pre- vs post-treatment measurements do not demonstrate the expected change, the measurement may yet be valid; the intervention may have been ineffective.

Social Validity

Social validity refers to the extent to which an observation system yields scores that are consistent with those in the patient's normative group or with the subjective evaluations of people in the patient's social environments. These strategies make it possible to determine whether a measurement process yields socially meaningful information. Kazdin described two forms of social validation: social comparison and subjective evaluation.[32] Social comparison involves determining the correlation or concordance between observations of the patient before and after clinical care with the average values in the patient's normative group. For instance, patients in a weight reduction program are measured before and after treatment, and their weights are compared to standard or "ideal" weights established by height and gender. To the extent that weight losses bring patients from an "abnormal" (pretreatment) to a "normal" value (eg, within plus or minus one standard deviation of the mean for a normally distributed group), confidence in the ability of the measurement system to recognize socially significant change is increased.

Blanchard and co-workers[33] offer an example of the subjective type of social validation for the headache diary, which is a patient self-recording form widely used in headache research. The diary requires patients to rate the intensity of cephalalgia four times daily on a scale from 0 to 5, where 0 equals no pain and 5 equals incapacitation pain. These investigators determined the difference for each patient between average daily pain rating during the seventh and eighth week of progressive relaxation therapy and the average daily pain rating during the last four weeks of baseline (pre-treatment) recording. They then compared these difference scores to ratings made by significant others (eg, roommate, spouse) of the patients' improvement on a 100-mm visual analogue scale, where 0 equaled unchanged or worse and 100 equaled markedly improved or cured. The resulting correlation ($r = 0.44$) suggested a weak, but significant ($p < .002$), association between changes in patients' self-ratings and significant others' perceptions of these changes.

Evaluation of Clinical Interventions

If valid and reliable measurement procedures are available, it is possible to evaluate the clinical effectiveness of intervention methods systematically. Among the questions that can be explored are: is the intervention effective, is the treatment more or less effective than other forms of intervention, what is the expected clinical course under care, and what are the costs and comparative costs of the therapy? These various questions involve differing research strategies, although several research questions can sometimes be addressed within a single project.

Clinical Effectiveness

The purpose of clinical effectiveness evaluations is to determine whether a particular form of treatment produces a dependable, beneficial clinical effect over and above the natural history (ie, no treatment) of the health problem. Effectiveness is most rigorously evaluated by clinical experiments that control for or eliminate threats to (rival explanations for) the validity of a clinical intervention.

There are usually a great many untested rival (null) hypotheses to the claim that a particular form of intervention is effective. For instance, based on private observations or clinical lore, a doctor may believe that adjusting subluxated vertebrae will reduce bed-wetting in children. Such beliefs can be challenged in many ways, however.[34,35] The patients may not have had the condition for which treatment was applied (eg, bed-wetting due to subluxations vs bed-wetting due to visceral pathology), or the doctor may selectively recall those cases in which clinical improvement followed treatment, but overlook those cases in which patients failed to improve or deteriorated. Reduction in bed-wetting frequency during adjustive care may represent maturation (most children "outgrow" their bed-wetting) or spontaneous remission in patients with a cyclical disorder.

Some threats to the validity of clinical intervention techniques are exacerbated by the particular research methods used to evaluate the clinical procedure. Misdiagnosis, for example, is a much more serious error source in single-subject and small-group experiments than in large-scale control group designs. Control group experiments, however, in which each patient may be measured only once or a very few times, are more susceptible to errors due to statistical regression (the tendency for an extreme score to change toward the mean on retest) than are time-series experiments. In clinical trials that lack a no-treatment control comparison, but that show a specified intervention to be more effective than is a placebo, investigators may be tempted to conclude that the experimental intervention is effective; in fact, patients who received neither the experimental nor the sham would have shown greater clinical improvement.

Thus, different experimental designs control or eliminate different kinds of invalidity/error, and no single experiment nor type of experiment is likely to rule out all rival hypotheses. Among the variety of clinical trial designs that may be of value in determining the clinical utility of interventions are time-series reversals,[35] multiple baselines across subjects,[35,36] and randomized control group trials[37]—with and without placebo conditions. These experimental-clinical designs are among the least frequently reported types of research in the chiropractic refereed literature,[38,39] but they are essential to the validation (and invalidation) of chiropractic methods of healing.

Clinical Course

The temporal distribution of clinical improvement (or lack thereof) during or following an intervention is the clinical course of patients who are receiving the intervention. Somewhat surprisingly, third-party payers of chiropractic care have shown more interest in this area of clinical evaluation than in the documentation of effectiveness. Although priorities for professional and economic accountability may well change in coming years, third-party payers are particularly eager to have quantitative studies (even uncontrolled studies, such as clinical series) that indicate how many clinic visits are required to produce some specific clinical marker (eg, 50% improvement or latency to return to work).

Although experimental designs are capable of providing descriptive information about patients' probable course under a particular intervention regimen, the more common strategy is to employ a large-scale uncontrolled clinical series. Cox and Shriener provided an example of an uncontrolled chiropractic series in 23 private practitioners' offices.[40] They prospectively studied 576 consecutive cases of low back pain to determine, among other things, the typical number of treatment visits necessary to produce 50% through maximal improvement from manipulation for various diagnostic subclassifications (eg, annulus fibrosis injury, nuclear bulge, nuclear protrusion, and nuclear prolapse). Although their data provided no basis for a conclusion that the observed improvements were due to chiropractic manipulation (since no control comparisons were available), they did provide a basis for a prediction of clinical outcome in future chiropractic patients with similar health problems.

The clinical course of patients under manipulative care for low back and related musculoskeletal syndromes is still unclear.[41] On the basis of meta-analysis, Ottenbacher and DiFabio suggested that the benefits of spinal manipulation amount to little more than short-term analgesia and that longitudinal investigations are necessary.[42] On the other hand, Meade and associates' recent contrasted (relative effectiveness study) chiropractic care vs hospital-based outpatient medical care (including mobilization and manipulation) of patients with low back pain by means of evaluations at 6, 12, and 24 months after the initiation of treatment their data suggested more durable effects of chiropractic manipulative interventions.[43] Resolution of this dispute (ie, short- vs long-term value of spinal manipulation) will ultimately require controlled clinical investigations that permit better contrasts of short- vs long-term clinical outcomes and clearer descriptions of intervention methods.

Relative Effectiveness

Some studies focus on the comparative benefits of one type of intervention vs another. Such relative effectiveness studies always provide a basis for comparison, but may or may not constitute genuine experimental designs. For example, a number of investigators have reported retrospective comparisons of medical vs chiropractic clinical outcomes and costs of care for patients with low back pain syndromes and related musculoskeletal conditions.[44] These retrospective surveys, however, do not rule out the rival explanation that patients who choose chiropractic care may have less severe health problems than do those who choose medical care and, therefore, that any apparent advantage for chiropractic services may reflect patient differences rather than greater relative effectiveness.

Experimental comparisons of the relative effectiveness of a chiropractic intervention vs other types of health care interventions could control for the self-selection bias if patients are randomly assigned to chiropractic vs alternative care and followed prospectively to evaluate any differential outcomes. The disadvantage of group experimental comparisons is that they require very large samples in order to detect differences in effectiveness between intervention methods when both methods have merit. Single-subject experimental comparisons, on the other hand, require the not always justifiable assumptions that the effects of one treatment do not add to the effects of the other and that the combination of methods does not constitute a qualitatively different (third) form of care.

The relative effectiveness of chiropractic adjustive and physiological therapeutics vs medical care is likely to become an increasing focus of concern. Rapidly rising health care costs encourage closer scrutiny of all health care. For example, in the absence of quantitative demonstrations that adjustive care is more effective than is the use of analgesics and short-term bed rest for low back pain patients, many insurers may prefer to pay for a medical examination and prescription rather than for 12 visits to the chiropractor. If an economic advantage can be demonstrated for chiropractic vs medical care (eg, a decrease in the likelihood of expensive surgery), however, third-party payers may be more willing to underwrite chiropractic services. Alternatively, if relative effectiveness studies were to suggest a clinical advantage for chiropractic vs alternative care, chiropractors may well have a moral responsibility to press for inclusion in health insurance policies, irrespective of greater relative costs.

Experimental study of the relative effectiveness of several treatments can be combined with investigation of the simple effectiveness of each method if a no-treatment comparison is added to the research design (Figure 2-2). The combined design requires at least three groups (or experimental conditions): treatment A, treatment B, and a waiting-list control comparison. This design permits three contrasts: treatment A vs no treatment, treatment B vs no treatment, and treatment A vs treatment B. Although administratively more demanding, designs such as this provide very strong tests of the merits and relative merits of various clinical strategies.

Efficacy Studies

Although designed to determine the effective components of clinical interventions, efficacy studies differ from effectiveness studies. Effectiveness designs seek to determine whether a therapeutic intervention has made a

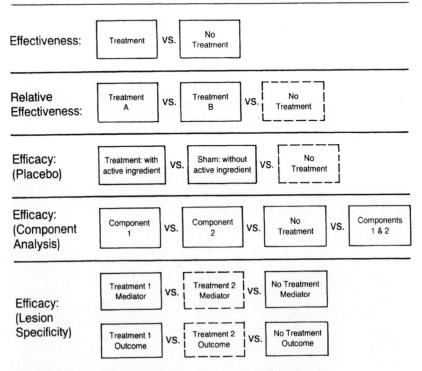

Figure 2-2 Experimental comparisons for various types of clinical questions.

difference (eg, a beneficial effect compared to no treatment), without asking what the active ingredient(s) of the treatment may be. This distinction seems especially important to the chiropractic profession, which has many times heard the criticism that chiropractic care is "all placebo." Such criticism (if and when justified) does not address the issue of patient benefit, but rather the cause(s) of the benefit received from chiropractic care.

Placebo-controlled clinical trials are examples of efficacy designs. In these designs patients' responses to the treatment in question are compared to responses to a sham treatment that contains all the components of treatment except the "active ingredient" (see Figure 2-2). Waagen and colleagues, for example, studied the short-term effects of spinal adjustments for low back pain.[45] They compared pain responses in patients who received an osseous adjustment (ie, high-velocity, low-force, segment-specific, manual thrusts) to pain responses in patients who received the sham procedure. (ie, bilateral manual pressure applied with sufficient force to release a drop-piece, plus paraspinal massage). The results indicated an advantage for those who received adjustments, which suggests that the adjustment has analgesic potency beyond what might be expected from nonspecific and/or psychosocial factors in the doctor-patient relationship (eg, patient expectations, laying on of hands).

The separate and combined effects of two (or more) components of a treatment package may be evaluated by factorial designs. For example, a chiropractor may hypothesize that appropriate care for patients with a particular disorder involves a spinal adjusting plus pre-adjustive massage of paraspinal soft tissues. If the responses of patients who receive no care are compared to responses under each of the components individually (ie, adjusting only, massage only) and the combination (see Figure 2-2), the relative effectiveness of the parts vs the "whole" may be assessed.

In many clinical situations, doctors expect a beneficial clinical outcome (eg, reduced symptoms, improved patient functioning) only if some biological mediator can be changed. Because the traditional chiropractic "mediating variable" is the subluxation,[46] efficacy studies in which the effects of adjustive care on subluxation and clinical outcome are compared in patients who are adjusted and those who are not adjusted would be helpful (see Figure 2-2). To the extent that beneficial outcome parallels change in subluxation status (and fails to occur if subluxations are not reduced or eliminated), confidence in the importance of subluxation reduction will be increased.

Fielding provides an example of how this mediator/outcome specificity may fail to be supported.[47] Clinicians in urology and psychology have long suspected that bed-wetting in children is mediated by functional bladder capacity (the ability of the urinary vesical to distend/accommodate sufficiently to retain its contents throughout the sleep cycle). Fielding found that,

among enuretics whose bed-wetting was reduced or eliminated through behavior therapy, significant increases in bladder capacity either were not seen,
or occurred only after a number of dry nights were achieved. In this case,
although the effectiveness of the intervention was supported, the hypothesized mechanism was not. The efficacy of Fielding's behavior therapy for
bed-wetting awaits the discovery of some mediator other than bladder
capacity.

Might the same be true for adjustive care of some or all of the disorders
that chiropractors see? Might adjustive care have beneficial effects, irrespective of the presence and reduction of subluxation? At this time we simply do
not know.[19]

RESEARCH FINDINGS VS CLINICAL IMPLEMENTATION

Research-derived standards of quality care in chiropractic are but a means
to an end: patient benefit. Accordingly, it is essential to take a step back from
the research process at this point to recognize that standards for health care
professionals should not be based exclusively on the results of clinical and
experimental investigations. This is true for several reasons, not the least of
which is the reality that patient-responses studied under the relatively con-
trived circumstances of a clinical investigation may not be representative of
what will happen in the real world. Despite the best efforts of investigators,
the process of recruiting patients may introduce factors not encountered in
actual practice, where patients seek out doctors rather than vice versa. Efforts to standardize therapeutic interventions so as to permit valid comparisons among methods may alter the nature of the services provided, and
thereby limit generalizations from the laboratory to the field. Too, clinicians
will often be confronted with patients and health problems for which there is
little relevant clinical research from which to extrapolate.

Even under ideal circumstances, research findings and the standards derived from them should be considered tentative. A clinical method that is
effective for 90% of research patients may be considerably less useful for the
practitioner (Figure 2-3). Moreover, it may not be possible to replicate the
findings from a well-designed investigation in subsequent studies or to implement them in the doctor's office. Newer information may contradict previous findings or contribute factors that make simple translation from the
science journal to the doctor's office difficult or impossible. The converse, of
course, is equally possible; extrapolations from the field to the clinical laboratory must be made with great care if reasonable approximations to the real
world are to be operationalized.

Accordingly, highly controlled clinical investigations described in this
chapter should be considered but a prelude to the efforts of practitioners to

replicate procedures in the real world. Not only must clinicians be involved in the consensus process that leads to research-derived standards of care, but also they must provide feedback in the form of case reports and small-scale, practice-based clinical trials to college- and university-based investigators.

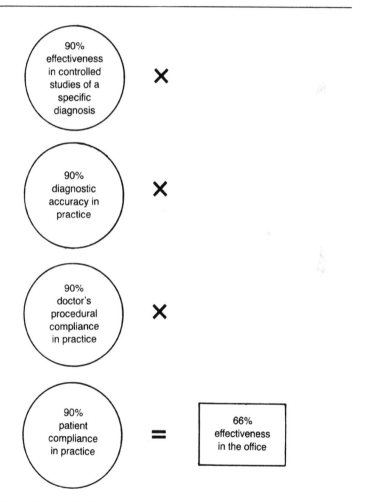

Figure 2-3 Generalization of findings from clinical research settings to implementation in the field. As each factor is added (multiplicatively), the expected effectiveness for the field practitioner diminishes.

ROLE OF THE PRACTITIONER

The establishment of quantitative, empirically based standards by chiropractors is a responsibility of the profession: the colleges, accrediting agencies, membership associations, licensing boards, research foundations, clinical specialty boards, and the field at large. Although the responsibility of educational institutions to take the lead in these efforts is widely recognized, the role of the individual practitioner in fostering chiropractic science is less widely appreciated. Yet, there are three roles that individual clinicians can play to make significant contributions to these efforts.

Financial Supporter

Perhaps the easiest and least time-consuming way for the practitioner to contribute to the scientific and standard-setting activities of the profession is by donating funds to the colleges and research-funding agencies, such as

- American College of Chiropractic Radiologists (ACCR); Bryan Gatterman, D.C. (President), Life Chiropractic College-West, 2005 Via Barrett, San Lorenzo, CA 94580, USA
- Australian Chiropractic Research Foundation (ASRF); Charlotte Leboeuf, D.C. (Coordinator), School of Chiropractic, Phillip Institute of Technology, Plenty Road, Bundoora, Victoria 3083, Australia
- Chiropractic Foundation for Spinal Research (CFSR); Ali Raizman, D.C. (Chair, Board of Trustees), 1056 St. Mary's Road, Winnipeg, Manitoba R2M 359, Canada
- Foundation for Chiropractic Education & Research (FCER); Steve Wolk, Ph.D. (Executive Director), 1701 Clarendon Boulevard, Arlington, VA 22209, USA
- Foundation for the Advancement of Chiropractic Tenets & Science (FACTS); (c/o International Chiropractors' Association), 1110 N. Glebe Road, Suite 1000, Arlington, VA 22201, USA
- International College of Applied Kinesiology (ICAK); Marc Rosen, D.C. (Director of Research), 1086 Walden Avenue, Cheektowaga, NY 14211, USA
- Lincoln College Education & Research Fund (LCERF); Edward L. Maurer, D.C. (Chair, Board of Trustees), 2330 Gull Road, Kalamazoo, MI 49001, USA
- National Institute of Chiropractic Research (NICR); Paul J. Osterbauer, D.C. (Research Administrator), 3714 East Indian School Road, P.O. Box 80317, Phoenix, AZ 85060-0317, USA

- Consortium for Chiropractic Research (CCR); Robert Jansen, Ph.D. (Executive Director), Palmer College of Chiropractic/West, 1095 Dunford Way, Sunnyvale, CA 94087, USA

Research in the science of chiropractic is a woefully impoverished enterprise. It is the rare chiropractic college that devotes 5% of its resources to research, as most are tuition-dependent for more than 80% of their operating budgets. The colleges must rely on the profession at large for the seed monies necessary to attract private and government support for scientific studies. Support for research from the membership organizations has to date been rather meager, however. For example, the annual contribution of the American Chiropractic Association, the world's largest chiropractic membership association, to research (via the FCER/Foundation for Chiropractic Education & Research) amounts to barely $25 per member per year.

It is thoroughly unrealistic to expect that the chiropractic profession could afford to underwrite all the research activities necessary to develop standards of quality of care; moreover, other health care professions are not expected to do so. Indeed, the federal government's annual contribution to the wider biomedical research effort in the United States typically amounts to some $10 billion in the form of research and training grants to medical schools, the military, and the Veterans Administration.[48-51] Efforts have been initiated recently to recruit federal assistance for chiropractic investigations through request of earmarked federal funding for chiropractic research and training.[52]

Without substantial increases in seed monies available for college-based chiropractic research, very meager progress, at best, can be expected from the poverty-stricken institutions. The colleges' ability to attract external (eg, federal) funding for chiropractic science is determined in part by chiropractors' ability to demonstrate commitment and expertise in scientific investigations. Without the support of the field, the credibility of the chiropractic research enterprise will be difficult to establish. Likewise, the ability of chiropractic research-funding organizations to support the research activities of the colleges and others depends on the willingness of the profession to underwrite the applied science of chiropractic.

Research Consumer

The conduct of research and the development of quality standards can have little practical significance unless doctors of chiropractic choose to regularly and critically read, evaluate, and selectively implement the findings of chiropractic science. Regular subscription to and review of the scholarly literature in chiropractic is essential to the implementation of scientifically sound, enduring chiropractic standards, for it is only through critical analysis and debate that science progresses. Furthermore, only through reading can the chiropractic physician keep up-to-date with this knowledge base. The currently meager circulation of legitimate chiropractic scientific periodicals (eg, approximately 5,000 *JMPT/Journal of Manipulative & Physiological Therapeutics* subscribers in a profession of more than 40,000) must be greatly increased.

A number of chiropractic periodicals currently provide high-quality critical reviews of research manuscripts. Critically reviewed chiropractic scientific, historical, and education journals:

- *Chiropractic History* (Ed: Russell W. Gibbons); 207 Grandview Drive South, Pittsburgh, PA 15215, USA
- *Chiropractic Sports Medicine* (Ed: Robert Hazel, D.C.); 220 Vroom Avenue, Spring Lake, NJ 07762, USA
- *Journal of Chiropractic Technique* (Ed: Thomas F. Bergmann, D.C.); 735 Keokuk Lane, Mendota Heights, MN 55120, USA
- *European Journal of Chiropractic* (Ed: Simon M. Leyson, D.C.); 16 Uplands Crescent, Swansea SA2 OPB, United Kingdom
- *Journal of Chiropractic Education* (Ed: Grace E. Jacobs, D.A.); 590 N. Vermont Avenue, Los Angeles, CA 90004, USA
- *Chiropractic (Research Forum)* (Ed: Robert J. Wagnon, Ph.D.); 741 Brady Street, Davenport, IA 52803, USA
- *Journal of Manipulative & Physiological Therapeutics* (Ed: Dana J. Lawrence, D.C.); 200 E. Roosevelt Road, Lombard, IL 60148, USA
- *Chiropractic Journal of Australia* (Ed: Mary Ann Chance, D.C., and Rolf E. Peters, D.C.); P.O. Box 748, Wagga Wagga NSW 2650, Australia
- *Journal of the Canadian Chiropractic Association* (Ed: Allan Gotlib, D.C.); 1396 Eglinton Avenue West, Toronto, Ontario M6C 2E4, Canada

Although their circulations are small, their contents are often quite significant.

To encourage the habit of regular review of the chiropractic knowledge base among practitioners considerably greater efforts in the colleges and the field will be necessary. Doctors and students will require instruction in the rudiments of research design and statistical analysis in order to be able to interpret the publications in scientific journals.[53] Social reinforcement, perhaps in the form of journal clubs,[54] will be important in this habit development. More widespread inclusion of research workshops and paper sessions at the conventions of the various membership organizations (ACA, ICA) could aid in raising research consciousness and consumption, as could the granting of relicensure credit for journal-based continuing education. The looming legal significance of the profession's scientific literature also needs to be more widely recognized.[55]

Research in Practice

Chiropractic needs the continuing contributions to the literature of its skilled clinicians in private practice.[38] Full-time practitioners have vital roles to play in identifying significant clinical phenomena; in proposing diagnostic and treatment hypotheses; in reporting clinical observations, both controlled and uncontrolled; and in field-testing the results of large-scale, college- and university-based clinical trials.[56,57] Indeed, the job of testing clinical methods cannot be considered complete until the typical clinician can replicate laboratory and college-based large-scale trials.

The full spectrum of research methodologies (eg, observation, prediction, experimentation) is available to the clinician, although the full-time practitioner will usually choose the more modest, small-scale projects, that do not disrupt a busy practice:

- descriptive case reports: uncontrolled; may focus on assessment/diagnosis or treatment/intervention; may involve time-series methodology[58]
- time-series clinical trials: controlled; may involve one or many patients who are measured/monitored repeatedly; experimental controls embedded in designs, such as the reversal, and multiple baselines across subjects[59]
- clinical series: uncontrolled (descriptive) quantitative reports of characteristics and outcomes of two or more patients[40]
- intra- and interobserver reliability: typically require little or no continuing clinical responsibility to subjects[26]

Unfortunately, the chiropractic practitioner frequently misunderstands the value of small-scale, uncontrolled clinical reports (such as case studies). Perhaps because such studies rarely provide "proof" of the clinical value of chiropractic methods and perhaps because of the exceedingly harsh and humiliating criticisms that chiropractic case reports (and their poor cousins, anecdotes and testimonials) have sometimes received from elements of the medical community, practitioners often dismiss these observational projects. Ironically, the medical literature shows the profound effects that single-case reports can have on health care practice.[60]

Significant changes in attitude will be necessary before private practitioners will believe in the viability of their contributions to the chiropractic knowledge base.[11,18,61] Ironically, there are few more noble kinds of gifts that practitioners can make to the science and art of chiropractic than contribution of new knowledge or perspectives to the data base. So long as the typical doctor fails to question the value of particular clinical methods for specific health problems, however, the critical attitude that characterizes the clinician-investigator cannot emerge. The idea that "we already know it works" undermines the motivation to raise critical questions. The mistaken notion that purpose of research is to "prove" the value of some clinical method has already been suggested as a barrier to the conduct of quality observational reports (eg, case studies) as well as controlled trials.

Skilled clinicians will also be important participants in the formal development of research and consensus derived standards of care. Few would argue that meaningful standards of quality care can be formulated without the active participation of those who must implement them. The profession needs to recruit its most astute diagnosticians and its most skilled adjustors to collaborate with chiropractic scholars and investigators in the formulation of standards of quality. The process of standard setting has recently begun; whether the profession (through its membership associations) will adequately support these efforts remains to be seen. Encouragingly, there does seem to be a growing awareness among doctors that standards will be determined by chiropractors or will be determined for chiropractors by third-party payers.

CONCLUSION

Standards of quality of care are ideally based upon the consensus of those who investigate and implement clinical care. The determination of the clinical value of particular methods for particular types of patient problems requires careful, systematic, and controlled observations. In chiropractic, no less than any other health care profession, the data that standard setters need to form opinions requires familiarity with procedures of critical evaluation, that is, clinical research methodology. Moreover, the implementation of data based standards of quality health care requires the practitioner to function as a sophisticated consumer of the scientific literature. Clinical research methodology is well established in other disciplines, but still somewhat novel in the chiropractic profession.

The motivation for chiropractors to become familiar with clinical research methods has, until recently, been limited. There is a risk that pressure for greater volumes of clinical outcome data may provoke the profession to engage in clinical research for the wrong reasons. While economic viability (derived from data-based standards of care) is essential to chiropractic's future, it will be unfortunate if chiropractors come to view research merely as a means of furthering its political and financial stability. Care must be taken so that the profession does not see research as a means of "proving what we already know is true." The primary purpose of chiropractic investigations should be the determination of what works best, whether or not such research determination supports or refutes current practices.

Growth in research sophistication in the profession must not be limited to some elite group of full-time chiropractic scientists. While the specialized skills of researchers are needed for the conduct of large-scale clinical trials, the prerogative and duty of the individual chiropractic clinician to contribute to research should be emphasized. The field doctor can contribute through financial donations, through more knowledgeable and regular reading (and selective implementation) of the chiropractic and related literature, and by contributions to scholarly chiropractic journals.

REFERENCES

1. Kusserow RP. *State Licensure and Discipline of Chiropractors*. Washington, DC: Office of Analysis and Inspections, US Department of Health and Human Services; 1989.

2. Lamm L, Wegner E. Chiropractic scope of practice: What the law allows. *American Journal of Chiropractic Medicine*. 1989; 2(4):155–159.

3. Chassin M, Brook R, Park RE, et al. Variations in the use of medical and surgical services by the Medicare population. *N Engl J Med*. 1986;314:285–290.

4. Eddy DM. Clinical decision making: From theory to practice. The challenge. *JAMA*. 1990;263(2):287–290.

5. Flanagin A, Lundberg GD. Clinical decision making: Promoting the jump from theory to practice. *JAMA*. 1990;263(2):279–280.

6. Kaminski M, Boal R, Gillette RG, et al. A model for the evaluation of chiropractic methods. *Journal of Manipulative & Physiological Therapeutics*. 1987;10(2):61–64

7. Vear HJ. Standards of chiropractic practice. *Journal of Manipulative & Physiological Therapeutics*. 1985;8(1):43.

8. Hansen DT. Letter to the editor. *Journal of Manipulative & Physiological Therapeutics*. 1989;12(3):237–239.

9. Keating JC, Hansen DT. Closing the research gap in chiropractic: A 1% solution. *Chiropractic Technique*. 1989;1(2):62–64.

10. Keating JC. Philosophical barriers to technique research in chiropractic. *Chiropractic Technique*. 1989;1(1):23–29.

11. Watkins CO. Clinical research as the basis for chiropractic practice, March 7, 1966. Distributed to the ACA Committee on Research, Committee on Accreditation, and accredited colleges. (Posthumously published in *Dynamic Chiropractic*, November-December 1986).

12. Budden WA. Comments on a proposal. *National Chiropractic Journal*. 1948;18(12):5.

13. Palmer DD. *The Chiropractor's Adjuster: The Science, Art and Philosophy of Chiropractic*. Portland, Ore: Portland Printing House; 1910.

14. Stephenson RW. *Chiropractic Textbook*. Davenport, Iowa: Palmer School of Chiropractic; 1927/1948.

15. Strang VV. *Essential Principles of Chiropractic*. Davenport, Iowa: Palmer College of Chiropractic; 1984.

16. Homewood AE. What price research? *Dynamic Chiropractic*. March 15, 1988: 32–33.

17. American Chiropractic Association Council on Technic. The evaluation of chiropractic technique. *ACA J Chiro*. 1986;23(3):64–65, 68, 70, 72–73.

18. Watkins CO. *The Basic Principles of Chiropractic Government*. Sidney, Mont: Author; 1944. Available from Dr. Ted Shrader, 17017 Via Media, San Lorenzo, CA 94580.

19. Keating JC. Several strategies for evaluating the objectivity of measurements in clinical research and practice. *Journal of the Canadian Chiropractic Association*. 1988;32(3): 133–138.

20. Rosner B. *Essentials of Biostatistics*. Boston: PWS Publishers; 1986.

21. DeBoer KF, Harmon R, Tuttle CD, Wallace H. Reliability study of detection of somatic dysfunctions in the cervical spine. *Journal of Manipulative & Physiological Therapeutics*. 1985;8(1):9–16.

22. Mootz RD, Keating JC, Kontz HP, Milus TB, Jacobs GE. Inter and intra-examiner reliability of passive motion palpation of the lumbar spine. *Journal of Manipulative & Physiological Therapeutics*. 1989;12(6):44.

23. Sigler DC, Howe JW. Inter- and intra-examiner reliability of the upper cervical x-ray marking system. *Journal of Manipulative & Physiological Therapeutics*. 1985;8(2):75–80.

24. Jackson BL, Barker W, Bentz J, Gambale AG. Inter- and intra-examiner reliability of the upper cervical x-ray marking system: A second look. *Journal of Manipulative & Physiological Therapeutics*. 1987;10(4):157–163.

25. Jackson BL, Barker WF, Gambale AG. Reliability of the upper cervical x-ray marking system: A replication study. *Chiropractic*. 1988;1(1):10–13.

26. Boline PD, Keating JC, Brist J, Denver G. Interexaminer reliability of palpatory evaluations of the lumbar spine. *American Journal of Chiropractic Medicine*. 1988;1(1):5–11.

27. Mior SA, King RS, McGregor M, Bernard M. Intra- and interexaminer reliability of motion palpation in the cervical spine. *Journal of the Canadian Chiropractic Association*. 1985;29(4):195–198.

28. Zachman ZJ, Traina AD, Keating JC, Bolles ST, Braun-Porter L. Interexaminer reliability and concurrent validity of two instruments for the measurement of cervical ranges of motion. *Journal of Manipulative & Physiological Therapeutics*. 1989; 12(3):205–210.

29. Brunarski DJ. Chiropractic biomechanical evaluations: Validity in myofascial low back pain. *Journal of Manipulative & Physiological Therapeutics*. 1982;5(4):155–161.

30. Meeker WC, Gahlinger PM. Neuromusculoskeletal thermography: A valuable diagnostic tool? *Journal of Manipulative & Physiological Therapeutics*. 1986;9(4):257–266.

31. Nansel D, Cremata E, Carlson J, Szlazak M. Effect of unilateral spinal adjustments on goniometrically assessed cervical lateral-flexion end-range asymmetries in otherwise asymptomatic subjects. *Journal of Manipulative & Physiological Therapeutics*. 1989;12(6):419–427.

32. Kazdin AE. *Single-case Research Designs: Methods for Clinical and Applied Settings*. New York: Oxford University Press; 1982.

33. Blanchard EB, Andrasik F, Neff DF, Jurish S, O'Keefe DM. Social validation of the headache diary. *Behav Ther*. 1981; 12:711–715.

34. Haldeman S. Basic principles in establishing a chiropractic clinical trial. *ACA J Chiro*. 1978;12(5):S-33–S-37.

35. Keating JC, Seville J, Meeker WC, Lonczak RS, et al. Intrasubject experimental designs in osteopathic medicine: Applications in clinical practice. *J Amer Osteo Assoc.* 1985;85(3):192–203.

36. Center DB, Leach RA. The multiple baseline across subjects design: Proposed use in research. *Journal of Manipulative & Physiological Therapeutics.* 1984;7(4):231–236.

37. Campbell DT, Stanley JC. *Experimental and Quasi-Experimental Designs for Research.* Chicago: Rand McNally; 1966.

38. Keating JC, Booher J, Door FA. JMPT: A 1987–88 update. *Chiropractic Technique.* 1989;1(4):146–149.

39. Keating JC, Larson K, Stephens M, Mick TJ. *The Journal of Manipulative & Physiological Therapeutics*: A bibliographic analysis. *Journal of Manipulative & Physiological Therapeutics.* 1989;12(1):15–20.

40. Cox JM, Shreiner SS. Chiropractic manipulation in low back pain and sciatica: Statistical data on the diagnosis, treatment and response of 576 consecutive cases. *Journal of Manipulative & Physiological Therapeutics.* 1984;7(1):1–11.

41. DiFabio RP. Clinical assessment of manipulation and mobilization of the lumbar spine: A critical review of the literature. *Phys Ther.* 1986;66(1):51–54.

42. Ottenbacher K, DiFabio RP. Efficacy of spinal manipulation/mobilization therapy: A meta-analysis. *Spine.* 1985;10(9):833–837.

43. Meade TW, Dyer S, Browne W, Townsend J, Frank AO. Low back pain of mechanical origin: Randomised comparison of chiropractic and hospital outpatient treatment. *Br Med J.* 1990;300:1432–1437.

44. Johnson MR, Ferguson AC, Swank LL. Treatment and cost of back or neck injury: A literature review. *Research Forum.* 1985;1(3):68–78.

45. Waagen GN, Haldeman S, Cook G, Lopez D, DeBoer KF. Short-term trial of chiropractic adjustments for the relief of chronic low back pain. *Man Med.* 1986;2(3):63–67.

46. Keating JC, Miller CW. The science of chiropractic and the big idea. *Dynamic Chiropractic.* March 1986;14-5, 20-1, 37.

47. Fielding D. The response of day and night wetting children and children who wet only at night to retention control training and the enuresis alarm. *Behav Res Ther.* 1980;18:305–317.

48. Keating JC. Science and politics and the subluxation. *American Journal of Chiropractic Medicine.* 1988;1(3):107–110.

49. Taskel L, Jolly P, Beran R. US medical school finances. *JAMA.* 1989;262(8):1020–1028.

50. Durenberger D. Perspectives: A senator. *Health Affairs (Millwood).* 1988; 7(2 suppl): 39–44.

51. Medical education programs sponsored by government agencies (Section VI). *JAMA.* 1989; 262(8):1068–1072.

52. Keating JC. The National Institute of Chiropractic Research speaks to Congress. *Dynamic Chiropractic.* May 23, 1990: 1, 20,21,37.

53. Keating JC, Calderon L. Clinical research preparation for chiropractors: Implementing a scientist-practitioner model. *Journal of Manipulative & Physiological Therapeutics.* 1987;10(3):124–129.

54. Hildebrandt RW. Chiropractic continuing education: A critical review (Editorial). *American Journal of Chiropractic Medicine.* 1989;2(3):89–92.

55. Hildebrandt RW. Reply to Dr. Ray. *American Journal of Chiropractic Medicine.* 2(4):177–178.

56. Keating JC. The chiropractic practitioner-scientist: An old idea revisited. *American Journal of Chiropractic Medicine*. 1988;1(1):5–11.

57. Keating JC, Meeker WC, Mootz RD. The role of the practitioner in the science of chiropractic. *ICA Rev Chiro*. 1986;73,75,77–80.

58. Lowden TA, Keating JC, Meeker WC. A multivariate time-series descriptive case study of chiropractic care in the treatment of cervical pain. *Journal of Manipulative & Physiological Therapeutics*. 1986; 9(4):267–277.

59. Meyer JJ, Zachman ZJ, Traina AD, Keating JC. Effectiveness of chiropractic management for patello-femoral pain syndrome's symptomatic control phase: A single-subject experiment. *Journal of Manipulative & Physiological Therapeutics*. 1990;13(9):539–549.

60. American Medical Association. *51 Landmark Papers*. Chicago: AMA; 1985.

61. Keating JC. Why shouldn't chiropractic be a first class clinical science? *American Journal of Chiropractic Medicine*. 1989;2(2):67–71.

3

Scope of Chiropractic Practice

Herbert J. Vear

Since its beginning in 1895, chiropractic has passed through a catalog of scope-of-practice statements, each in its time alleged to be the definitive determination for the chiropractic care of the sick. Unfortunately, many such statements have been couched in metaphysical terms with global and even heavenly aspirations far beyond all reality, while others have been limited to the most simplistic of healing concepts. Scope of practice implies clinical investigation of health and disease by orthodox diagnostic methods and the domain in which chiropractic clinical care can be a benefit.[1] Two classifications for scope of practice exist today: statute (political) and scientific (educational and research).

Statutory scope-of-practice definitions form part of every chiropractic practice act. There is a lack of consensus among chiropractic practice acts, however, concerning diagnostic and treatment procedures and, most important, description or definition for scope of chiropractic practice[2(p10),3-5] The failure of statutes to define chiropractic consistently reflects the serious lack of agreement within the chiropractic profession. Consequently, statutory scope-of-practice statements (definitions) cannot be used as a basis for chiropractic education, research, or standards of practice and quality care.

The very survival of the profession as practiced today may be threatened if the divided political arm of the profession fails to reach agreement on definitions critical to chiropractic education, research, and practice. Yessian recommended intraprofessional consultation to "develop guidelines for state chiropractic practice acts" and "to develop a standard definition of the scope of chiropractic practice."[2(pp24-25)] The American Chiropractic Association passed several resolutions in July, 1989 as a welcome step in that direction.[6] For example, Resolution #22 "encourages the academic, scientific and clinical components of the profession to direct research toward further defining the terms "subluxation," "vertebral subluxation," and "vertebral subluxation

49

complex" in view of the clinical history of the profession and in a manner that may be validated scientifically. . . ." and of more current concern Resolution #23 "the ACA in order to prevent practice standardization from being dictated by entities from outside the profession, commit itself to a leadership role in promoting acceptable uniform practice guidelines for the profession." A report of the American Chiropractic Association issued in August, 1989 further recognized the need for a "unified front to the outside world [for]. . . standards, scope, education, legislative goals, etc."[7]

The preferred method for defining the scope of chiropractic practice is to base the definition on acceptable clinical and scientific criteria, through consensus. The following statements provide a foundation for the construct of such criteria:

- Chiropractic is not a philosophy, but a health science discipline consisting of a philosophy, principles (hypotheses and theories), and practice.
- Chiropractic clinical care is not a panacea, but a health care delivery system that addresses the multifactorial cause of disease. (It would not be necessary to include this statement if there were political and ideological unanimity.)[8,9]
- Chiropractic clinical care is based on the biological sciences, behavioral sciences, clinical sciences, and research.[10,11]
- Chiropractic physicians do not provide a comprehensive health care service,[12-17] but are a portal of entry to the health care system.[15(p4)]
- Chiropractic clinical care is a limited health care delivery system.[16,17]
- Chiropractic health care is not used to its clinical potential in any society.

In an early attempt to evolve an educational/research scope-of-practice statement, Vear developed the concepts of primary, secondary, and tertiary scope of chiropractic practice.[18] The primary scope of practice focuses on functional disease or disorders characterized by aberrant physiology of the body's different systems, more particularly those disorders that are brought about through the detrimental effects of subluxations or joint dysfunctions upon the nervous system and may become pathological if not treated effectively.

The secondary scope of practice involves pathological conditions of the neuromusculoskeletal systems that tend to interfere with the normal physiological integrity of the body, but are not sufficiently developed or of such a nature as to contraindicate spinal adjustments (manipulation) of subluxation or conservative adjunctive treatment. Chiropractic physicians are cognizant of the limitations of body tissues and of human skills to alter the natural and relentless progression of most pathological conditions.[19] The clinical benefits offered by the chiropractic physician's spinal and accessory adjustive/manipulative procedures have been demonstrated empirically, however. It is postulated that the pathomechanics of the vertebral column commonly result in a neurological insult to neurologically dependent organs and other structures, which appear as clinical disorders.[20,21]

The tertiary scope of practice focuses on pathological conditions of the body that are known not to be amenable to spinal adjustment/manipulation, but whose symptoms may be amplified or extended because of the involvement of the spine and nervous system and whose symptoms may be ameliorated by the improvement of the physiological mobility of the spine, nerves, and related structures. Many terminal pathological diseases have disturbing secondary somatic symptoms that justify the conservative chiropractic care approach. Although their effectiveness is poorly documented, chiropractic clinical procedures provide palliative relief to many of these patients. The objective is to assist body function despite the relentless progression of the disease process.[19]

In a study of patients who were seeking chiropractic care, it was found that the primary scope of practice covered 80% of the patients; the secondary scope of practice, 18%; the tertiary scope of practice, only 2%.[22] Significantly, the majority of patients covered by the tertiary scope of practice were referred to either a primary care medical physician or a secondary care medical specialist. Several studies of a similar nature conducted during the late 1970s and throughout the 1980s produced similar findings.[15(p26),23] This approach to defining scope of practice was considered too theoretical and applicable only to education in courses on chiropractic principles, however.

In 1973, the European Chiropractic Union adopted a scientific definition for chiropractic as a health discipline that Illi, Grillo, and Sandoz of Switzerland had developed.

> Chiropractic is a discipline of the scientific healing arts concerned with pathogenesis, diagnostics, therapeutics, pain syndromes and neurophysiological effects related to the statics and dynamics of the locomotor system, especially of the spine and pelvis.[24]

The faculty of the Canadian Memorial Chiropractic College deemed this definition appropriate for the development of a scope-of-practice statement for educational and research purposes. It was their belief that an agreed upon definition for the scope of chiropractic practice and education would have social, political, and professional benefits for chiropractic organizations and colleges worldwide.

- statute conformity based on consensus

- a standard for the profession to use in socioeconomic and legislative matters
- a guideline for chiropractic physicians in matters of diagnosis, therapeutic goals, interdisciplinary cooperation, and other professional responsibilities
- a reference and guideline for the monitoring and development of chiropractic education (undergraduate and graduate) by accredited chiropractic colleges
- a guideline for chiropractic scholarship, research, and technology development

SCOPE OF PRACTICE FOR CHIROPRACTIC EDUCATION

In 1974, the Canadian Memorial Chiropractic College converted the European Chiropractic Union definition of chiropractic as a health care discipline into a scope-of-practice statement for education.[25] The following is a revised version with the key words italicized:

1. Primary chiropractic practice means any *professional* service usually performed by a chiropractic physician, the aim of which is to restore and maintain health; it includes
   a. the *diagnostics, treatment,* and *prophylaxis* of *functional disturbances, pathomechanical states, pain syndromes,* and *neurophysiological effects* related to the *statics* and *dynamics* of the *locomotor system,* more particularly the spine and pelvis
   b. the treatment of such conditions by *adjustment* and/or *manipulation* of the spine and other anatomical structures
   c. *counseling,* the realization that genetic, emotional, sociological, economic, workplace, and environmental factors are significant and common causes of interference with the normal function of the nervous system in the whole person
   d. the use of diagnostic imaging, such as roentgenography, computed tomography, magnetic resonance imaging, and thermography
   e. *consultation* and *referral,* duties when the patient requests, when a diagnosis cannot be determined, when clinical trial care is without evidence of improvement, and if treatment is beyond the skill, knowledge, and scope of practice of the chiropractic physician.
2. Adjunctive physical procedures involve the use of supportive measures, including rehabilitative exercise, heliotherapy, thermotherapy, hydrotherapy, electrotherapy, and mechanotherapy (eg, traction; sup-

portive collars, tape, and braces; heel or sole lifts; foot stabilizers), as required.

3. Nutrition focuses on dietary regimens and nutritional supplementation to influence the physiological processes by which the living organism receives and uses the materials necessary for the maintenance of its functions and for growth and renewal of its components.

4. Other diagnostic and treatment procedures may be included as provided by statute.

The primary chiropractic practice statement describes the minimum standard for the scope of chiropractic practice to be provided to all patients and is the basis for standards of practice applied to diagnosis and treatment. In many jurisdictions, such a statement represents the entirety of the statutory scope of chiropractic practice. Unfortunately, the practice acts of a few jurisdictions limit the scope of chiropractic diagnostic and treatment privileges so that they are well below the primary care currently taught in and through accredited colleges. Patients in these jurisdictions are being denied access to many diagnostic and clinical procedures used in the responsible practice of chiropractic. Many legislative events have been complicated by this professional discrimination, for example, restrictions placed on chiropractic care in the 1973 Social Security Act.[26]

Most chiropractic practice acts provide for the additional therapeutic advantages of adjunctive physical procedures and nutrition. Practice beyond core chiropractic is frequently interpreted as "broad scope of practice," however, a designation that serves no useful purpose.

The defining of key words is imperative if a policy statement is to receive general acceptance. To provide scientific and clinical support for each key word, in their definition, the Canadian Memorial Chiropractic College faculty conducted a comprehensive search of the chiropractic, osteopathic, medical, and scientific literature from 1900 to 1975. More than 2,000 papers were reviewed in the search for suitable scientific support for the key words.

Profession

The generally accepted criteria for all professions weigh heavily on education, knowledge, skills, privilege, and ethics. Brandies noted that

a profession's educational process is characterized by:
   i. an undergraduate program requiring a high level of entrance to the program and a superior level of academic achievement within the program.

ii. a graduate program which prepares the better academics to serve in a teacher-scientist role.

iii. a program of research which is directed by the senior faculty with some participation by undergraduates and more particularly assistance by graduate students.[27]

In addition to education, all professions should have the following characteristics, according to Brandies:

1. a highly complex body of knowledge combined with the ability to use intellectual processes which are, at least to some extent, peculiar to the profession;
2. certain practical skills and professional techniques without which this knowledge cannot be applied in the practice of this profession;
3. the capacity to use knowledge, from day to day, in the service of other people's interests and to solve, or help to solve, practical problems arising within the sphere of the profession;
4. a particular kind of relationship with clients or patients, arising from the complexity of the subject matter which deprives the client or patient of the ability to make informed judgments for himself and so renders him, to a large extent, dependent upon the professional man; and
5. a self imposed code of professional ethics intended to correct the imbalance inherent in this relationship and to resolve inevitable conflicts between the interests of the client or patient and the interests of the professional man himself or of the community at large.[27]

Diagnostics

The Council on Chiropractic Education (CCE) and its member institutions established clinical competency objectives in 1984 for the measurement of those chiropractic diagnostic skills necessary for the accepted practice of chiropractic.[28] Because the introduction of clinical competency measurement in most chiropractic colleges is so recent, the skills of the majority of practicing chiropractic physicians have not been evaluated by these more stringent standards. The CCE has required colleges to maintain high standards for clinical experience since 1974,[29] however, which covers the majority of chiropractic physicians in practice.

Chiropractic practice is a specialized domain of health care that requires its practitioners to possess the clinical judgment and procedural diagnostic skills distinctive of the discipline. A chiropractic physician's diagnostic skills need not be the same as those of a medical or osteopathic physician, however. For example, a medical differential diagnosis may be defined as "the determination of which one of several diseases may be producing the symptoms"[30] or as "the distinguishing between two diseases of similar character by comparing their symptoms."[31] A chiropractic differential diagnosis, on the other hand, means the recognition of indications and contraindications for chiropractic care. It includes the following:

1. the determination of whether the presenting signs and symptoms are vertebrogenous or nonvertebrogenous in origin and, if the latter, whether to refer at this stage
2. the determination of whether vertebrogenous syndromes are due to dysfunction or to visceral pathology (ie, a tentative diagnosis)
3. the identification of visceral pathologies sufficient to make an appropriate referral
4. the identification of functional and pathomechanical vertebral syndromes sufficient to arrive at a clinical diagnosis and plan adequate therapy
5. the application of a therapeutic trial, following which a definitive diagnosis is made

The chiropractic physician employs orthodox clinical diagnostic procedures and instrumentation, along with specialized chiropractic diagnostic methodologies accepted by a majority of the chiropractic profession and taught in and through accredited colleges of chiropractic.

Most chiropractic patients complain of back pain and/or symptoms related to the locomotor system.[32] The pain may be located anywhere between the cranium and the coccyx, and it may or may not radiate to the extremities. In this case, the chiropractic physician first determines whether the pain is vertebrogenous in origin and whether there are any contraindications for chiropractic care. This involves the clinical diagnostic procedures of history taking, physical examination, spinal and neuromusculoskeletal examination, clinical and laboratory examination, and diagnostic imaging. Diagnosis by deduction and exclusion leads to a clinical impression or initial working diagnosis. Patients who require specialized diagnostic examinations that are not available as routine office procedures are referred to providers or facilities that specialize in such procedures.

The chiropractic physician must grasp the degree of urgency for referral to other health care providers, as indicated by the patient's symptoms and general condition. If the disorder is nonvertebrogenous and beyond the chiropractor's scope of practice, diagnostic probing extends to the point of reaching a tentative diagnosis. The patient is then referred to an appropriate specialist. If the disorder appears to be vertebrogenous in origin, the chiropractic physician must then determine whether the symptoms are due to a functional or pathomechanical disorder of the spinal column and/or locomotor system. If so, the chiropractor proceeds with a comprehensive differential diagnostic procedure specific to chiropractic practice. This procedure includes specialized techniques such as static and dynamic motion palpation, postural mensuration, and diagnostic imaging. The examination sometimes reveals contraindications to chiropractic care that require the patient's being referred to another health care discipline. On the other hand, if the examination indicates the need for chiropractic care, the chiropractor proceeds with a definitive therapy plan and/or clinical trial.

Treatment

As defined by *Dorland's Illustrated Medical Dictionary*, treatment is "the management and care of a patient for the purpose of combating disease or disorder."[30(p1635)] Treatment involves consideration of maneuver, method, technique, tests, and therapy. Modern chiropractic therapeutic procedures consist of a wide array of techniques and auxiliary procedures. According to the CCE,

> the following categories constitute acceptable avenues for patient care when in accordance with the chiropractic physician's clinical judgment. He/she is expected to render care in accordance with the patient's need, and in the public interest.
> 1. Spinal adjusting
> 2. Manipulation
>   a. Spinal
>   b. Articular
>   c. Soft Tissue
> 3. Adjunctive physical procedures
> 4. Nutritional and psychological counseling
> 5. Supportive procedures
> 6. First aid and emergency procedures
> 7. Patient education
> 8. Consultation and/or referral[33]

Prophylaxis

Boyd defined prophylaxis as "that branch of applied biology which seeks to reduce or eradicate disease by removing or altering the responsible etiologic factors."[34] In chiropractic practice, prophylaxis can be described as primary or secondary.[35]

Primary prevention includes the early identification of any static and dynamic mechanical disrelationships of the neuromusculoskeletal system to prevent the occurrence of such disrelationships due to poor postural hygiene, inadequate physical fitness, and faulty (acquired or anomalous) body mechanics. For secondary prevention, the recurrence of problems is of prime concern. It focuses on maintenance and rehabilitation care. Many disrelationships are not correctable, but may become quiescent with chiropractic treatment; the reason for follow-up care is to prevent the development of further pathology or, at least, to retard the progress of the pathomechanical process.

Functional Disturbances

In chiropractic practice, the term *functional disturbances* refers to aberrant joint biomechanics, including the classic chiropractic subluxation, with attending clinical disorders. In allopathic medicine, the term *functional* suggests a psychological factor as a cause or contributor to disorders in which no organic change to account for the symptoms is evident. In other instances, allopathic medicine extends the term *functional disturbances* to include such common disorders as asthma, paroxysmal tachycardia, peptic ulcer, primary dysmenorrhea, enuresis, and countless other idiopathic conditions. For statutory purposes, it would be appropriate for the chiropractic profession to do likewise, especially if the term *functional disturbances* is the only manner in which visceral disorders are to be included in the scope of chiropractic practice. Otherwise, all forms of aberrant physiological disorders (functional) etiologically related to or caused by disturbed biomechanics are best included in the term *neurophysiological effects*.

Pathomechanical States

In 1950, Schmorl and Junghanns described the vertebral motor segment as a viable model for studying vertebral mechanics.[36] Since that time, there has been an acceleration of research and a phenomenal accumulation of knowledge in the field of spinal pathomechanics and pathophysiology. Because of its very nature, chiropractic clinical practice has had a long and unique experience with this challenging field of study. Pathomechanical states, defined as structural changes in the joints, are the scars of imbalanced motion and weight bearing, trauma, and biomechanical changes associated with aging and deficiency states.

Pain Syndromes

The relationship between abnormal spinal mechanics and the elaboration of pain remains a mystery in spite of heroic attempts to clarify it. Numerous pain syndromes have sufficient uniformity and consistency in their clinical appearance to be diagnosed frequently on that basis alone.[37] The evaluation of pain is generally made difficult, however, by the fact that it is a subjective phenomenon. Pain syndromes caused by spinal joint and nerve root insult or injury are relatively easy to diagnose, but the actual mechanism that creates the painful syndrome can remain elusive. As Gitelman stated, "I have presented data which would indicate that manipulation is effective in relieving pain and other complexes, which result from vertebral dysfunction. The exact mode of action of manipulation is not known. In this regard, I have presented questions, not answers."[38]

Neurophysiological Effects

The term *neurophysiological effects* denotes functional or aberrant disturbances of the peripheral or autonomic nervous systems. It designates nonspecific clinical and physiological responses related to

1. motor and sensory functions of the peripheral nervous system
2. vasomotor activity, secretomotor activity, and motor activity of smooth muscle initiated by the autonomic nervous system
3. trophic activity of both the peripheral and autonomic nervous system

The essence of chiropractic practice is found in this field of clinical interest. It is reasoned that spinal pathomechanical states and functional disturbances become clinically evident through this mechanism. The clinical literature is abundant with empirical evidence to support this view. On the other hand, pathophysiological studies of spinal nerve irritation are characterized by a substantial lack of supporting research data.

Statics, Dynamics, and Locomotor System

Statics may be defined as "that phase of mechanics that deals with the action of forces and systems of forces on bodies at rest"[30(p1468)] or "the science that deals with bodies at rest or at equilibrium relative to some given state of reference."[39(p858)] Dynamics deals with "the motion of material bodies taking place under different specific conditions"[30(p481)] or the "science that treats of matter in motion."[39(p736)] The locomotor system is "that group of organs and body parts concerned with progressive motion (locomotion);[39(p388)] "of or pertaining to locomotion; pertaining to or affecting the locomotive apparatus."[30(p887)] Locomotorium is "the locomotive apparatus of the body."[30(p887)]

These terms are important for the chiropractic physician, who must comprehend the diagnostic value of integrating static and dynamic findings in all assessments of a patient's body mechanics. However subjective the findings may appear, a significant correlation of clinical biomechanical findings has been found between clinicians. The skill must be refined further.[40,41]

Adjustment and Manipulation

The terms *adjustment* and *manipulation* continue to plague chiropractic politics, education, and practice.[42] Before the February, 1975 National Institutes of Health conference on spinal manipulative therapy, the use of the term *manipulation* was guarded and uncommon in the chiropractic literature. The focus of chiropractic treatment was primarily on "adjustment," although some early chiropractic authors did discuss manipulation.[43,44]

Since 1975, the word *manipulation* has been creeping into chiropractic literature at an accelerated rate. It is a generic term that embraces all forms of spinal, extremity, and soft tissue manipulation. Adjustment (spinal) is a major division of manipulation, which is limited to chiropractic education and practice. The American Chiropractic Association Council on Technic has defined manipulation and adjustment as

> Manipulation—therapeutic application of manual force. Spinal manipulative therapy broadly defined includes all procedures where the hands are used to mobilize, adjust, manipulate, apply traction, massage, stimulate or otherwise influence the spine and paraspinal tissues with the aim of influencing the patient's health.[45(p52)]

> Adjustment—a specific form of direct articular manipulation utilizing either a long or short leverage technique with specific contacts and is characterized by a dynamic thrust of controlled velocity, amplitude and direction.[45(p46),46]

Definitions for manipulation and adjustment cannot be left in a "vacuum"; there remains the question of their application and skills. Chiropractic colleges have a responsibility to ensure that students reach at least an 80% psychomotor skill level for chiropractic spinal care before graduation. All clinical applications of manipulation, more particularly spinal adjustment, should be preceded by an evaluation of the patient's clinical state and an intellectual analysis of the spine, pelvis, other articulations, and soft tissues. This should be based on scientific criteria, not on untested theories.

Counseling

The chiropractic profession has always stressed patient counseling as an important component of patient care. Traditionally, this procedure occurs during a chiropractic physician's summary of clinical findings to the patient. Counseling on diet, life style, exercise, alcohol, tobacco, drugs, and ergonomics forms the basis for this interaction with the patient.

Chiropractic educational institutions place great emphasis on patient counseling, requiring students to take courses in the social sciences and humanities. All CCE-accredited colleges provide at least one course in clinical psychology.[11] Considerable emphasis is also placed on patient counseling in applied science and clinical science courses, as well as during the clinical experience. Although chiropractors do not receive patients directly for psychological assessment or counseling, it is not uncommon for them to refer patients to clinical psychologists.

Consultation and Referral

Consultation with another health care provider is indicated when there is any doubt about the diagnosis or the most effective therapy. Chiropractic physicians are encouraged to take advantage of consultation. Patients will interpret this as the decision of a prudent physician. The chiropractic physician has a duty of referral to all patients when examination and diagnosis indicate that the primary therapy for the complaint is beyond the chiropractor's clinical skill and scope of practice.

SCOPE OF PRACTICE FOR CHIROPRACTIC DIAGNOSTICS

The diagnostic scope of chiropractic practice is based on the chiropractor's legal and ethical responsibility, as a primary health care provider, to diagnose conditions correctly, provide appropriate treatment, and consult or refer the patient to another health care provider when necessary. It is essential that chiropractors definitively diagnose, *to the eightieth (80th) percentile*, all disorders that fall within their scope of practice. Similarly, it is essential for them to distinguish, but not definitively diagnose, *to the eightieth (80th) percentile*, those disorders that fall outside their scope of practice and for which patients should be referred to other health care providers. [10,46]

Chiropractors can not function within a diagnostic vacuum if they are to be held responsible by the courts and by society for their actions in treating or referring patients. As science and technology advance, so should the components of chiropractic diagnostic knowledge and skill. Chiropractic physicians will not need to own and operate new diagnostic equipment, especially without certified education and training in the technology that it uses, [47] but they will need equal access to facilities that provide the required diagnostic services.

SCOPE OF PRACTICE FOR CHIROPRACTIC THERAPEUTICS

Traditionally, the manual adjustment or manipulation of the spine, pelvis, and extremities to effect the neurological, muscular, articular, and vascular functions of the body in health and disease is the basis of chiropractic therapy. Although chiropractic health care is viewed as a single therapeutic modality, most chiropractors regularly use a wide range of therapies. [11]

The American Chiropractic Association has provided an interpretation of scope of chiropractic treatment. [48]

> Chiropractic treatment methods are determined by the scope of practice authorized by state law. In all areas, however, these methods do not include the use of prescription drugs or surgery. Chiropractic prides itself on being a drug-free, non-surgical science. Essentially, treatment methods include chiropractic manipulation, necessary dietary advice and nutritional supplementation, adjunctive physiotherapeutic measures, and professional counsel.
>
> The most characteristic aspect of chiropractic practice is the correction (reduction) of a subluxated vertebral or pelvic segment(s) by means of making a specific, predetermined adjustment. The purpose of this correction and its determination is to normalize the relationships of segments within their articular surfaces and relieve any attendant neurological, muscular, and vascular disturbances.
>
> The corrective structural adjustment by a chiropractic physician should not be confused with other forms of manipulation. Manipu-

lative therapy in one form or another is used in all the healing arts. Allopathic manipulation is usually little more than putting a joint through its normal range of motion, by a therapist, in order to stretch muscles and break adhesions. Osteopathic manipulation is designed to increase joint motion and relieve fixations. On the other hand, chiropractic corrective adjustment is made only after careful analysis, delivered in a specific manner, to achieve a predetermined goal. It is a precise, delicate maneuver, requiring special bio-engineering skills and a deftness not unlike that required for other specialties. Rarely is the process painful.

Most chiropractic corrective adjustments involve the articulation of the spinal column and extremities. Some techniques, however, are light-touch reflex adjustments which involve the neurovascular, neurolymphatic, and neuromuscular systems, gentle manipulation and passive mobilization.

Vitamin and mineral food supplementation can, if professionally supervised, serve to prevent the onset or assuage the existence of some types of dysfunction of the nervous system and other tissues. If deemed necessary in case management, dietary regimens and nutritional supplementation are often advised as adjunctive therapy.

Physiotherapeutic methods and procedures are frequently used as adjunctive therapy to enhance the effects of the chiropractic adjustments. Such procedures may include the use of diathermy, galvanic currents, infra-red and ultra-violet light, ultrasound, traction, paraffin baths, hot or cold compresses, acutherapy, hydrotherapy, heel and sole lifts, foot stabilizers, and other commonly utilized modalities when indicated. Taping and strapping and other forms of first aid are often used in injuries of the extremities. Injuries of the neck, lower back, elbow, knee and ankle may call for the use of supportive collars and braces during recuperation, to guard against re-injury, and to assist healing and strengthening. Rehabilitative exercises, as a physical therapy, comprise an important aspect of professional counseling to assist recovery and prevent further strain.

Counsel is often given in such areas as dietary regimens, physical and mental attitudes affecting health, personal hygiene, occupational safety, lifestyle habits, posture, rest, work, and the many other activities of daily living which would enhance the effects of the chiropractic adjustment. Chiropractic is concerned with the total individual: his or her health, welfare, and survival.

It is apparent that chiropractic therapeutics is not only of a broad scope but also is accepted as such by a majority of the profession.

SCOPE OF PRACTICE FOR CHIROPRACTIC CLINICAL EFFECTIVENESS

The scope of chiropractic clinical effectiveness has not been defined, although neuromusculoskeletal complaints represent the largest percentage by far of clinical situations seen by chiropractors today (Table 3-1).[15,22,49]

There is a pool of clinical trial evidence suggesting that chiropractic treatment is effective for many conditions. Regardless, the efficacy of care will continue to be an area of debate and contention. It is also the most important field for research. The scope of practice for chiropractic education includes pathophysiological interests of sufficient breadth to challenge the profession's research resources well into the next century. Allopathic medicine has efficacy problems as well. Several medical critics agree with this quotation from Rachlis and Kushner: "As many as 80% of all treatments, including surgeries, have never been scientifically tested to prove their worth. Medical history is littered with abandoned therapies that were once common practices but are now utterly discredited."[50] Chiropractic appears to be in good company.

CRITERIA FOR A VALID SCOPE-OF-PRACTICE STATEMENT

It is reasonable to assume that the scope of chiropractic practice will be a prominent issue in the future of the profession as society and its agencies

Table 3-1 Percentage of Practice by Conditions Treated

	1988	1987	1986	1985	1984	1983
	%	%	%	%	%	%
Conditions						
Neuromusculoskeletal	86.4	87.5	87.2	86.8	85.3	84.2
Viscerosomatic	8.6	8.0	8.9	8.9	9.2	10.4
Vascular-related	3.7	2.9	3.0	2.9	4.0	4.0
Nutrition	0.3	0.3	0.3	0.4	0.4	0.4
Other	0.9	1.2	0.6	1.0	1.1	1.0
TOTALS	99.9	99.9	100.0	100.0	100.0	100.0

Courtesy of American Chiropractic Association

become increasingly aware of the capabilities, responsibilities, and limitations of the major disciplines that make up the health care system. All health care professions must accept the public sector's right to study appropriate roles for each discipline based on each profession's experience and clinical research data. Such studies will have a far-ranging effect on health care planning worldwide. In 1982, Canada's Minister of Health appointed a Health Professions Legislative Review Board "to examine health disciplines legislation worldwide." He said, "For the first time anywhere, as far as I am aware, the profession of medicine has been asked to define its scope of practice."[51] It would be foolish for any health care discipline to assume that it is immune to sociological change.

A valid scope-of-practice statement should meet several criteria. For example, it must be rational. All health care disciplines have certain broad limitations of practice, which should be identifiable within the scope-of-practice statement either by inclusion (negative) or exclusion (positive). It is far better, for example, to use a phrase such as "neurophysiological effects" to identify a broad area of clinical involvement than to list neurological disorders included or excluded. The chiropractic profession needs to reaffirm its primary role in health care, its secondary and tertiary health care roles in interdisciplinary cooperation, and its support for proved public health measures.

Any inference that a treatment modality has therapeutic value should be supported by clinical research or, preferably, by clinical trial data. Efficacy should not be based on theoretical considerations. If chiropractic therapy is effective in a specific clinical situation, an effort should be made to demonstrate this through well controlled research and to share the information through professional publications. Original research by chiropractic researchers published in refereed journals becomes even more critical, in this context, to defend the primary care role of chiropractic clinical care. The profession cannot rely on the research findings of others to defend the scientific basis of chiropractic health care. A nucleus of superbly qualified chiropractic researchers is active at all chiropractic colleges, adding to the pool of scientific knowledge.

Society will continue to demand accountability of all health care professions, as well as of the legal machinery necessary for the enforcement of practice privileges. The growing complexity of the social order creates its own bureaucracy, part of which concerns health care—particularly if public funds are involved (eg, Medicare). It will be difficult to be credible and accountable if each health care discipline does not have appropriate statements that clearly define the principal field of interest. As Chapman-Smith stated,[51] the Ontario Health Professions Legislative Review Board asked questions of the major health care professions such as

- Should a statute define your scope of practice and, if so, what should it be?
- What mechanisms should be used to assess the continuing competence of members?
- Why do medicine and dentistry (and USA osteopathy) assert that only they have proper training for diagnosis?
- How do you define spinal manipulative therapy?
- Why do medical practitioners require a 1-year, full-time postgraduate course of study to be capable of performing safe and effective spinal manipulative therapy?

There were dozens of similar questions for all health care disciplines. The important observation is that they were asked of medicine as well as chiropractic by an independent team of experts from the private sector.

Chiropractic is a distinctive type of health care profession. The description of the scope of practice implies that chiropractic physicians will have a primary role in the overall pattern of health care services. Therefore, chiropractors must acquire not only technical skills in diagnosing and treating disorders of spinal origin, but also a knowledge of the biological and behavioral sciences that will allow them to build on their experiences and to incorporate scientific advances into their practice. Clinical chiropractic consists of skills, knowledge, diagnosis, therapy planning, and patient management. The competent practitioner also has a duty to keep abreast not only of developments in chiropractic, but also of relevant socioeconomic factors and related community services.

REFERENCES

1. Sandoz R. A perspective for the chiropractic profession. *Journal of Canadian Chiropractic Association.* 1977;4:151–153.

2. Yessian MR. *State Licensure and Discipline of Chiropractors.* Washington, DC: Office of Inspector General, US Department of Health and Human Services; 1989:10,24–25.

3. *ACA Legal Handbook: Vol. II. Scope of Chiropractic Practice by Statute, Board Rule/Regulation.* Arlington, Va: American Chiropractic Association; 1985.

4. Preiss CE. *Official Directory of Chiropractic Examining Boards with Licensure and Practice Statistics, 1986–87.* Glendale, Calif: Federation of Chiropractic Licensing Boards; 1986.

5. Lamm LC, Wegner E. Chiropractic scope of practice. *American Journal of Chiropractic Medicine.* 1989;2:4,155–159.

6. Harris RL. 1989 ACA convention report. *Journal of the American Chiropractic Association.* 1989;8:43.

7. Pammer JC. Memo to members of council of delegates, American Chiropractic Association. Arlington, Va: 1989.

8. Hildebrandt RW. Reflections on a failed chiropractic association merger effort and its aftermath (Editorial). *American Journal of Chiropractic Medicine.* 1989;2:47–49.

9. Donahue JH. A proposal for the development of a contemporary philosophy of chiropractic. *American Journal of Chiropractic Medicine.* 1989;2:51–53.

10. *Scope of Practice and Educational Requirement for Chiropractors in Ontario—1973.* Toronto: Ontario Council of Health; 1973: Appendix D, 38–39.

11. *Educational Standards for Chiropractic Colleges.* Des Moines, Iowa: Council on Chiropractic Education; 1989.

12. Kranz KC. Chiropractic in the health care system with respect to primary care and the components of primary care. Presented to American Public Health Association Convention; November 18, 1985; Washington, DC.

13. MacDonald MJ, Morton L. *Chiropractic Evaluation Study—1985.* Aurora, Colo: US Department of Defense OCHAMPUS; 1986. MRI Project No. 8533-D.

14. Jamison JR. Chiropractic within the orthodox health care system. In: Campbell SA, Dillon NJ, Jamison J, eds. *Proceedings of a Conference on the Development and Needs in Education and Social Science Research of Chiropractic.* Armidale NSW Australia:UN of New England; 1984:53–66.

15. *Chiropractic State of the Art—1989-90.* Arlington, Va: American Chiropractic Association; 1989.

16. Vear HJ. Anatomy of a policy reversal. *Chiropractic History.* 1987;7:17–22.

17. Medical Practice Act of 1987, Ch 111, §2, amended 1989, General Assembly, State of Illinois, 1989–1990.

18. Vear HJ. An approach to the chiropractic scope of practice. *Journal of the Canadian Chiropractic Association.* 1973; 17:12–16.

19. Vear HJ. A pathological basis for prognosis. *Journal of the Canadian Chiropractic Association.* 1959;3:1,8–10.

20. Grice AS. Pathomechanics of the upper cervical spine. In: Vernon H, ed. *Upper Cervical Syndrome: Chiropractic Diagnosis and Treatment.* Baltimore: Williams & Wilkins; 1989:103–112.

21. Wyke B. Articular neurology and manipulative therapy. In: Glasgow E, Twomey L, Scull E, Kigynhans AM, Idezak R, eds. *Aspects of Manipulative Therapy.* Melbourne: Churchill Livingstone; 1985:72–80.

22. Vear HJ. A study into complaints of patients seeking chiropractic care. *Journal of the Canadian Chiropractic Association.* 1972; 16:9–13.

23. Phillips RB. A survey of Utah chiropractic patients. *Journal of the American Chiropractic Association.* 1981;15:113–134.

24. Juan G. Scope of practice, Membership memo. European Chiropractic Union; Paris; 1973.

25. Vear HJ. The status of chiropractic in Canada, 1976. *Journal of the American Chiropractic Association.* 1976;13:7, 23–26.

26. 42 U.S.C.100, 1395R, 1395U; 1973.

27. Brandies L. *Business-A Profession.* Boston: Hale, Cushman and Flint; 1914.

28. *Clinical Competencies.* Des Moines, Iowa: Council on Chiropractic Education; 1984.

29. *Educational Standards for Chiropractic Colleges: 1974-1988.* Des Moines, Iowa: Council on Chiropractic Education.

30. *Dorland's Medical Dictionary,* 25th ed. Philadelphia: WB Saunders; 1974:435.

31. *Blackiston's Gould Medical Dictionary.* 4th ed. New York: McGraw-Hill; 1979: 384.

32. Brennan MJ. Department of statistics completes 1988 survey. *Journal of the American Chiropractic Association.* 1989;26:52-54.

33. Position/policy paper on diagnosis, treatment and referral, adopted 1979. In: *Educational Standards for Chiropractic Colleges.* Des Moines, Iowa: Council on Chiropractic Education; 1988: IV-17.

34. Boyd W. *Preventive Medicine.* 7th ed. Philadelphia: WB Saunders; 1960: preface.

35. Vear HJ. The role of chiropractic in preventive health care. *Journal of the Canadian Chiropractic Association.* 1974;18:10-13.

36. Schmorl G, Junghanns H. *The Human Spine in Health and Disease,* 2nd ed. New York: Grune & Stratton; 1971:35-39.

37. Travel J, Simons D. *Myofascial Pain Dysfunction—the Trigger Point Manual.* Baltimore: Williams & Wilkins; 1983.

38. Gitelman R. The treatment of pain by spinal manipulation. In: Goldstein M, ed. *The Research Status of Spinal Manipulative Therapy.* Bethesda, Md: US Department of Health, Education and Welfare, 1975. NINCDS Monograph No. 15.

39. *Oxford English Dictionary-Compact Edition.* Oxford: Oxford University Press; 1971: Vol I:388.

40. Shambaugh P, Schafani L, Faneslow D. Reliability of the Derifield-Thompson test for leg length inequality, and use of the test to demonstrate cervical adjusting efficacy. *Journ Manip Physiol Therap.* 1988;11:396-399.

41. Herzog W, Read L, Conway J. Shaw L, McEwen M. Reliability of motion palpation procedures to detect sacroiliac joint fixations. *Journ Manip Physiol Therap.* 1989;12:86-92.

42. Vear HJ. Chiropractic spinal manipulation. In: *Introduction to Chiropractic Science.* Western States Chiropractic College; 1981:164-173.

43. Levine M. *The Structural Approach to Chiropractic.* New York: Comet Press; 1964.

44. Beatty H. *Anatomical Adjustive Technic,* 2nd ed. Denver: Author; 1939:20,25.

45. Peterson DH. Chiropractic terminology: a report. *Journal of the American Chiropractic Association.* 1988;46-57.

46. Vear HJ. Standards of chiropractic practice. *Journ Manip Physiol Therap.* 1985;1:33-43.

47. Puta FP. Nurse-physician collaboration toward quality. *Journal of Nursing Quality Assurance.* 1989; 3:2, 11-17.

48. *The Practice of Chiropractic—Treatment Methods. Chiropractic State of the Art, 1989-90.* Arlington, Va: American Chiropractic Association; 1989:16-17.

49. American Chiropractic Association. ACA department of statistics completes 1989 survey. *Journal of Chiropractic.* 1990; 27:2, 80.

50. Rachlis M, Kushner C. *Second Opinion.* Toronto: Collins; 1989:10.

51. Chapman-Smith D. Legislation for health care: Experience from Ontario. *Journal Australian Chiropractic Association.* 1987;17:4.

4

Objectives and Standards for Practice

Herbert J. Vear

A chiropractic physician who accepts a patient for any professional reason has a duty and a responsibility to perform an appropriate clinical evaluation and to arrive at a clinical impression or diagnosis of the patient's complaint before proceeding with care, consultation, or referral. This is a premise required by the profession, wherever chiropractic physicians practice,[1,2] and it is prescribed in the educational standards of all chiropractic accrediting agencies.[3-5]

> The doctor of chiropractic has the legal and ethical responsibility as a primary health care provider, to adequately diagnose and render treatment and/or referral commensurate with his findings and education.[3(p66)]

The construct of objectives for chiropractic practice, standards of care, and quality of care is the responsibility of the profession, through its associations, its accredited colleges, and the consensus of its practitioners. Although the objectives and standards of practice may be based primarily on what is taught in and through chiropractic colleges, they must be consistent with those of the scientific community and with the usual and customary practices of the profession. For example, the chiropractic adjustment is the usual and customary therapeutic modality used by all chiropractors. Science has not adequately evaluated this therapy except in a few clinical situations, however. Regardless, clinical trials have demonstrated unequivocally that there is an important clinical value for chiropractic adjustment beyond that expected by random chance or obtained through a placebo.[6] On the other hand, there is an undisputed scientific basis for analysis of urine and blood for the differential diagnosis of certain diseases. This distinction between "usual and customary" and "scientific basis" for therapeutic and diagnostic modalities applies also to allopathic medicine, as it is estimated that 80% of all medical therapies are scientifically untested.[7,8]

In the evaluation of the clinical judgment used in applying the accepted standards of chiropractic practice, a dichotomy presents itself. Clinical (ie, diagnostic and therapeutic) procedures that are primary to clinical chiropractic (eg, spinal adjustment) are interpreted and judged by chiropractic physicians. Clinical procedures that are not primary to chiropractic practice (eg, electrodiagnosis and clinical psychology), however, are interpreted and judged by those in whose professional domain these procedures are primary. In many situations, two or more health care professions share a domain (eg, diagnostic imaging), although the perspectives may differ (eg, biomechanical findings and pathological findings).

There are two sources for standards of chiropractic practice. The standards of practice taught by accredited colleges and accepted as usual and customary by the profession represent the highest level of standards, eclectic and ethical. Chiropractic practice acts also dictate standards of practice, however. Some of these are at a level below what the profession and its educational institutions have mandated as minimal. There is little uniformity from one practice act to another in determining a statutory "usual and customary" practice protocol.[9]

It is essential for standards of practice to be rational and defensible; they must not place artificial barriers in the way of clinical progress. As science and technology advance, so should the components and standards of chiropractic practice. Not to be forgotten is the fact that standards of practice represent the "patient's Bill of Rights" in all matters of health care and, as such, must be under constant review to reflect the changing scope of practice and technology.

ORTHODOX, EXPERIMENTAL, AND ANECDOTAL CLASSIFICATIONS

Orthodox/mainstream procedures, technologies, and equipment include all categories and classifications of procedures, technologies, or equipment that are widely used and accepted within or among individual branches of the health care disciplines; their use is generally based on the scientific method.

Experimental/investigational procedures, technologies, or equipment do not have widespread use and acceptance within or among individual branches of health care disciplines, but they are nevertheless of such a nature that, based on testing and clinical trial, there is no organized scientific opposition to their use in health care. Although not orthodox, such items are not considered quackery. Anecdotal procedures, technologies, or equipment have not been adequately evaluated by the experimental method or clinical trials. Items included in this category originate and depend on experience and observation. *Post hoc, ergo propter hoc* (after this, therefore, because of this).

Accredited colleges should make every effort possible to present course material in chiropractic clinical sciences with due regard for these three categories. Critical and discriminatory analysis of diagnostic and therapeutic procedures according to these categories will increase the credibility of chiropractic education and stimulate meaningful research into clinical chiropractic.

ANALYSIS OF CHIROPRACTIC OBJECTIVES

Objective 1

To establish a satisfactory and confidential relationship with the patient and determine the nature of the patient's health problem.

There is little argument that the failure of a chiropractic physician to establish a satisfactory relationship with a new patient from the very beginning of the doctor-patient association is a major source of grievance later. The emphasis placed on the initial interview with the patient by the courts, by practice management consultants, and by clinical writers is evidence of the importance of this event.

No single attribute is more difficult to acquire and more exacting to maintain than the doctor-patient bond. Effective interpersonal skills do not just happen, nor are they inherited; they are learned. Because clinical practice requires a great deal of interaction with other people, the ability to relate to other individuals in productive and meaningful ways is essential. Positive human relationships and patient cooperation can be achieved by showing concern and consideration for patient distress and attempting to relieve anxiety, tension, and discomfort by listening, understanding, and communicating. The confidentiality of the clinical interaction is also imperative. Violation of confidentiality or improper disclosure of the patient's record may subject the chiropractic physician and his or her staff to civil and criminal liability. Patient records can be released only if the patient has authorized the release or if statutory, regulatory, or other legal authority prevails.[10]

The establishment of a doctor-patient relationship is not the only outcome of the first meeting with a patient. It cannot automatically be assumed that every patient who seeks chiropractic care will require or benefit from such care. A patient is entitled to an interview of reasonable duration to enable the chiropractic physician to determine whether to proceed with the case history and the clinical review. Thus, the outcomes of the initial interview should be

- establishment of a doctor-patient relationship with a continuing goal to build trust, communication, and understanding
- an appreciation of the patient's chief complaint and the reasons for consulting with the chiropractor
- a determination by the chiropractic physician either to proceed further with the patient or to make a referral to another health care provider

In meeting Objective 1, the chiropractor must comply with certain professional standards of practice. As a primary health care provider, the chiropractic physician shall

1. accept responsibility for the chiropractic care of the patient
2. recognize his or her own professional capabilities and limitations
3. during the initial patient interview and consultation, employ measures of observation to profile the patient's health problem
4. continue to provide care for the patient and/or refer the patient to another health care provider
5. provide the patient with confidentiality and the assurance that clinical records shall be released only with the patient's authorization

Objective 2

To elicit from the patient a case history to determine if the patient has a health problem amenable to the application of chiropractic therapeutic procedures or whether referral to another primary health care provider is indicated.

As a primary health care provider, the chiropractic physician has imposing professional, ethical, and moral responsibilities to provide the patient with a quality clinical evaluation, which is permanently recorded in the patient's case record. The confidentiality of the case history contributes to the doctor-patient bond. History taking provides the chiropractor with an opportunity to increase rapport with the patient through empathy, understanding, and patience.

It is a primary responsibility of the chiropractic physician to take a detailed case history before performing a diagnostic examination or providing health care. The case history is a record of the patient's past and present health pattern, and it is the basis for the physical examination and the ordering of specific radiologic and laboratory tests. The importance of the case record is never greater than in the defense of a malpractice suit.

When information on examination findings, diagnosis, treatment plan, and patient progress have been added to the history, the case report becomes a valuable data base for purposes of a practice audit and clinical research beyond the basic patient management needs. A justifiable and consistent criticism leveled at the chiropractic profession is the lack of clinical data that support the professed scope of practice, competency claims, and cost containment for therapeutic and maintenance care. Lane added support to this viewpoint.

> Medical records serve a variety of purposes. Their principal purpose is to memorialize by documentation the patient's symptoms and history, examinations and tests conducted, findings, diagnosis, treatment and progress. This would of course be true whether the patient receives medical attention while hospitalized or as an outpatient or during office visits. Medical records serve as a means of transmitting information between health care providers. This is of course absolutely essential to medical personnel who have the responsibility of evaluating a patient's condition and planning medical care. Medical records are also important because they serve to provide information for researchers and those involved in continuing medical education programs.[11(p302)]

Often it is difficult or impossible to communicate with the patient because of age (eg, infants and children), language, disease (eg, cerebrovascular accident), conscious state, and lack of cooperation. Under such circumstances, it is the chiropractor's duty to obtain information from other sources before beginning diagnostic or treatment schedules.

A standard of practice also applies to Objective 2. For example, the chiropractic physician shall do a thorough case history on each patient and provide a permanent record of the findings, including

1. an understanding of the patient's chief complaint, past and present health pattern, and psychosocial factors
2. a basis for the specific physical, laboratory, and radiologic examinations needed
3. recognition that in the best interest of the patient, referral or consultation may be necessary before further clinical investigation takes place

Objective 3

To arrive at a provisional diagnosis by evaluating evidence obtained through differential diagnostic assessment, diagnostic tests, diagnostic imaging, and an attempt to identify any unrecognized problems.

As stated earlier, the case history is one basis for determining the appropriate depth and direction of the physical and laboratory examination of the patient. Such a clinical evaluation, involving diagnostic procedures usual and customary to chiropractic practice, should focus on the system(s) most affected in or by the patient's chief complaint. As the examination continues, indications for further specific diagnostic imaging and clinical laboratory tests are likely to become evident.

The failure of a chiropractic physician to perform a comprehensive physical examination could result in a malpractice claim if, by omission, clinical findings go undiscovered and the patient suffers harm through diagnostic or treatment negligence. In this regard, chiropractors have two additional duties. First, it is imperative that diagnostic procedures (and treatment) be consistent with scientific knowledge, with the usual and customary practices of a majority of the profession, and with the teachings of accredited colleges. Second, under the doctrine of informed consent, a patient has the right to know the risks, consequences, or side-effects that may arise from a diagnostic (and treatment) procedure. These two concerns are of particular importance in chiropractic because of the many untested, quasi-scientific diagnostic (and therapeutic) procedures used in the discipline, many from entrepreneurial sources.

Testing procedures used in chiropractic practice should be based on anatomical and physiological fact, and the chiropractor should use orthodox instrumentation to perform the physical examination. Experimental and anecdotal procedures and/or instrumentation, if used, should be explained to the patient as such. The attitudes of chiropractors vary on charging for experimental and anecdotal procedures. It does not seem completely ethical, however, to charge for experimental or anecdotal methods unless a prior agreement has been reached with the patient or guardian.

Many examination procedures are anecdotal at best, but chiropractic physicians have sufficient clinical expertise and acumen in orthodox orthopedic and neurological testing, with clinical value judgments based on the specific needs of chiropractic practice, not to venture into uncharted waters. For example, test and examination procedures researched and developed by the chiropractic profession to evaluate spinal biomechanics for subtle and difficult deviations from normal are orthodox to the profession, regardless of their use or acceptance in other health care professions.

There can be no restrictions on a chiropractic physician's ability to order the laboratory examinations necessary to arrive at a clinical impression for chiropractic care or to make an appropriate referral. Of course, there is societal concern about the overutilization and abuse of laboratory examinations by those in all health care professions. The free exchange of patient clinical data among health care professionals would reduce many costs. The educational program approved by the Council on Chiropractic Education (CCE) and all member colleges includes the clinical indications for using and interpreting the test results of appropriate laboratory procedures. The importance of laboratory tests to successful care is frequently forgotten by the busy physician, an omission that will not be forgotten in a malpractice lawsuit.

It is incumbent on the chiropractic physician to use reasonable judgment in arriving at a diagnosis or clinical impression before initiating a treatment program or making a referral to another provider. In determining a diagnosis or clinical impression, for example, the chiropractor must use the principles of differential diagnosis. The chiropractic physician uses not only the diagnostic skills, procedures, and terminology peculiar to chiropractic, but also the procedures and terminology of generic medicine. The courts recognize that diagnosis of human ailments is an art, but they require adherence to usual and customary procedures.

In accomplishing Objective 3, the chiropractor again considers the standards of practice. For example, the chiropractic physician, within the statutory scope of practice, shall

1. use the diagnostic procedures, techniques, and instrumentation used in the academic and clinical training received in and through accredited colleges of chiropractic
2. perform and interpret appropriate physical examination procedures and techniques, recording the findings
3. use selected and/or appropriate laboratory tests and procedures, interpret the test results, and record the findings
4. arrive at and record a provisional diagnosis objectively by evaluating evidence and using differential diagnostic assessment
5. recognize concomitant conditions, establishing any interrelationships, directing their proper referral, and recording them in the case record

Objective 4

To use reasonable judgment in deciding on the appropriate chiropractic care, taking into account any specific or general contraindications to the planned therapy.

Although chiropractic is a drugless, nonsurgical approach to health care, the array of therapeutic procedures available to the chiropractic physician for patient care is impressive. The primary therapeutic modality and common denominator of chiropractic care is the correction of a subluxation-fixation complex by specific adjustment to a vertebral or pelvic segment(s). In recent years, the designation *spinal manipulative therapy* has become common usage throughout the world.[12] The chiropractic profession and its educational institutions prefer to distinguish between chiropractic adjustment and manipulation, however (see Chapter 3).

Because the majority of state and provincial chiropractic practice statutes permit chiropractic physicians to use reasonable judgment in selecting a variety of therapeutic procedures in a supportive role to spinal manipulation (adjustment), these adjunctive procedures must be identified and codified—along with the right to add procedures as need and new discovery require. Reasonable judgment is based on the education, clinical skills, and experience of the physician. Physician awareness of medical necessity, as defined by Schaffer, is imperative to quality practice.

> Once a patient is accepted by the doctor, the physician automatically acknowledges that the patient's condition will be diagnosed if possible (at least differentially diagnosed) and that the examination, tests, and therapy to be used will be based on scientific studies and principles that are generally accepted by the profession at large as being necessary and appropriate to properly diagnose and treat patients with the particular condition presented.
>
> The relationship between condition and procedure is termed the "medical necessity," and the third party contracts usually call for a direct relationship between covered services and medical necessity. It also underscores why office documents are necessary to substantiate the services rendered.[13]

To avoid making poor judgments, clinical decisions must be made at the higher cognitive level of evaluation in the taxonomy of educational objectives.[14] Gronlund defined evaluation as

> concerned with the ability to judge the value of material for a given purpose. The judgments are to be based on definite criteria. These may be internal or external criteria. Learning outcomes in this area are highest in the cognitive hierarchy because they contain elements of all the other categories, plus conscious value judgments based on clearly defined criteria.[15]

It is a tradition in chiropractic practice to provide new patients with a report of clinical findings before beginning chiropractic care. This report includes not only the chiropractor's clinical impression of the patient's complaint, but also the kind and frequency of treatment recommended, an estimate of the number of treatments required, and the projected cost. What has not been traditional, but is of growing importance, is informed consent. The chiropractic physician has the duty to obtain the patient's consent to proceed with treatment. It is essential that common language is used. If there are reasonable alternative therapies available of risks inherent in the application of chiropractic care, the patient must be informed of these possibilities. The probability of success and the result to be anticipated if nothing is done should also be explained to the patient.

Each procedure included in the treatment plan (eg, therapy rehabilitation, prevention, or maintenance) must be recorded in the patient's case record file. All additions or deletions to the plan must be recorded, along with patient response. It is a serious error of omission not to record therapeutic procedures in view of the dangers of litigation. To summarize, reasonable judgment in diagnosis and treatment is based on the physician's ability to criticize, discriminate, justify, interpret, relate, and support clinical action—the application of scientific protocol.

There is a standard of practice that is relevant to Objective 4. The chiropractic physician, in deciding on appropriate care, shall

1. provide patients only with those appropriate treatment methods that fall within the scope of practice authorized by state or provincial law and/or medical necessity
2. identify any contraindications or nonindications to chiropractic therapeutics and make a proper referral
3. apprise the patient in nontechnical terms about all anticipated practices and procedures, including the probability of success and the results to be anticipated if nothing is done; receive the patient's informed consent for chiropractic therapeutics; and record this in the patient's case record
4. record and date the treatment plan in the patient's case record file, together with any conditions or deletions that may occur

Objective 5

To monitor the patient to ensure that the patient is progressing as expected and to make appropriate changes in management as required.

Not all health care results in the relief of discomfort or the alleviation of causal factors. The application of reasonable judgment to a therapeutic plan is no guarantee to the patient or the physician that a clinical improvement will follow. The use of acceptable clinical care and repeated evaluations of the patient's condition provide a better opportunity for clinical success. Controlled clinical trial is a valid approach to patient care. Quite likely, a large percentage of all health care falls into this category, largely because of lack of clinical outcome data.

Reasonable judgment in deciding on appropriate chiropractic care should include consideration of the needs of individual patients. For example, it may be necessary to adapt chiropractic treatment for pregnant patients, bedridden patients, osteoporotic patients, physically handicapped patients, injured patients, geriatric patients, or pediatric patients. The manual dexterity required to provide satisfactory adjustments and other modalities of treatment must also receive consideration. Although chiropractic practice is dependent on the manual skills of the chiropractor, it is not possible for colleges or licensing boards to measure the manual dexterity needed for all manipulative and adjustive procedures available for patient care. The responsibility for the chiropractic care of the patient remains with the chiropractic physician, who must recognize his or her capabilities and limitations.

It is not uncommon for a patient to receive health care from more than one health care provider at the same time. In fact, interdisciplinary cooperation in providing health care is increasing and should be encouraged. The chiropractic physician has the responsibility to recognize the consequences of delayed treatment, particularly treatment that is not within the chiropractic domain.

As for the other objectives, there is a relevant standard of practice. The chiropractic physician, in providing appropriate care, shall

1. institute the appropriate chiropractic management and treatment, including treatment of the disorder; the relief of discomfort; and the alleviation of environmental, casual, and irritating factors, where possible
2. modify treatment to the needs of individual patients
3. use only those manipulative and adjustive techniques for which a manual dexterity competence has been achieved
4. use only those modalities of treatment for which competence has been achieved

Objective 6

To discharge the patient at the end point of treatment or when no further improvement in the patient's condition can be expected.

This responsibility includes follow-up care of the patient, where necessary.

At no time is it more important to maintain a good relationship with a patient than during a course of treatment, no matter how many days or weeks the treatment may take. Pain and anxiety may change patients' moods and attitudes toward themselves and their doctor dramatically, even during a single office visit. Once again, the chiropractic physician is called upon to exercise sound and reasonable judgment. The chiropractor has a responsibility to provide a reasonable amount of time for the care of each patient, not only for the chief complaint, but also for those less explicit, but nevertheless essential, services to the total person. This requires patience, understanding, concern, and, above all, empathy.

As mentioned earlier, it is essential for the chiropractor to make adequate and intelligible progress notes in the patient's case record. These notes should include verbatim patient statements of reaction to treatment or improvement, nature of the treatment, home care counseling, and other pertinent facts (eg, telephone calls of concern for progress and reaction, and canceled appointments). The CCE succinctly stated that

> the doctor of chiropractic is expected to keep and maintain adequate records clearly showing the progression of events under the clinical review, diagnosis or clinical impression, chiropractic care and case management. These records and/or reports should be available to the patient or other appropriate designee.[3(p67)]

The chiropractor must monitor the patient's progress in order to assess the effects of treatment, upgrade the working diagnosis and prognosis, and report these to the patient as a part of continuing informed consent. The point at which consultation or referral is necessary depends primarily on the clinical experience of the chiropractor. In general, some evidence or measurable clinical improvement (objective or subjective) should be noted in most cases within eight visits or 2 to 4 weeks. Jaquet suggested a slightly lower figure of 4 to 6 visits, however.[16] The total number of visits to reach a medically stationary condition is not a factor for standards of practice, but it is a consideration for standards of care and quality assurance (process and outcomes).

Monitoring the patient's progress requires frequent reassessment by means of appropriate examination procedures. It is a good practice to reevaluate the patient's condition at each visit, by appropriate examination procedures including static and dynamic palpation as an indicator for the clinical need of spinal manipulation. Of course, the extent and depth of reexamination is entirely dependent on individual circumstances. A patient who is not making satisfactory progress requires a more extensive examination, however; as Osler noted, "Listen, the patient is telling you the diagnosis."[17] Jaquet noted four possible reasons for little or no clinical progress: (1) the original diagnosis is not correct; (2) the treatment is not appropriate; (3) the doctor-patient relationship is not satisfactory; and (4) the doctor has not understood why the patient sought chiropractic care in the first place.[16] Thus, reexamination sometimes leads to referral to another health care provider for consultation or care. When it has been determined that chiropractic care is ineffective for a patient, referral to another primary or secondary health care provider is a duty.

Health insurers generally will not pay for health care (therapeutic) beyond medical necessity or beyond the patient's attainment of a stationary clinical state; insurance plans are not health plans intended to cover maintenance and casual care, but a means to underwrite the cost of sickness and injury. This is an important consideration when a chiropractor must decide on the end point of treatment, which is not always an easy task. The chiropractor again must use reasonable judgment. The patient should be given an appropriate exit examination to confirm that the end point of treatment has been reached and that no further clinical improvement can be expected by continuing an active therapeutic regimen. Not infrequently, the patient makes the decision to discontinue treatment for one of a number of reasons.

• a return to health or preclinical status
• no improvement beyond a certain point, as the patient has reached stationary status
• an impression that treatment is being continued only for monetary reasons
• lapse of insurance coverage
• financial burden
• an impression that the chiropractor has lost interest in the case, is too busy to provide quality care, ignores telephone calls or office questions, and does not respond to emergency situations

Although these reasons may not be germane to the standard objective, they are important to quality of care.

Maintenance care, a regimen designed to provide for the patient's continued well-being or to maintain the optimum state of health while minimizing recurrence of the clinical problem,[18] is a clinical reality for all health care professions, but there must be a scientific rationale for such care. Maintenance and preventive care, treatment procedures considered necessary to prevent the development of clinical status,[18] are enigmas to chiropractic practice. There are no clinical studies to support the validity of either form of intervention for nonspecific or ambiguous clinical situations. Furthermore, there is a marked difference between maintenance or preventive care directed to the general and nonspecific health status of the patient and follow-up care directed to the clinical stationary status of a patient who has undergone therapeutic care for a specific clinical problem.

It is the responsibility of the chiropractor to justify follow-up maintenance care, using scientific or clinical trial rationale whenever possible. Such treatment requires the patient's informed consent, however. According to Schaffer, a charge of abandonment leading to a malpractice claim can be made if "the doctor fails to provide adequate follow-up care, and an adverse event happens to the patient that would probably have been prevented by reasonable follow-up skill and care."[19] This implies that, once a patient reaches a chiropractic clinical stationary status and some clinical problem remains, it may be necessary to refer the patient to another health care provider for additional follow-up care. Palliative care (ie, treatment that relieves the symptoms of exacerbations, but results in no net improvement in the patient's stationary condition[20]) is a reasonable and valid clinical approach, however, to which the chiropractic physician can resort when a patient experiences recurring symptoms or exacerbations caused by the original complaint.

The 12-treatment service cap instituted by Medicare in 1984, allegedly to control overutilization of chiropractic care, does not serve the continuing health care needs of Medicare patients. Because of excessive care by a small percentage of the profession, all Medicare patients lose access to palliative chiropractic care. Therefore, it is in each patient's best interest to learn about preventing either a recurrence of the complaint or a new disability. The chiropractor can help by providing the patient with the basic principles of spinal care for primary and secondary prevention of clinical problems.[21]

Two standards of practice follow from Objective 6. The chiropractic physician, during the course of providing care, shall

1. monitor and assess the patient's progress resulting from treatment and record such information in the patient's case record file
2. recognize the need for reassessment of the patient regarding treatment, diagnosis, and prognosis, including consultation and referral
3. modify treatment and management appropriately, based on reassessment

The chiropractic physician, in determining limits to a patient's therapeutic care, shall

1. evaluate the patient's clinical progress and, by examination and other means, decide on the end point of treatment
2. plan effective follow-up care by referral; by maintenance care; by palliative care; by counseling; and by instructing the patient and the family, if necessary, regarding the cause, management, and prognosis for the problem, including preventive measures

CONCLUSION

The "patient's Bill of Rights" represents a continuation of efforts by the educational and political arms of the chiropractic profession to give formal recognition to standards of practice and quality care,which are concerned more with process and outcome than structure. As chiropractic practice acts are revised, the profession must expect legislators to pay more attention to economic issues, scope of practice, standards of care, and quality assurance. The profession must be prepared for such legislative activity.

REFERENCES

1. *Code of Ethics.* Arlington, Va: American Chiropractic Association; 1988.

2. *Code of Ethics.* Mississauga, Ontario: Ontario Chiropractic Association; 1989.

3. *Educational Standards for Chiropractic Education.* Des Moines, Iowa: Council on Chiropractic Education; 1989.

4. *Educational Standards for Chiropractic Education.* Toronto: Council on Chiropractic Education (C); 1990.

5. *Accreditation Procedures and Standards for Chiropractic Education.* Mornington: The Australasian Council on Chiropractic Education; 1988.

6. Egli AB. Spine and heart, vertebrogenous cardiac syndrome. *Annals of Swiss Chiropractic Association.* 1969;4:95–105.

7. Rachlis M, Kuschner C. *Second Opinion.* Toronto: Collins Publishers; 1989:10.

8. *Assessing the Efficacy and Safety of Medical Technologies.* Springfield, Va: National Technical Information Service, US Department of Commerce; 1978.

9. Kusserow RP. *State Licensure and Discipline of Chiropractors.* Washington, DC: Office of Inspector General, US Department of Health and Human Services; 1989.

10. Roach WH, Chernoff SN, Esley CL. Liability for improper disclosure of medical records. In: *Medical Records and the Law.* Gaithersburg, Md: Aspen Publishers; 1985;156.

11. Lane F. Purpose and importance of medical records. In: Lane F, ed., *Medical Litigation Guide.* Wilmette: Callaghan & Co; 1984; 1:3–4.

12. Goldstein M, ed. *The Research Status of Spinal Manipulative Therapy.* Bethesda, Md: US Department of Health, Education and Welfare; 1975. NINCDS Monograph No. 15.

13. Schaffer RC. *Developing a Chiropractic Practice.* Arlington, Va: American Chiropractic Association; 1984;6–7.

14. Bloom BS, ed. et al. *Taxonomy of Educational Objectives: Cognitive Domain.* New York: David McKay Co; 1956.

15. Gronlund NE. *Stating Behavioral Objectives for Classroom Instruction.* New York: Macmillan; 1970:20.

16. Jaquet PF. *An Introduction to Clinical Chiropractic.* Geneva: Grounauer; 1974:25.

17. Osler W. *Principles and Practice of Medicine.* Philadelphia: Lippincott; 1892.

18. *Manual of Chiropractic Peer Review Information.* Des Moines, Iowa: American Chiropractic Association; 1973.

19. Schaffer RC. *Clinical Malpractice: Basic Preventive and Defensive Procedures.* Des Moines, Iowa: National Chiropractic Mutual Insurance Company; 1983:16.

20. Hansen DT, ed. *Chiropractic Standards of Practice and Utilization Guidelines in the Care and Treatment of Injured Workers.* Olympia, Wash: Chiropractic Advisory Committee, Department of Labor and Industries; 1988:14.

21. Vear HJ. The role of chiropractic in preventative health care. *Journal of the Canadian Chiropractic Association.* 1970;12:10–13.

5

Quality of Care and Chiropractic Necessity

Daniel T. Hansen

[The chiropractic profession] must exactingly define the role that it can best play in the present day health world on the basis of good clinical evidence it presently has, not on what it may hope to scientifically prove at some indefinite time in the future.

. . . It must be recognized that ultimately it will be the professional competency of its practitioners that will prevail, not the politicolegal acquisition of constitutional rights.

R. Hildebrandt

Ever since the chiropractic profession entered the insurance reimbursement arena more than three decades ago, there has been a growing interest in the use of chiropractic services. The concern of public and private reimbursement agencies about the "necessity of chiropractic care" and the composition of "reasonable and necessary" services has paralleled the chiropractic profession's rapid expansion into reimbursement schemes. As the chiropractic inclusion in insurance programs has matured, so has the expectation that chiropractic providers will respond to health care industry initiatives in quality assurance and standards of care. Reimbursement managers have orchestrated this movement in response to the uncontrolled escalation of health care costs over the past 10 years with no significant improvement in general health. More and more physician groups, including specialty societies, are establishing practice parameters, partly to prevent the purchasers of health care from establishing such parameters.

Past attempts at physician monitoring and cost controls have done little in holding down the rapid rise of costs associated with hospitalization, physician services (including chiropractic services), ancillary services, and the purchase of durable goods. Many of the increased costs may be due to technological advancement and defensive medicine, but a significant portion of the increase in costs is attributable to the purchase of inappropriate care.

The contemporary rhetorical questions are, why is the public and private reimbursement system expected to pay for unnecessary surgical procedures, hospital stays, and excessive physical therapy or chiropractic care? What guidelines for utilization or standards of care exist for provider groups that can be used in controlling costs and ensuring the purchase of quality and cost-effective care? Who are the authorities in these provider groups that can be counted on to establish those guidelines?

QUALITY ASSURANCE: HISTORY OF ITS DEVELOPMENT

"Until the 1970's practitioners, hospitals, [health care] researchers and medical schools enjoyed a broad grant of authority to run their own affairs."[1] Health care came under socioeconomic pressure in the 1970s, however, and mandates for reform began with the Nixon Administration. When health care reforms at the national level proved ineffective, emphasis shifted to the individual states. Now the states are looking to big business for assistance in comprehensive health care planning and management strategies.

The impetus for this shift from governance by the practitioner to monitoring by "Big Brother" is the rising cost of health care, which continues to punish society. This is evidenced by the cutbacks on basic health coverage in public sector programs and the increases in insurance premiums at the private level. The public has become sufficiently disgusted with this disproportionate escalation to demand that the health care system develop strategies for the purchase of cost-effective care and eliminate duplication and waste. Although there is still a need to improve access to efficient and effective care, the movement for reducing costs has become stronger than ever.

The key to the shift of the control of health care during the past 20 years has been the development of competition and quality assurance in the health care market. Both concepts have been slow in their maturation, but, with the coming of the 1990s, each will play significant roles in the distribution of and reimbursement for health care resources. Competition is manifested by managed care schemes, such as health maintenance organizations (HMOs) and preferred provider organizations (PPOs). Quality assurance developed slowly, first as research efforts and later in programs implemented by various public and private reimbursement agencies.

Development of Quality Assessment

Modern health care quality assessment is attributed, for the most part, to one person—Avedis Donabedian, known in the industry as the "father of the academic enterprise of quality assessment in health."[2] The pillar of his accomplishments is his delineation of the "methods of quality assessment," including structure, process, and outcome.[3] These categories provide the fundamental framework of quality assessment.

Structure is the study of the total assemblage of resources or the environment for health care, such as health care delivery personnel, credentials of providers, health care facilities, and collected protocols of health care procedures. If measures of structure of care are used alone, however, it is difficult to infer anything about the quality of care actually provided. As a result, structure measures have fallen in disfavor in recent years.

Process involves factors related to the delivery of care, such as normative behavior associated with diagnostic evaluation, access to care, rate of utilization, and choice of therapeutic procedures. Both technical and art-of-care dimensions can be assessed when evaluating process of care. The art-of-care measures may include the degree to which patients feel that the physician is compassionate, listens carefully to their complaints, and explains the reasons for the tests ordered and the treatment prescribed.

Donabedian defined outcomes as the end products of health care, determined by health status indicators, morbidity/mortality ratios, and patient satisfaction. The health status indicators include not only the usually emphasized physical and physiological measurements, but also social and psychological functions. Outcomes should not be used exclusively in measuring quality of care for three reasons: (1) it is difficult to attribute specific outcomes to specific episodes of care; (2) outcomes of interest are usually difficult to measure, except mortality; and (3) outcome measures do not provide information that is directly useful in quality assessment.[4] Good outcome measures can be tied to process measures directed at specific steps that can be taken to improve care, however.

Another key figure in the development of quality assessment has been John Wennberg. More than 20 years ago, Wennberg did a "small area analysis" in which he examined surgery rates in various geographical sites in Vermont. He found that the frequency of common surgical procedures varied significantly in different geographical areas. The sudden exposure of variation in the delivery of health care raised doubts about the appropriateness of certain procedures.[5] Since then, the interest of quality in health care has mushroomed, and health care economics has become a more significant component to health care quality assessment and quality improvement.

Methods of Investigation

The evolution of quality assessment also includes the maturation of methods of investigation, both inside and outside the health care professions.

Over the past 40 years, but especially within the past 20 years, there have been three general methods of investigation explored: implicit review, explicit review, and the use of sentinels (ie, "red flags").[6]

The *implicit review* process depends on the use of intraprofessional experts who can recognize good care. This may involve peer review or similar professional review panels. Implicit measurement techniques have several documented disadvantages.

1. The reliability of judgments made by implicit raters is typically very low.
2. Different raters judge the same cases differently.
3. The credibility of implicit raters is difficult to support.
4. Unadorned implicit judgments fail to provide specific guidance about why specific episodes represented poor quality of care.[4]

The advantages of implicit measurement techniques are that they are relatively inexpensive and they are useful in assessing all aspects of a particular episode of care.

Explicit review revolves around the creation of criteria for care and the subsequent review of records to determine whether the care conformed to those set criteria. The standards or criteria for care must be established and accepted by consensus. This method is well suited for use by appropriately trained nonprofessionals. The disadvantages of explicit measurements are that they

1. are much more difficult than implicit measurements
2. tend to be highly specific to an individual topic
3. are not easily applied to complex conditions

The *sentinel method* of investigation has been used in recent years for quality assessment of the chiropractic profession. With this approach, quality assurance managers attempt to define unacceptable events or procedures as "red flags." Once one or more of these events has occurred, a more detailed implicit or explicit investigation may be undertaken. In one such contemporary system, the statistical "outliers" are identified according to the rates of utilization, and the providers involved are subsequently reviewed for those previously determined sentinel "flags."

CONSIDERATIONS IN QUALITY OF CARE

From the quiet arrival of the Donabedian and Wennberg era, the health care professions have now entered a never before realized period of accountability that should, at the very least, touch physicians (including chiropractors), administrators, regulators, purchasers of care, and patient advocates. It can be hoped that a nurturing of further interest in improving the quality of care will cause leaders in these groups to become quality assessment experts within or on behalf of their particular professional group. Presently, there is a paucity of such experts in the chiropractic profession.

The primary components in the definition of the quality of care remain excellent technical care and favorable health status outcomes. The former is assured through proof of professional competency, technological assessment, and adherence to standards of care; the latter, through outcomes assessment. Other measurements of quality include access to care, appointment access, waiting time in waiting rooms, ambience, support staff warmth, provider warmth, provider skill, continuity of care, patient's sense of sharing in the control of care, and patient satisfaction.[6] Although the evaluation of these other elements of "caring" may not weigh as heavily with some investigators, they are nonetheless important.

Factors That Contribute to Poor Quality

A recent report from the Congressional Office of Technology Assessment (OTA) evaluated information available to consumers on quality of care. OTA subsequently adopted the following definition of quality of care:

> The quality of a provider's [health] care is the degree to which the process of care increases the probability of desired patient outcomes and reduces the probability of undesired outcomes, given the state of medical knowledge.[4(p9)]

A multidisciplinary panel and task force of the National Institute of Medicine also evaluated concepts of quality of care, especially to the elderly, and determined that there is a significant "burden of poor quality." They listed three contributing factors, each of equal importance.

1. improper care, that is, poor performance of physicians in technical skills or interpersonal relations. This care would have been appropriate if it had been properly performed.
2. overuse of health care services. There is substantial evidence that overutilization exists and poses a risk to patients.
3. underuse of health care services. This is believed to be considerable, but is harder to detect; it also poses risks to patients.

Each of these three kinds of problems calls for different measurement techniques and different quality improvement mechanisms.

The first-line strategy of health care quality control managers who must ensure the purchase of quality care is the elimination of unnecessary care. In the design of HMOs, for example, patients receive fewer services; in PPOs, where there is a co-payment, patients have fewer physician visits and hospitalizations without apparent deleterious effects on health.[6]

According to Chassin and colleagues,[4] as much as 30% of health care is inappropriate as overuse of services. In this context, overutilization includes not only higher numbers of treatments, but also increased use of expensive or inappropriate diagnostic tests; furthermore, it carries substantial cost implications. This is one of the few areas in which the twin goals of cost containment and quality assurance converge. The benefits of solving overuse problems can be measured in dollars saved as well as in unnecessary risks averted.[4]

On the opposite end of the spectrum is the underutilization problem, the failure to employ appropriate health care services.[7] Underutilization is likely when treatment "lids or caps" are placed on a benefit, such as chiropractic services. These caps are typically overly prescriptive, and they do not adequately take into account medical or chiropractic necessity. It is not uncommon for a health plan to have a limit of five or ten visits for chiropractic services, which undoubtedly denies some patients needed care. If there is a request for an extension of chiropractic care, a nonchiropractor typically determines the necessity. Underuse is a difficult problem to investigate, because the effort requires an examination of events that should have occurred, but did not. Moreover, underuse is a problem that will be very costly to remedy.[4]

Factors That Contribute to Unnecessary Care

The traditional fee-for-service reimbursement programs encourage increased services, because physicians and other providers are reimbursed for *each* service provided. The tendency of PPOs to discount fees is a further incentive for physicians to increase the volume of services in an effort to preserve their revenues or earning capacity. Successful PPOs have strong mechanisms for evaluating the appropriateness of the care that they provide.

On the other hand, fee-for-service plans also contribute to underuse. The large deductibles and co-payments may discourage patients from seeking needed care. Failure to cover or the underuse of important services, such as screening examinations and preventive services, may lead to more serious problems later.[4] The incidence of problems caused by improper use may also be increased in fee-for-service settings because of the encouragement of higher rates of utilization; with greater volumes of service come more opportunities for errors in clinical performance.

An alternative to fee-for-service systems is the "capitated" or "prospective payment" system of reimbursement. Underuse problems are of greater concern in capitated settings, and the kinds of underuse, whether patient-initiated or physician-initiated, are broader for all categories of services than in the fee-for-service plans. If patients have limited access to physicians or other health care services, patient visits obviously will be low. Virtually no quality-of-care research has yet been conducted with the newer independent practice associations or in HMOs with novel payment structures, such as the primary physician gatekeeper approach.[4]

Eisenberg described several factors that contribute to the delivery of unnecessary services by physicians, such as personal characteristics of the physician and patient, peer opinion, tradition, organization and practice, financial incentives, and expectations of patients.[8] Making process changes for each of these factors can decrease variations in care. For example, quality assurance and improvement strategies can

- change physician attitudes and characteristics through the publication of standards of care for certain procedures
- change peer opinion and dependence on tradition by education in the latest advances in care
- change practice organizations (eg, clinics and group practices) through financial incentives
- change patients by educating them about their health so that they become better consumers of health care services

More research is necessary in the area of physician behavior, especially as it relates to the specific effects of individual financial incentives or groups of incentives. Chiropractors should join other health care providers to investigate the questions posed by Hillman.[9]

1. Which financial incentives distort physicians' judgments rather than influence them merely to practice cost-effective [health] care?
2. Will certain contractual agreements encourage excess frugality independent of the context in which they are used—or do they depend on synergy with other financial arrangements?
3. What is the threshold at which specific financial incentives reduce quality of care?
4. How do non-financial measures magnify or counterbalance financial incentives?

In this "era of accountability," the health care professions must ensure that reasonableness and patient safety are not sacrificed for the sake of improving the health care purchaser's balance sheet. The economic tools used in the present-day management of health care are conversions of economic instruments currently used in business and industry. The health care professions will need personnel trained not only in the provision of health care, but also in these socioeconomic programs.

Coile suggested that the physician of the future must be proficient at health care forecasting, quality assessment, and outcomes management.[10] Nash predicted that new roles for physicians within the health care business community will include director of clinical outcomes, vice president of quality care, director of clinical effectiveness, and director of health policy.[11] Partly because of the history of quality assessment, but mostly because of present-day and future needs, there will be many professional opportunities for such experts. In December, 1989, for example, the US Congress established the Agency for Health Care Policy and Research and directed it to "enhance quality and appropriateness of health care services and enhance the access to such services."[12] This is an intellectually honest attempt by government to assess health care—regardless of costs. This new agency will conduct and support research, demonstration projects, evaluation, training, guideline development, and dissemination of information. It will be vital for the chiropractic profession to be a part of this process.

CHIROPRACTIC QUALITY OF CARE: HISTORICAL PERSPECTIVE

Although the chiropractic profession is nearly 100 years old, it has not been a unified profession. Early in its history, there was a splintering of its ideology, and many different "schools of thought" developed. The survivors were termed the "straights" and the "mixers," with each group having its own proprietary concepts or belief systems.

The fundamental difference between straights and mixers rested on the definition of the chiropractic lesion, the subluxation. Before 1972, the working definition of this defect was a source of considerable debate and controversy. With the movement into federal reimbursement for chiropractic services through the Medicare program, it became necessary for the various factions to agree on an operative definition of subluxation that could be presented to the federal government. The result of a "consensus" conference held to develop such a definition was a classification of the radiographic manifestations of vertebral subluxation that demonstrated the necessity of chiropractic care for Medicare beneficiaries. Subsequently, reimbursement for Medicare services was allowed, provided that the presence of a subluxation was documented on x-ray film. So by default, the standard of care for treatment of the Medicare population was to take spinal x-ray films before chiropractic treatment.

There was no provision for the chiropractic physician to be reimbursed for these "necessary" x-ray films or even for the "optional" chiropractic examination. The Medicare patient was to pay for these expenses. This early line of logic contributed to the lingering dependence on invasive radiation to determine chiropractic necessity, while failing to take into account other valuable clinical information that could substantiate subluxation findings. The real tragedy here was that the desire for reimbursement motivated the effort to reach a consensus on the definition of subluxation. There was essentially no research-guided impetus for the creation of the Medicare definition of subluxation; now, it has come back to haunt the chiropractic profession. [13]

Peer Review Systems

The national chiropractic associations complied with the federal requirements for the creation of peer review systems, seen originally as a method to assess the necessity of care when there was a potential dispute. Much organizational energy went into review efforts at the association level, leading to the publication of peer review manuals. [14] This effort trickled down to the state organizations and specialty councils, which were each required to establish peer review committees and protocols for review and corrective action. By the mid-1980s, this activity had ceased in almost all jurisdictions, however, because increased liabilities to the peer review organizations resulted in lawsuits and many judgments against the review organizations and associations. One such deep pocket exposure (*Bartholomew v Virginia Chiropractic Association*[15]) touched a national association and has radically changed association-based peer review. Even state associations against which there had been no legal action dropped out of the peer review business because of the inflated rate of liability insurance premiums or even the lack of available coverage.

Unfortunately, although their request for radiographic criteria to confirm the presence of a subluxation had been satisfied, Medicare officials were still looking for agreed upon standards regarding the appropriate number of chiropractic services (manipulations) required to treat a given acute or chronic condition. The Inspector General of the United States has chastised the national associations for not approving or endorsing utilization review criteria. [13] Because the chiropractic profession did not design its own "brakes on costs and utilization," a 12-service per year cap was instituted on Medicare reimbursement for chiropractic services. The government report suggested that the "impact of a 12 service cap on patients would be minimal" and explained that 12 visits "would allow patients with chronic conditions one treatment per month and would encompass the number of services provided to a majority of the patients needing acute care." This overly prescriptive 12-visit limitation has found its way into other public sector reimbursement systems. Unless the national chiropractic associations act as a common chiropractic authority and take the initiative to develop reasonable guidelines, the profession will continue to be confused and misguided. There really are no reasonable guidelines created implicitly by the chiropractic profession for use in programs such as peer review.

Peer review in chiropractic has been resurrected with the establishment of state agency–based peer review boards that are defined by statute. These groups are typically governed by the state chiropractic examining board or by similar licensing authorities. They have statutory authority in determining appropriateness issues regarding the delivery of chiropractic care and are protected from legal action by immunity clauses, because they are acting as "agents" for the state. The reviewers are licensed professionals who may or may not have experience in quality assessment, but are placed in the position to make judgments on chiropractic necessity.

Independent Review

The 1980s also saw other attempts at chiropractic quality assurance. Mostly because of the influence of the auto casualty insurance carriers, "paper review" firms and independent chiropractic examiners emerged. The paper review firms contract with insurance carriers to render opinions of the necessity of care, based on a review of charts and chiropractic billings. They have established explicit guidelines that are, for the most part, proprietary. They operate by retrospectively comparing chiropractic utilization on a claim against these explicit criteria. Insurance companies deny reimbursement for chiropractic care that exceeds the anticipated amount of care for the injury or condition, based on the review of their "chiropractic experts."

The second opinion examination is used to the greatest extent by private sector insurance companies, but public sector programs have been put in place as well. Independent chiropractic examiners must have received sufficient training to qualify as independent examiners according to established standards of education and behavior. Such standards exist in the states of New York, California, and Washington. Paramount to these established review standards is the prerequisite of postgraduate education necessary to achieve excellence in clinical decision-making skills and to determine appropriate levels of chiropractic care or the need for interdisciplinary referral.

Exhibit 5-1 Indications for Second Opinion Consultations

Chiropractic Consultation
 —Daily treatment exceeding two weeks
 —3x/week treatment exceeding 4 weeks
 —Temporary disability for longer than 4 weeks
 —No objective signs of improvement, condition worsening in first two weeks of
  care, or no perception of change by the injured worker
 —No improvement in any one month of care
 —Extended office visits for more than two weeks or more than 6 in number
 —Diagnosis is inconsistent with mechanism of injury
 —Conservative or chiropractic care extending past one hundred twenty days fol-
  lowing initial visit
Radiologic Consultation
 —Suspected fracture or dislocation
 —Suspected bone pathology
 —Uncertain soft tissue findings on osseous film
 —Suspected spinal motion unit instability
 —Questionable significance of anomaly
 —Inadequate progress of patient in response to treatment
 —Second opinion on questionable biomechanical significance
 —Second opinion as to contraindication to skeletal manipulation
 —Second opinion as to necessity for referral for further diagnostic imaging pro-
  cedures or for other diagnosis or treatment
Medical/Surgical Consultation or Special Examination
 —Evidence of systemic disease or infection
 —Second diagnostic opinion
 —Closed head injury
 —Fracture/dislocation
 —Conditions where chiropractic care is contraindicated

Source: Reprinted from *Chiropractic Standards of Practice and Utilization Guidelines in the Care and Treatment of Injured Workers,* (p. 41) by DT Hansen, Washington State Department of Labor & Industries, 1988.

The criteria used to decide the necessity for a second opinion examination are called "flags" or utilization review "edits." Once a claim triggers one or more of the flags, the claim adjudicator may then establish the need for a second opinion examination. A sample of these "sentinel" edits is found in Exhibit 5-1.

Development of Standards of Care

New in the 1980s was the advent of chiropractic standards of care. Although the topic was first discussed in the literature in 1985,[16] chiropractic institutions, accrediting agencies, and national associations had been having informal discussions and making plans for documenting practice standards. The more progressive chiropractic institutions and state/national associations have since embarked on this process, leading to the development of documented standards and protocols. The impetus for this sudden push is the search of public and private purchasers of health care for a "quick fix" to perceived problems of overutilization and increased costs. One such effort in Washington state resulted in the hasty assemblage of a standard-of-practice document that was never used for its intended purpose,[17] although many states and provinces used the same document as an outline for similar efforts.

The most rigorous project to date is a joint venture of the Consortium for Chiropractic Research, the Foundation for Chiropractic Education and Research, the RAND Corporation, and the California Chiropractic Association to determine the appropriateness of chiropractic health care intervention by using state-of-the-art consensus methodology. Current approaches include a critical review of the literature, the convening of inter- and intradisciplinary expert panels, and the consensus methodology used by RAND in previous ventures.

In the spring of 1991, the Consortium for Chiropractic Research issued a policy statement that addressed the necessary components in the development and evaluation of chiropractic practice guidelines (Appendix A). This statement is a good tool for any organization to use in evaluating the process of chiropractic guideline development and ensuring the accountability of that process. The attributes discussed in the statement are consistent with those of other policies found in the health care professions, as they have been modeled after the guidelines established by the Agency for Health Care Policy and Research, the National Institute of Medicine, and the American Medical Association Specialty Society Practice Parameters Partnership.

Future efforts in chiropractic quality assurance will combine the attributes of appropriateness research with prospective and concurrent assessment of chiropractic necessity. With the arrival of rapid information technology, reimbursement agencies will be able to follow claims closely and to prevent the provision of unnecessary care. Quality improvement paradigms will bring increased educational opportunities for both chiropractors and patients, which will lead many patients who had previously been shielded or denied access to chiropractic care to use these services.

CHIROPRACTIC NECESSITY

The determination of whether a patient requires the services of a chiropractor drives chiropractic necessity. Conservative schools of thought favor determining if a subluxation is present by simple means. Historically, a basic assessment has included the use of x-ray line drawing schemes, static and motion palpation interpretations, measurement of leg length, muscle testing, measurement of skin temperature differential, and postural analysis. Unfortunately, investigators have found that many of these procedures are not statistically reliable between examiners or even with the same examiner,[18-20] raising concern about the clinical validity of these assessment procedures.

Other schools of thought emphasize clinical outcome by subjective appraisal through case history; objective assessment through physical, orthopedic, neurological, laboratory, and chiropractic examination; radiographic assessment; and the use of other devices and techniques, such as vasculizers (plethysmography), thermograms (thermography), dual and quadrant weight scales, and Moire photography. The reliability and validity of some of these devices and procedures in the determination of chiropractic necessity have also been suspect, however.

The key to chiropractic treatment is the chiropractic adjustment, also termed spinal manipulative therapy. Almost all chiropractors possess the art and skill of this treatment modality, clearly setting them apart from other health care providers. Studies have suggested that the manipulative skills possessed by chiropractors exceed those of the other physical medicine practitioners.[21,22] Chiropractic practitioners also emphasize other conservative measures and life styles that are now being embraced by traditional medicine, such as stretching and exercise, nutritional counseling, physiological therapeutics, weight control, smoking cessation, and instruction in daily activities and proper body mechanics.

Utilization Trends

As with traditional medical care, chiropractic has variations in the delivery of care—even among chiropractors practicing in the same locale. Although there has been no study in chiropractic parallel to Dr. Wennberg's work in medicine, there has been more opportunity recently to obtain claims data from public sector health care purchasers.[23] Pertinent data available from Washington state, for example, make it possible to study utilization trends. The data for purchased chiropractic services through a state-operated workers' compensation system for the 3 consecutive years since 1986 show a significant increase in the number of injured workers treated by chiropractors; all indexes of utilization (eg, units of service per patient, months of treatment time per patient, and payment allowed per patient) demonstrate a downward trend. Calculating the chiropractors' average number of services per claim and graphing them produces a bell-shaped distribution curve with a long tail extending to the right beyond the first (+1) standard deviation (Figure 5-1). This outlier "tail" represents approximately 10% of the practitioners. The standard deviation is one way of identifying variation. The higher the standard deviation value, the more variation in this aspect of practice. Quality has improved when variation decreases, or when the bell shape of the curve becomes narrower.

Table 5-1 shows what has occurred in the delivery of chiropractic services to injured workers in Washington state. All indexes of utilization have declined over this 3-year period, even though no rigid quality assurance or quality improvement program was in place. Not only was there a decrease in the respective mean values, but the standard deviations continued to decline, indicating a matched decrease in practice variation. During 1987, the chiropractic providers had been alerted to the fact that their utilization of services would be compared statistically and that corrective action might be taken on persistent outliers. The subsequent significant decrease in utilization is typical of a sentinel effect, which is better known and documented as the Hawthorne effect. Past investigations in both industry and health care show that worker/provider behavior and production improve when the workers/providers "know" that they are being observed.

During this period of investigation, there was no effort by the payer or chiropractic trade associations to educate the providers on issues of quality

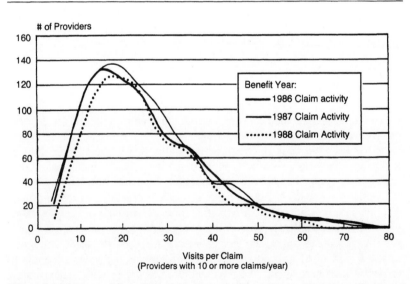

Figure 5-1 Visits per claim—1986: chiropractic providers. *Source:* Data from Washington State Department of Labor & Industries.

Table 5-1 Chiropractic Profile per Provider

	1986		1987		1988	
	mean	SD	mean	SD	mean	SD
Units of service/claim	24.53	22.40	22.79	13.87	21.88	13.90
Days of service per claim	129.99	95.12	117.59	56.51	111.52	54.21
No. of months per claim	4.81	3.03	4.41	1.81	4.22	1.76
Payment allowed per claim	$654.26	781.41	464.45	282.63	445.74	264.85

Note: SD, standard deviation.

Source: Data from Washington State Department of Labor & Industries.

management and quality improvement. Thus, the demonstrated decrease in utilization and variation is behavioral. This exercise demonstrates the need for "second guessing" the determination of chiropractic necessity. Other health care professions have seen a Hawthorne effect occur with contemporaneous review of procedures. Once the review mechanisms were removed, however, the aberrant behavior returned, and practice variation increased.[8]

Questionable Chiropractic Necessity Strategies

Some chiropractic management entrepreneurs support the concept of increased utilization in the treatment of injuries (workers' compensation and personal injury) in order to obtain maximum return from the insurance benefit. At one time, "success seminars" were in vogue; "successful" practitioners would boast about a patient visit average over 100 and a per patient charge average over $1,000. There typically is no sensitivity to appropriateness issues in the context of these programs.

Other factors leading to questionable chiropractic necessity strategies include the use of a monocausal diagnosis and/or nonstandardized terminology and protocol. Many purchasers of health care do not accept the singular use of the term subluxation as a diagnosis on the ground that it does not adequately describe the condition of the patient who requires care. One large Midwest health care "think tank" stated, "Claims using the term *subluxation* without a complete explanation of specific symptoms, physiologic involvements, pathologies, etc., should be denied until such explanations are provided."[24] Ironically, the same criticism has been made of medical physicians—that every condition is diagnosed as a "virus" or "arthritis." Both professions need to improve.

It has been suggested that the legal profession also contributes to questionable utilization and determination of chiropractic necessity. Haddad found that workers' compensation claims in which an attorney was involved resulted in significantly greater utilization of health care resources, at higher cost, and longer temporary disability periods than did those in which an attorney was not involved. His conclusion was that "iatrogenic and 'jurisgenic' factors have a direct effect on promulgation of medical care, and delay in returning to gainful employment, and, consequently, contributing to the high cost."[25]

Likely, the determination of chiropractic necessity will hinge on the use of reliable and valid measures of health and illness (dysfunction), including physical, physiological, and functional measures. Other outcome measures will include paper-and-pencil questionnaires that will address health and functional status, and dysfunction arising from pain and disability.

MEASUREMENT OF QUALITY OF CHIROPRACTIC CARE

Analyses of economic data, such as total dollars billed per claim and average number of visits per claim, and comparisons of individual practitioners to the computed statistical "norms" are crude, but expedient, appraisals of quality. These data are the most common quality assessment measures used in the health care reimbursement industry. Unfortunately, they are not sensitive to demographic variations and are not typically weighted to consider high-risk occupations or other environmental exposures. Newer claim management systems now make it possible to measure the utilization of or referral patterns for expensive and invasive procedures by provider and to compare these values to statistical "norms." High rates of utilization of these procedures would not be considered prudent delivery of health care.

Educational and licensing systems are the early filters for the quality of chiropractic care, as each of these entities test the competency of the practitioner. No jurisdictions have as yet imposed continuing competency assessments for relicensure, such as self-testing. In general, chiropractors can keep their license active simply by maintaining a certain level of continuing chiropractic education. Only those chiropractors who choose to pursue their education by enrolling in postgraduate specialty programs undergo further competency testing. Those who voluntarily and actively participate in comprehensive continuing education activities demonstrate their commitment to staying current with contemporaneous knowledge—an important structural measure of quality of care. Successful completion of these programs will appear on curricula vitae and then be accessible for credentialing purposes.

Chiropractors who have performed negligently are investigated by the disciplining body within their licensing board or through the civil court system. There are national disclosure laws that allow a credentialing body access to information about adverse actions. Public and private reimbursement agencies can screen chiropractors who provide negligent care and restrict them from providing care to their beneficiaries.

Health care purchasers place great significance on the outcome measure of patient satisfaction. Patients/customers who are satisfied are likely to continue their enrollment in the plan of a particular insurance company, for example, and may even encourage others to use it. The insurance industry is very competitive, and benefits managers want that repeat business. There are well-developed research models of patient satisfaction for use in a variety of specific circumstances. Some are available as commercial products. There is a considerable amount of health services research under way on this topic.

There is also a need for more chiropractic study in health status assessment by patient survey techniques. In the treatment of back pain, chiropractic physicians have been shown to score higher in patient satisfaction than do family physicians and internal medicine specialists.[26,27] Cherkin, an expert in patient satisfaction instruments, offered several questions that can be used in the development of evaluation-of-care subscales.[28]

- questions included in the information subscale:
  1. The doctor gave me enough information about the cause of my back pain.
  2. The doctor did not give me a clear explanation of the cause of my pain.
  3. The doctor told me what to do to prevent future back problems.
- questions included in the caring subscale:
  1. The doctor seemed to believe that my pain was real.
  2. The doctor did not understand the concerns I had about my back problem.
  3. The doctor did not seem comfortable dealing with my back pain.
  4. The doctor was not concerned about what happened with my pain after I left the office.
- questions included in the effectiveness subscale:
  1. The treatment the doctor prescribed for my back was effective.
  2. The doctor seemed confident that the treatment she/he recommended would work.

3. The doctor gave me a clear idea of how long it might take for my back to get better.

- questions not included in any subscale:

1. After seeing the doctor, I did not know what I needed to do for my back.
2. The doctor did not listen carefully to my description of my back problem.
3. The doctor made me feel less worried about my back problem.
4. The doctor performed a thorough examination of my back.
5. The doctor did not understand what was wrong with my back.
6. The doctor should have ordered more tests or x-rays.
7. The doctor should have referred me to a back specialist.

If patients are consistently more satisfied with the outcome of the chiropractic service, the purchaser will want to continue with this benefit. These measures of patient satisfaction and caring can become questionnaires that health care purchasing entities use routinely to assess delivery of quality care.

Corrective action models from the manufacturing industry and their quality assurance philosophy have entered the health care management scene in recent years. They apply an ordered sequence for finding aberrancies and determining how best to correct them without disrupting production elsewhere. Although most professional peer review systems may be considered corrective action models, they are implicit for the most part, and it may be difficult to "blind" against bias. Figure 5-2 illustrates a public sector agency corrective action model that incorporates explicit review criteria and blinding of the peer reviewers.

Blinding a peer reviewer involves the "sterilization" of the file by completely blacking out data such as names and addresses so that the reviewer cannot identify the patient or the attending physician. In double blind review, two reviewers investigate the same claim/physician, but are blinded from each other; a third reviewer then summarizes the review from the results of the first two.

Study is warranted into the causes of variation in chiropractic practice and the extent to which it is due to patient populations, available resources, patient preferences, clinician uncertainty, or other clinician qualities.

DEVELOPMENT AND USE OF CLINICAL ALGORITHMS

The decade of the 1990s will find the health care professions solidly entrenched in the development of practice guidelines and standards of care.

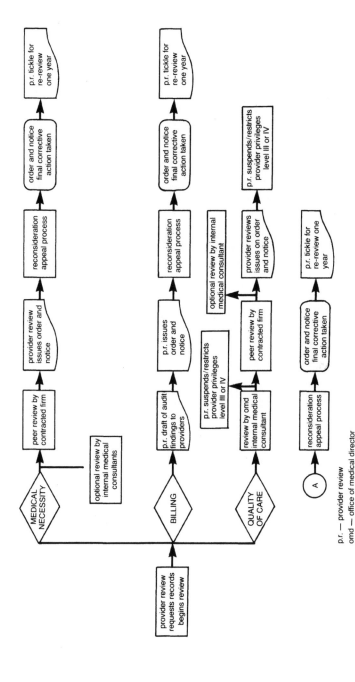

Figure 5-2 Provider review corrective action model. *Note:* p.r. = provider review; o/n = order and notice; omd = office of medical director. *Source:* Presented by Nancy Peterson to the Chiropractic Advisory Committee, State of Washington Department of Labor & Industries, September 1989.

The sudden explosion of interest in the development of clinical guidelines is the result of social mandates to ensure the purchase of cost-effective, quality health care. National and state health care purchasing agencies are providing the strongest push of all. It is expected that guidelines and standards will assist in both quality assessment and quality improvement and yet will be sensitive to outcomes. Until recently, the chiropractic profession has not recognized appropriate intraprofessional authorities to define clearly the process of developing implicit chiropractic standards.

For the chiropractic profession, the appropriateness research that produces a body of knowledge to be referenced in establishing and fine-tuning guidelines for treatment is expanding, despite the lack of funding from federal sources. From the foundation of basic clinical knowledge comes the development of guidelines. These treatment guidelines can take the form of a clinical algorithm that sets forth a stepwise procedure for making decisions about the diagnosis and treatment of clinical problems. Because algorithms are clear and concise and can be represented graphically, they provide an excellent basis for communicating and representing specifications of optimal clinical care. Gottlieb, Margolis, and Schoenbaum of the Harvard Community Health Plan stated that "clinical algorithms may both improve quality and decrease costs by guiding clinicians toward more standardized, clinically optimal, cost-effective strategies and by facilitating more valid measurement of clinical process and outcomes."[29]

Although much is known about the various methodologies for developing clinical guidelines and criteria for evaluating the process of guideline development have been published, little is known about decreasing inappropriate variations in clinical practice and improving the quality of clinical practices through the use of these guidelines. As a result, most past and current efforts to establish guidelines have failed to have significant impact.[30] This failure is due to a variety of factors, such as an undue focus on individual clinicians in the tail of the quality curve ("bad apples"), the use of "boundary guidelines" rather than optimal care guidelines,"[30] failure to link guideline efforts to decision support and measurement, failure to consider system or process capabilities, lack of practitioner involvement, and inadequate attention to local adaptation and development. Incorporating clinical guideline development in a quality improvement model which can overcome these shortcomings.

As clinical guidelines, algorithms make it possible to analyze the causes of variation and poor quality more thoroughly; to give attention to system, process, and individual causes of variation; to generate new knowledge; and to link the implementation of solutions with continuous quality improvement activities. The development of clinical algorithms for specific health care settings should involve the practitioners for whom they are designed. The algorithms will then be based both on research reports and on the clinical experience or perspectives of practitioners from the many clinical specialties that may be involved in managing a patient with a given problem. Because the clinicians who will use the guidelines are their developers, the guidelines are uniquely adapted to the clinical setting. Thus, an algorithm for uncomplicated low back pain in a teaching clinic of a chiropractic college may differ from one found in an HMO that has an employee chiropractor.

Several criteria should be considered when choosing clinical algorithm topics.

1. common clinical conditions
2. unexplained variation in clinical practice (perceived or documented)
3. unexplained variation in utilization of limited or costly resources
4. unexplained variation in internal or external referral patterns
5. general clinical uncertainty or controversy
6. uncertain indications for risky or costly intervention
7. internal resource access or supply constraints
8. apparent risk management problem
9. introduction of new diagnostic test, therapeutic procedure, or medication
10. quality of care problem perceived by patients, clinicians, or managers[29,(p81)]

As a part of curriculum development at the Los Angeles College of Chiropractic, the staff evaluated and scored 62 conditions against 6 selection criteria: (1) high prevalence, (2) frequent management by chiropractic, (3) high morbidity, (4) manageability, (5) preventability, and/or (6) usefulness as a model to teach important concepts (written communication, A.H. Adams, DC, November 10, 1990). Among the clinical entities found to be worthy of critical study were

- osteoarthritis
- chronic pain
- hypertension
- lumbosacral strain/sprain,
- intervertebral disc syndrome
- sacroiliac syndrome
- cervical strain/sprain
- scoliosis
- thoracic strain/sprain

- torticollis
- lateral stenosis—lumbar
- acute cervical pain
- osteoporosis
- subluxation

Eventually, each of these topics should be scrutinized through a quality improvement paradigm that would then be available to the profession as a quality guideline.

Following is a model of the process used in algorithm development at the Harvard Community Health Plan, a Boston-based HMO:

Project Planning
  1. Identification of topic
  2. Identification of intended users
  3. Determination of suitability for "local" or "central" consensus
  4. Identification and selection of group leader
  5. Identification and selection of members of consensus group

Consensus Algorithm Development
  6. Literature search and summary
  7. "Seed algorithm" construction
  8. Review of literature and seed algorithm by consensus group members
  9. Brief algorithm and consensus development training session
 10. Consensus development via nominal group process and/or Delphi method

Algorithm Review
 11. Identification of "essential nodes" for possible measurement
 12. Identification and selection of "algorithm keeper"
 13. Selection of date for next review and revision
 14. Review and approval of algorithm by affected clinical managers

Implementation
 15. Distribution of algorithm with request for feedback
 16. Design of implementation strategies[29,(p82)]

Key features in this model are the participation of clinical groups that will be affected by its application, the use of nominal group and/or Delphi consensus process, and continuous monitoring once the guideline is implemented. Oftentimes, this process unexpectedly reveals that some components of the practice environment need to be modified in order to provide the care designated by the guideline. This process may also make it possible to identify specific practice recommendations that should be quantitatively measured to assess the algorithm's impact on practice variation, cost of care, and patient outcome. Algorithms can be created even with diagnostic or therapeutic controversy, as when there is no clear clinical consensus for the appropriateness of a procedure or treatment. If there is no consensus, the use of an algorithm becomes an opportunity for a specific clinical outcomes study on those controversial factors.

Currently, the chiropractic literature yields clinical algorithms in the management of scoliosis (Figure 5-3) and back pain.[31,32] Henderson has generated an algorithm for the management of vertebral artery syndrome (see Chapter 6). More study and development are necessary to improve these models and to investigate the possibility of developing algorithms for other clinical entities. More chiropractic practitioners must become competent in the development of algorithms so that chiropractic authorities can depend on this process when considering quality improvement strategies.

METAMORPHOSIS INTO MANAGED HEALTH CARE

Although the idea of managed care has been around for more than 20 years, its influence on the health care marketplace has never been as significant as it is now. Managed care is the opposite of the classic indemnity fee-for-service care with no controls. Formally defined as any prepaid health plan or insurance program in which beneficiaries receive health services in a coordinated manner to eliminate unnecessary medical services, managed care places emphasis on the selection of physicians, the monitoring of physician performance and behavior, the pre-authorization of expensive procedures, case management, and utilization review.

Managed care entities (eg, HMOs) are implementing quality improvement and utilization management models to enhance their quest for effective and efficient care. Business and industry are purchasing these managed care services and expect these quality paradigms to be in place and functional. This trend of business/employer influence on the purchase of health care is one reason that traditional health care coverage, including indemnity, is rapidly disappearing.

Slowly, chiropractic is finding entry into these managed care schemes. The chiropractic provider applying to these managed care panels may have to expend more energy and money to be qualified, however. A chiropractic provider who wishes to become part of this managed care movement will be exposed to concepts in management that were not part of the chiropractic undergraduate curriculum.

In order to become a member provider in a managed care program, a practitioner must generally go through a "credentialing" process that in-

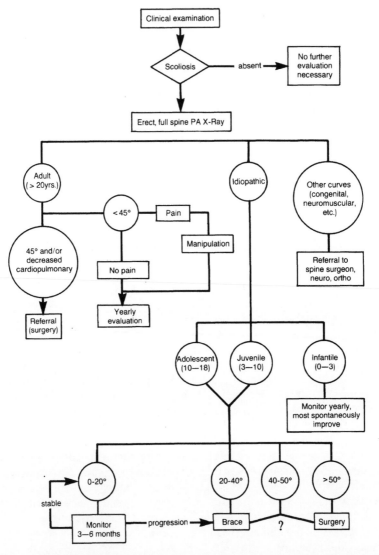

Figure 5-3 Nykoliation/Cassidy algorithm on scoliosis. *Source:* Reprinted with permission from JW Nykoliation, JD Cassidy, BE Arthur, and JH Wedge, An algorithm for the management of scoliosis, in *Journal of Manipulative and Physiological Therapeutics* (1986; 9[1]:1–14), Copyright © 1986, National College of Chiropractic.

cludes a review of clinical experience and expertise beyond qualifying for state licensure; assurance that there has been no disciplinary or any other negative action taken against the practitioner's license or professional standing; and proof of professional liability insurance, typically at a level higher than the average. Once accepted into the managed care program, the practitioner may be required to be "recredentialed" at set intervals (eg, every 2 years). This subsequent process may involve proof of continuing competency or education and reaffirmation of the status of the license.

A practitioner who contracts with a managed care plan agrees to provide competent services at a predetermined discount in exchange for assurance of increased patient volume and publication of the practitioner's name as a *preferred* provider. Because of the current movement into prospective and concurrent utilization review, the practitioner has also agreed to comply with the utilization management techniques employed by that managed care program. Prospective review includes pre-authorization of care, based on explicit utilization guidelines or diagnosis-driven algorithms; concurrent review requires the submission of reports at designated intervals with documentation of the necessity of continued care.

Many HMOs that contract with chiropractic providers reserve the right to use their medical physician "primary care providers" as gatekeepers. As such, these physicians determine the necessity of chiropractic care, based on their own explicit criteria. This system is failing, however, mostly because patients are frustrated by the delayed outcome and the need to be "rechecked" frequently by the primary care provider.

On the horizon for chiropractic providers is the concept of "capitation." In a capitated arrangement, the managed care entity contracts with a provider or provider group (eg, independent practice association) to render all the chiropractic services that its beneficiaries need for the entire benefit year in exchange for a lump sum payment. Any money remaining at the end of the year is the provider's reward for performing efficiently; the provider is at risk for expenses over that coverage, however. With the capitated plan, there is no need for a primary care provider to act as a gatekeeper, and chiropractors determine chiropractic necessity. Many medical, dental, mental health, optometric, and podiatric groups currently have capitation agreements with managed care plans.

Another option for managed care plans is to hire in-house chiropractic physicians to be part of their "closed panel." Some chiropractors presently have this arrangement within HMOs, and they work side-by-side with the other health care professionals, serving on staff committees and participating in specialty rounds. These practitioners are not paid on a fee-for-service basis; instead, they are salaried and have the typical fringe benefits of other panel physicians.

As mentioned earlier, private business and industry are moving into the managed care arena, providing these more conservative and cost-saving options to their employees. The rate of employee enrollment in these managed care plans is growing exponentially, as the patient/consumer pays fewer out-of-pocket expenses in these plans. Similar events are taking place in the public sector models. The Department of Defense is investigating managed care options in two separate demonstration projects for CHAMPUS* beneficiaries. The early results of these demonstrations reflect a significant movement of families away from the traditional indemnity coverage in CHAMPUS to one of their "preferred" plans,[33] and an insignificant number have disenrolled from the managed care program because they were dissatisfied with the care received or with the program itself. Other federal agencies (eg, Medicare) and state health care purchasing agencies are developing managed care programs in which patients will have access to chiropractic care. Coile estimated that, by 1995, physicians will receive 40% to 50% of their revenues from managed care plans and will select patients on the basis of their managed care plans.[10]

Unfortunately, the current chiropractic college curriculum does not cover the social history of and current trends in health care purchasing. At the very least, the senior chiropractic student should learn about trends in health care economics and reimbursement, with emphasis on managed care and quality improvement principles. Without that cursory introduction, the graduating students appear in the "real world" unprepared for what health care economics has in store for them.

FUTURE OF THE CHIROPRACTIC PHYSICIAN

Chiropractors must learn about preferred provider programs that require physician selection, credentialing, discounted fee schedules, prospective and concurrent case review, review of physician outcomes, and corrective action. Quality assurance means that chiropractors will be monitored in their delivery of care and compared to their peers in practice performance measurements. Quality improvement paradigms will require providers to comply with standards of care and treatment guidelines. Proper use of guidelines will lead to reeducation and periodic monitoring of noncompliant providers rather than harsher sanctions.

---

*CHAMPUS (Civilian Health and Medical Program of the Uniformed Services) provides insurance for children and spouses of uniformed services members, as well as retirees and their families, when needed health care is not available from military health installations.

Clinical guidelines should be designed to assist practitioners by providing a framework for the evaluation and treatment of the more commonly encountered patient problems. They are not intended to replace either the clinician's judgment or to establish a protocol for all patients with a particular condition. Some patients will not fit the clinical conditions addressed by such guidelines. Furthermore, a guideline will rarely establish the only appropriate approach to the problem.

The chiropractic profession should move proactively in this new direction of health care assessment. Chiropractors will require additional training in the disciplines of health care administration and economics, public health, and health services research. One of the most sought after professionals of the future will be the management-trained physician.[10]

At the same time, interactions between field practitioners and clinical researchers should be enhanced so that contemporaneous data can be obtained. More information on the management of chiropractic cases, including the treatment of geriatric and pediatric populations, and on the value of preventive chiropractic care is needed. This information is critical for the development of appropriateness indicators, standards of care, and clinical algorithms.

The chiropractic profession has been vulnerable and gullible throughout its history, often depending heavily on its charismatic leaders. In the past 10 years, there has been a shift in the search for role models; the profession is obviously now seeking one common chiropractic authority, especially with the new challenges of mainstream health care reimbursement systems.[34] Through experience with modern quality improvement methods and contemporary managed care programs, new clinical role models will emerge.[35] Chiropractors will initially struggle philosophically and economically with these changes. Those who can adapt because of their ability to appraise the quality of care, to assimilate new knowledge, and to implement quality improvement methods will be the survivors. Those who continue to live in the idealism of the past and refuse to change will not find acceptance within this societal environment.

The stage is now set for the chiropractic profession to assume broad responsibility for its role in health care delivery. Legitimization can be gained through the quality assessment and quality improvement tools currently available to the health care industry. From these efforts will come a critical appraisal of the diagnostic and therapeutic methods unique to the chiropractic profession. Chiropractic education should respond by preparing students to be clinical scientists and by teaching them about likely future trends in the health care reimbursement system. Ultimately, global subscription to these processes will broaden the social acceptance of chiropractic and help secure the profession's place in mainstream health care.

REFERENCES

1. Starr P. *The Social Transformation of American Medicine.* New York: Basic Books; 1982.

2. Berwick DM, Knapp MG. Theory and practice for measuring health care quality. *Health Care Financing Review.* 1987; (suppl):49.

3. Donabedian A. *Explorations in Quality Assessment and Monitoring.* Ann Arbor, Mich: Health Administration Press; 1980; 1:80–84.

4. Chassin MR, Kosecoff J, Dubois R. *Health Care Quality Assessment.* Midwest Business Group on Health; 1990:2.

5. Wennberg J, Gittelsohn A. Small area variations in health care delivery. *Science.* 1973;182:11102–11108.

6. Berwick DM, Knapp MG. Theory and practice for measuring health care quality. *Health Care Financing Review.* 1987; (suppl):50.

7. Park RE, Fink A, Brook RH. Physician ratings of appropriate indications for six medical and surgical procedures. *Am J Public Health.* 1986;76:766–772.

8. Eisenberg JM. *Doctor's Decisions and the Cost of Medical Care.* Ann Arbor, Mich: Health Administration Press; 1986.

9. Hillman AL. Health maintenance organizations, financial incentives and physicians' judgments. *Ann Intern Med.* 1990;112:891–892.

10. Coile RC. *The New Medicine: Reshaping Medical Practice and Health Care Management.* Gaithersburg, Md: Aspen Publishers; 1990.

11. Nash DB. Practice guidelines for the business community. Presented to the Puget Sound Health Care Purchasers Association; March 1990; Seattle, Wash.

12. Agency for Health Care Policy and Research. *Clinical Guidelines Development.* (AHCPR Program Note). Rockville, MD: DHHS; August 1990:1.

13. Kusserow RP. *Inspection of Chiropractic Services under Medicare.* Chicago, Ill: Office of Analysis and Inspections, Region VII, Office of Inspector General, US Department of Health and Human Services; 1986:17.

14. *Manual of Chiropractic Peer Review Information.* Arlington, Va: American Chiropractic Association; 1976.

15. *Bartholomew v. Virginia Chiropractors Association.* 77-0062-R WD Va, May 18, 1978.

16. Vear HJ. Standards of chiropractic practice. *Journal of Manipulative and Physiological Therapeutics.* 1985;8(1):33–43.

17. Hansen DT, ed. *Chiropractic Standards of Practice and Utilization Guidelines in the Care and Treatment of Injured Workers.* Olympia, Wash: Chiropractic Advisory Committee, Washington State Department of Labor and Industries; 1988.

18. Phillips RB, Frymoyer JW, MacPhaerson BV, Newburg AH. Low back pain: a radiographic enigma. *Journal of Manipulative and Physiological Therapeutics.* 1986;9:183–187.

19. Boline PD, Keating JC, Brist J, Denver G. Interexaminer reliability of palpatory evaluations of the lumbar spine. *American Journal of Chiropractic Medicine.* 1988;1:5–12.

20. Triano JJ. The subluxation complex: Outcome measure of chiropractic diagnosis and treatment. *Chiropractic Technique.* 1990;2:114–120.

21. Commission to Study Chiropractic. *Chiropractic in New Zealand.* Wellington, New Zealand: Government Printer; 1979.

22. Meade TW, Dyer S, Browne W, Townsend J, Frank AO. Low back pain of mechanical origin: Randomised comparison of chiropractic and hospital outpatient treatment. *Br Med J.* 1990;300:1431–1437.

23. Nyiendo J. Economic measures used in determining effectiveness and efficiency of chiropractic methods. *Chiropractic Technique.* 1990;2:143–150.

24. MacDonald MJ, Morton C. *TASK-IV Report on Chiropractic.* Kansas City, MO: Mid-West Research Institute; 1986:20–21.

25. Haddad GH. Analysis of 2932 worker's compensation back injury cases: The impact on the cost to the system. *Spine.* 1987;12(6):765–769.

26. Cherkin DC, Mac Cornack FA. Patient evaluations of low back pain care from family physicians and chiropractors. *West J Med.* 1989;150:351–355.

27. Kane RL, Leymaster C, Olsen D, Woolley FR, Fisher FD. Manipulating the patient: A comparison of the effectiveness of physician and chiropractic care. *Lancet.* 1974;1:1333–1336.

28. Cherkin, DC. Patient satisfaction as an outcome measure. *Chiropractic Technique.* 1990;2:138–143.

29. Gottlieb LK, Margolis CZ, Schoenbaum SC. Clinical practice guidelines at an HMO: Development and implementation in a quality improvement model. *Quality Review Bulletin.* 1990;2:80–86.

30. Berwick DM. *Clinical Quality Improvement: Designing Care.* Syllabus. Brookline, MA: National Demonstration Project on Quality Improvement in Health Care, 1990.

31. Nykoliation JW, Cassidy JD, Arthur BE, Wedge JH. An algorithm for the management of scoliosis. *Journal of Manipulative and Physiological Therapeutics.* 1986;9:1–14.

32. Aker PD, Thiel HW, Kirkaldy-Willis WH. Low back pain: Pathogenesis, diagnosis and management. *American Journal of Chiropractic Medicine.* 1990;3:19–24.

33. Fant DJ, Pool CJ. The CHAMPUS reform initiative and fiscal intermediary managed care. *Journal of Ambulatory Care Management.* 1990;13(3):22–28.

34. Hansen DT. Searching for the common authority in validation and standardization of chiropractic methods. *Journal of Chiropractic Technique.* 1990;2:72–73.

35. Greganti MA. Commentary: Where are the role models? *Arch Intern Med.* 1990;150:259–261.

6

Vertebral Artery Syndrome

Donald J. Henderson

Less than 10% of the population consult chiropractors as primary care practitioners for a variety of physical complaints.[1] Those who do require the usual and expected standard of care and skill necessary to ensure that there are no contraindications to manipulative treatment. Fortunately, most problems are benign in origin, and the treatment outcome is usually positive. One particular area, however, demands that the chiropractor take extraordinary care and caution—the treatment of functional disorders related to the upper cervical spine. The rare, but disastrous, effects of stroke attributed to manipulation have resulted in successful claims of malpractice and substantial awards.

Vertebrobasilar artery insufficiency is the result of transient, partial, or complete occlusion of one or both of the vertebral arteries or its branches (Figure 6-1).[2] The signs and symptoms of vertebral artery syndrome arising from vascular occlusion/compression include vertigo; postural collapse, with or without disturbance of consciousness (drop attack); dystaxia; dysarthria; disequilibrium; visual disturbances, such as diplopia, paresis, blurred vision, and nystagmus; suboccipital headache; and paresis of a limb(s). In some cases, death has followed occlusion of one of the vertebral arteries or its branches within hours or days.

De Kleyn and Nieuwenhuyse noted that vertebral artery occlusion may be connected with head and neck movements.[3] Cadaveric,[3-5] clinopathological,[6-10] and angiographic[11-19] studies of the vertebral arteries confirm the characteristic size inequality and the influence of cervical position or movement on vertebral artery flow. In addition to these studies, there have been early reports of vertebral artery syndrome in association with manipulation.[20-21] Terrett has recently reviewed all the available literature on this subject.[22]

115

Figure 6-1 Vertebrobasilar vascular supply.

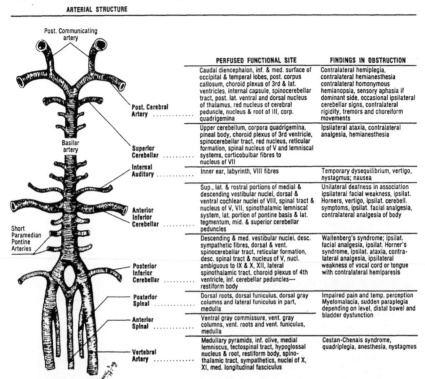

	PERFUSED FUNCTIONAL SITE	FINDINGS IN OBSTRUCTION
Post. Cerebral Artery	Caudal diencephalon, inf. & med. surface of occipital & temperal lobes, post. corpus callosum, choroid plexus of 3rd & lat. ventricles, internal capsule, spinocerebellar tract, post. lat. ventral and dorsal nucleus of thalamus, red nucleus of cerebral peduncle, nucleus & root of III, corp. quadrigemina	Contralateral hemiplegia, contralateral hemianesthesia contralateral homonymous hemianopsia, sensory aphasia if dominant side, occasional ipsilateral cerebellar signs, contralateral rigidity, tremors and choreiform movements
Superior Cerebellar	Upper cerebellum, corpora quadrigemina, pineal body, choroid plexus of 3rd ventricle, spinocerebellar tract, red nucleus, reticular formation, spinal nucleus of V and lemniscal systems, corticobulbar fibres to nucleus of VII	Ipsilateral ataxia, contralateral analgesia, hemianesthesia
Internal Auditory	Inner ear, labyrinth, VIII fibres	Temporary dysequilibrium, vertigo, nystagmus; nausea
Anterior Inferior Cerebellar	Sup., lat. & rostral portions of medial & descending vestibular nuclei, dorsal & ventral cochlear nuclei of VIII, spinal tract & nucleus of V, VII, spinothalamic lemniscal system, lat. portion of pontine basis & lat. tegmentum, mid. & superior cerebellar peduncles	Unilateral deafness in association ipsilateral facial weakness, ipsilat. Horners, vertigo, ipsilat. cerebell. symptoms, ipsilat. facial analgesia, contralateral analgesia of body
Posterior Inferior Cerebellar	Descending & med. vestibular nuclei, desc. sympathetic fibres, dorsal & vent. spinocerebellar tract, reticular formation, desc. spinal tract & nucleus of V, nucl. ambiguous to IX & X, XII, lateral spinothalamic tract, choroid plexus of 4th ventricle, inf. cerebellar peduncles—restiform body	Wallenberg's syndrome; ipsilat. facial analgesia, ipsilat. Horner's syndrome, ipsilat. ataxia, contra-lateral analgesia, ipsilateral weakness of vocal cord or tongue with contralateral hemiparesis
Posterior Spinal	Dorsal roots, dorsal funiculus, dorsal gray columns and lateral funiculus in part, medulla	Impaired pain and temp. perception Myelomalacia, sudden paraplegia depending on level, distal bowel and bladder dysfunction
Anterior Spinal	Ventral gray commissure, vent. gray columns, vent. roots and vent. funiculus, medulla	
Vertebral Artery	Medullary pyramids, inf. olive, medial lemniscus, tectospinal tract, hypoglossal nucleus & root, restiform body, spino-thalamic tract, sympathetics, nuclei of X, XI, med. longitudinal fasciculus	Cestan-Chenais syndrome, quadriplegia, anesthesia, nystagmus

Basilar Artery Obstruction Syndrome:
Headache, dizziness, coma, flaccid quadriplegia, areflexia, complete anesthesia, hyperpyrexia, miosis

Source: Reprinted with permission from DJ Henderson, "Significance of Vertebral Dyskinesia in Relation to the Cervical Syndrome" in *Journal of Manipulative and Physiological Therapeutics* (1979; 2[1]:3-15), Copyright © 1979 by National College of Chiropractic.

MECHANISMS OF VASCULAR INSUFFICIENCY

The vertebral arteries are vulnerable to mechanical compression, shearing, or stretching at a number of sites during head and neck movement, particularly on rotational motion.[22] Similarly, the internal carotid arteries may be subjected to mechanical strain by the atlantal transverse process in a small percentage of patients with preexisting vascular or osseous abnormalities.[23,24] Descriptions of vertebral artery insufficiency are more common in the literature, however. The three main potential sites of vertebral artery compression or injury are

1. the segment of the vertebral artery between the fixed intertransverse foramen of atlas and axis. The artery on the contralateral side of the neck rotation undergoes stretching and possible kinking. If healthy, the ipsilateral artery sustains blood flow requirements to the brain stem.
2. the C2-3 intersegmental level by the superior articular facet of C3. Arterial compression may occur during ipsilateral head and neck rotation.
3. within the area of the posterior atlanto-occipital membrane. Compressive strain may occur between the atlantal arch and the foramen magnum, or capsular expansion against the posterior membrane may have a stenosing effect during cervical extension coupled with rotation.

Some degree of arterial compression during cervical motion is physiological, and the risk of a vascular accident is undoubtedly increased when there are anatomical anomalies within the artery itself or the surrounding musculoligamentous and osseous structures. Acquired pathological or degenerative changes within the vessel wall (arterial disease), impaired hemodynamic factors (blood dyscrasias), and spondyloarthrotic changes of the apophyseal or uncovertebral joints makes the patient even more vulnerable. Structural changes evident on radiographs in cases of degenerative disk "disease" may shorten the cervical column, restricting motion, while the associated tortuous vertebral artery looping may increase the possibility of compression. Trauma to the artery wall leads to possible vasospasm, intimal tearing or dissection, thrombosis formation, embolization, and occlusive infarction of the basilar artery (the "locked-in" syndrome) and/or its branches, notably the posterior inferior cerebellar artery (ie, the dorsolateral medullary or Wallenberg syndrome).

INCIDENCE OF VERTEBRAL ARTERY SYNDROME ASSOCIATED WITH CERVICAL MANIPULATION

Most cases of arterial thrombosis and infarction in other areas of the body occur in the elderly, are spontaneous, and are unrelated to trauma. Vertebral artery syndrome attributed to cervical manipulation occurs in younger patients; the average age is just under 40. Furthermore, it occurs more often in women than in men.

The incidence of vertebral artery syndrome as a complication of cervical manipulation cannot be easily determined. Minor or reversible incidents may not be recognized or reported. Reliable, valid, and reasonable methods of identifying patients at risk have not been developed, making epidemiological study difficult. Well-documented, unbiased reports are necessary to determine the true extent of the problem and must be compared with a host of other activities that have reportedly resulted in vertebral artery syndrome.[25] A number of authors have provided information relating to the frequency of this manipulative complication, however.

Gutmann estimated two or three more or less serious incidents concerning the vertebrobasilar system per million manipulative treatments of the upper cervical spine.[26] Dvorak and Orelli, who surveyed the members of the Swiss Society for Manual Medicine, reported that slight neurological complications (eg, momentary dizziness or altered consciousness) occurred once in 40,000 manipulative procedures, while serious neurological complications (eg, stroke) occurred once in 400,000 manipulative procedures.[27] Maigne reported one death per several tens of millions of manipulations,[28] while Cyriax estimated the risk of death as one per ten million.[29]

In 1980, Jaskoviak estimated that 5 million treatments had been given at the National College of Chiropractic Clinics over a 15-year period without a single case of vertebral artery syndrome associated with manipulation.[30] Henderson found no incidents of vertebral artery syndrome at the Canadian Memorial Chiropractic College outpatient clinic over a 9-year period, during which an estimated 500,000 cervical treatments had been given.[31] The New Zealand Commission of Inquiry found historical evidence of only three cases of harm caused by chiropractic treatment in that country[32]; the nature of these incidents were not described.

In 1988, it was estimated that at least 100 million cervical manipulations were given worldwide annually by more than 60,000 full-time practitioners of manipulation, primarily chiropractors, osteopaths, physicians, and physiotherapists.[31] In the very rare instance, the manipulative adjustment—however delivered to the cervical spine of a vulnerable patient—becomes the final injurious act that, almost by chance, results in very serious consequences.

REPORTING AND DOCUMENTATION

Over the past two decades, there has been a rapid growth of literature on manipulation-induced vertebral artery syndrome.[25,33,34] Of the 126 reports studied by Terrett, 96 occurred after 1970, a time when practitioners had access to testing procedures and were generally more cognizant of the possible serious complications of cervical manipulation.[25] There can be no doubt that the elevated level of reporting is directly proportional to the generally increased awareness among all professionals interested in spinal manipulative therapy.

Anecdotal or polemic reports must be distinguished from those that objectively document evidence of true manipulation-induced vertebrobasilar vascular accidents. This differentiation is facilitated when rationally minded, unbiased chiropractic and medical specialists are consulted and/or when there has been a true test of documented inquiry through litigation. As in all fields of health care, this subject requires critical review by epidemiological investigators.[35,36]

It is necessary to establish a cooperative interprofessional forum in which those qualified to practice spinal (cervical) manipulation objectively document and analyze data concerning the incidence of vertebral artery syndrome. Although the effect of spinal manipulation on the vertebral artery has justifiably been the subject of recent study, certain other types of procedures in medical practice may similarly play a causative role in vertebral artery syndrome.[31] For example, the prolonged maintenance of an abnormal position during surgery[37-39] or at birth, which may involve unnatural, forced movements of the infant's neck,[40-41] may produce a lesion within the vertebral artery or its branches.

The significance of vertigo originating from the cervical spine must be recognized. More precise screening protocols, better outcome measures for patient selection, and more definitive standards for care will evolve from future cooperative investigations.

DETERMINANTS OF STANDARDS OF MANIPULATIVE CARE

The criteria used to evaluate a practitioner's compliance with a standard of care are based on elements common to all primary care practitioners. Measures used to decide the question of quality care and practice involve the case history and record keeping, examination procedures, diagnosis, patient communication and consent to treatment, management and treatment, and action taken in the event of an unfortunate incident. A practitioner is expected to act in the same manner that would be reasonably expected of a prudent practitioner of comparable professional training, experience, and standing under similar circumstances. Something more than mere error of judgment must be proved before a practitioner is found negligent and, hence, liable for patient harm.[42,43]

The average, reasonable practitioner is expected to be aware of the diagnostic and treatment procedures and standards currently described in the literature and taught at accredited colleges.[44,45] Learned jurists have stressed the importance of what ought to be done rather than what is done in establishing a standard.[42] It is sometimes most educational for the clinician to examine experiences in law related to standards of care. Claims of malpractice with respect to vertebral artery syndrome following spinal manipulation have emerged in many jurisdictions. In Canada, for example, statements of claim preparatory to litigation have alleged negligence because of

- failure to take a proper and relevant history, to make every reasonable effort to interview patients thoroughly prior to treating them (relevant history); failure to keep records
- failure to conduct a proper, relevant, and detailed examination
- failure to take proper radiographs
- failure to read or interpret the details of the history, examination, and radiographs correctly
- failure to arrive at an accurate diagnosis
- failure to administer or use proper or proved techniques
- failure to obtain proper and informed consent prior to manipulative treatment (The doctor has a strict duty to disclose fully information that may influence the patient's decision to proceed with treatment.)
- failure to refer or seek out a specialist in a timely manner
- failure to follow up on findings or test results
- application of force that is excessive or improperly directed during the manipulation
- failure to take proper, effective, or timely measures to remedy the injurious manipulation
- guarantee of results or wrongful claim of superior expertise in diagnosis or treatment
- suggestion that another practitioner's care was inferior, inappropriate, or inconsistent with orthodox and commonly accepted methods

Allegations are seldom, if ever, narrow in scope, which leaves the onus on the practitioner to defend every aspect of the doctor-patient encounter. This provides good reason, if not motivation, for reviewing office procedures that may be called into question sometime in the future.

Case History

Patients who seek health care from a chiropractor often do so for neuromusculoskeletal complaints that are benign and raise no unusual concern.[46-52] Not uncommonly, the patient's complaint has been treated elsewhere, perhaps with limited results. It is the duty of the primary care practitioner and the right of the patient to have the immediate problem investigated, regardless of prior consultations. A patient who has found chiropractic treatment helpful in the past will often consult the chiropractor first on the next occasion.

While a patient consults the medical physician primarily because of pain, a patient who sees a chiropractor often has the added feature of limitation of movement. The patient may be unable to function in the activities of daily living or to control the problem through home measures, such as medication, heat, rest, and massage. A "crick in the neck," a "twisted back," a "kink," or a "pinched nerve" in the back or neck are common descriptions of these problems, contrasting with descriptions that suggest an organic basis for the problems.

There are four fundamental reasons why any primary care practitioner must perform an adequate clinical evaluation in reaching a diagnosis.[53]

1. to identify the patient's health problem and correlate the subjective symptoms with the objective clinical findings
2. to determine whether the patient is a candidate for manipulative therapy or whether the patient's health problem could best be treated by another health care provider
3. to identify any unrecognized health problems
4. to determine how the patient's problem is to be managed and whether there are any contraindications to manipulative therapy

The correct sequence of questions may suggest the origin of the problem. A patient's stiff and painful neck may be the result of infection, inflammation, trauma, neoplasm, or some other condition. If the patient has experienced headaches, dizziness, nausea, or balance difficulties in association with the neck pain, the stiff and painful neck complaint that first appeared to result from cervical joint dysfunction becomes a more complex problem. It is then appropriate to rule out a vascular cause for what had originally seemed to be a routine or familiar problem.

Preliminary identification of individuals at high risk for stroke need not be a difficult task. Age, sex, history of cardiovascular disease, family history, relevant habits (eg, smoking, oral contraceptive use), and level of general health are simple historical data that can be obtained through interviews by trained staff or self-administered questionnaires (Exhibit 6-1). Although this method of history taking may fall within acceptable standard-of-care guidelines, it may be less than satisfactory where the doctor is not alert to "red flag" warnings.[54] The practitioner should personally pursue specific lines of questioning related to the cardiovascular system.

Exhibit 6-1 Patient Questionnaire Related to Signs and Symptoms of Vertebrobasilar Insufficiency

---

                                                                Case #_____
Patient's Name_____ Date_____ Age_____ Sex_____
                    Please Print

Instructions: Please circle the correct response. Sign and date when completed.

I. **Historical Information**   **Doctor's Notes**
    Have you ever been diagnosed or told you had any
    of the following?

    1. High Blood pressure (hypertension)   YES   NO

    2. Hardening of the arteries (arterio-   YES   NO
       sclerosis)

    3. Diabetes   YES   NO

    4. Heart or blood vessel diseases   YES   NO

    5. Bone spurs on the neck bones (cervical   YES   NO
       spondylosis)

    6. Whiplash injury (flexion-extension   YES   NO
       injury) (cervical sprain)

    7. Have any of your relatives ever suffered   YES   NO
       a stroke?

    8. Were you ever a smoker? From __ To __   YES   NO

    9. Do you take any medication on a regu-   YES   NO
       lar basis? What? (Coumadin, Heparin,
       Aspirin, Antihypertensive medicine,
       etc.) _____

    10. (Women Only) Have you ever taken   YES   NO
        oral contraceptives? From ____ To ____

    Have You Had Any of the Following,
    Even Short, Temporary Attacks, in the Last Year?

    11. Blurred vision?   YES   NO

    12. Double vision?   YES   NO

    13. Diminished or partial loss of vision in   YES   NO
        one or both eyes?

    14. Complete loss of vision in one or both   YES   NO
        eyes?

    15. Ringing, buzzing or any noise in the   YES   NO
        ear(s)?

16. Hearing loss in one or both ears?   YES   NO
17. Slurred speech or other speech   YES   NO
    problems?
18. Difficulty swallowing?   YES   NO
19. Dizziness?   YES   NO
20. Temporary lack of understanding?   YES   NO
21. Loss of consciousness, even momentary   YES   NO
    blackouts?
22. Numbness or loss of sensation in the   YES   NO
    face, fingers, hand, arms, legs or other
    parts of your body?
23. Any other abnormal sensations in any   YES   NO
    part of your body?
24. Weakness, clumsiness or loss of   YES   NO
    strength in the face, fingers, hands,
    arms or legs?
25. Sudden collapse without loss of   YES   NO
    consciousness?

_____
Patient's Signature   Date

NAME_____ CASE #_____ DATE_____

(The T.I.A. may occur many times a day, week, or a month for many years. The attacks
usually last for only a few minutes or seconds.)

Source: Palmer College of Chiropractic clinic form based on excerpts from PE George et al.,
Identification of the high risk pre-stroke patient in American Chiropractic Association *Journal of
Chiropractic* (1981;15:26–28).

Transient ischemic attacks signal the existence of significant cerebrovascular disease and clearly indicate the potential danger of cerebral or
brain stem infarction.[55,56] Vertigo, described by the patient as "dizziness,"
"disorientation," or "loss of balance," is the most common symptom of
vertebrobasilar ischemia (Table 6-1).[55] Unfortunately, based on a review of
the literature on vertebral artery syndrome associated with cervical manipulation, a past history of transient ischemic attacks or vertigo has not been a
notable complaint prior to the onset of stroke.[22,30] Any complaint of vertigo

Table 6-1 Incidence of Clinical Features of Transient Ischemic Attacks Referable to the Cerebral Vessels

Carotid Vessels		Vertebrobasilar Vessels	
Symptom	Incidence	Symptom	Incidence
Hemianesthesia	33%	Vertigo	48%
Hemiparesis	31%	Visual field disturbance	6–22%
Headache	25%	Drop attacks	10–16%
Dysphasia	20%	Dysarthria	11%
Visual field disturbance	14%	Hemianesthesia	9%
Monoparesis	7%	Hemiparesis	8%
Confusion	5%	Visceral sensations	8%
Facial paresthesias	4%	Diplopia	5–7%
Dysarthria	3%	Monoparesis	4%
		Headache	3%
		Tinnitus	1%

Source: Adapted from JJ Caronna, Transient ischemic attacks. *Postgraduate Medicine* (1976; 59[3]: 106–111), Copyright © 1976 by McGraw-Hill Book Company.

that develops during the course of treatment must be considered pathognomonic of stroke until proved otherwise, however.

The record of the patient history must document inquiry into the symptomatology of vertebral artery syndrome—even when the result is negative. There is an old saying that the doctor who cannot take a good history and the patient who cannot give one are in danger of giving and receiving bad treatment. Failing to record any unusual signs and symptoms or to assess their significance risks the patient's welfare and invites legal inquiry.[57]

Physical Examination

The physical examination takes the historical problem-solving task one step closer to diagnostic accuracy. A series of tests screen the patient's problem, based on the expected outcome for a particular condition. The predictive value of the examination is based on test sensitivity and specificity. There can be little doubt that the predictive value of screening tests for vertebral artery requires critical interprofessional evaluation. Having qualified this shortcoming, there are a few physical tests that may be helpful in identifying patients at unusual risk of vertebral artery compromise prior to considering manipulative intervention.

Since presenting complaints relating to functional disturbances of the cervical spine will be suspected, examination procedures routinely performed include neuro-orthopaedic and chiropractic tests and maneuvers. These will be described briefly given the relevancy of the cervical spine to the vertebral artery syndrome. However, since other problems attributable to the cardiovascular and the cerebrovascular system must be ruled out, specific tests thought to be helpful in this case will be described in more detail.

Testing for Mechanical Dysfunction

Establishing joint dysfunction is a necessary prerequisite to manipulation. Asymmetrical postural patterns or any restriction of active gross ranges of motion in any direction, with or without a pain pattern, provides the examiner with a sense of the mechanical origin of the problem. Testing movements first passively and then against resistance within the patient's tolerance isolates the general location and the tissues involved, whether they be joint or muscle tissue.

During static palpation, the examiner feels bony and soft tissue texture, noting any abnormality. Intensely tender soft tissues, called trigger points, or hyperirritable areas give rise to pain locally and/or remote from the site of digital pressure. Sensory, motor, and reflex testing helps distinguish radicular from referred pain. Other neurological and orthopedic testing will confirm the presence or absence of nerve root, disk, or other neuromusculoskeletal syndromes.

The mainstay of the chiropractic examination is the dynamic assessment of global segmental function through motion palpation.[58-60] Segmental mobility and end play are comparatively investigated, with a particular focus on restricted movement and degree of pain. Combined with the other information recorded, the findings of motion palpation make it possible to determine the level, direction, and amplitude of adjustive thrust necessary to "free" the motion segment restriction during treatment. Patient tolerance to motion palpation may best be described, in essence, as a test of manipulation.[2]

Segmental hypermobility or, more important, instability is best palpated through passive movement or resisted challenge. Upper cervical instability at the atlanto-axial level is palpated during resisted flexion and extension movements. Unusual crepitus may elicit a pseudo-articular "clunk," warranting radiographic assessment of the structural integrity of the atlantodental space and the odontoid peg. Congenital or acquired lesions (eg, os odontoideum, ruptured or agenic transverse ligament) contraindicate manipulative treatment. Any painfully strained movements on the patient's part should be carefully assessed; quite apart from the risk to the cord, serious injury to vertebral and internal carotid arteries may result from compression.

Testing for Cardiovascular Dysfunction

General cardiovascular information obtained from the case history may require objective corroboration. With the patient sitting, the examiner compares radial pulses bilaterally and notes the rate, rhythm, amplitude, and character of each pulse. Blood pressure readings in the left and right arm should be recorded. A relative 10 to 20 mm Hg difference in systolic pressure, along with any marked variation in the pulse, suggests an occlusive abnormality that may be reflected in the vertebral arteries.[54]

Arm activities, such as rapid arm circumduction with the head and neck held stationary, may trigger focal vertebrobasilar ischemia or cervicobrachial neurovascular distraction. If there is a stenotic lesion in the subclavian artery proximal to the origin of the vertebral artery, retrograde flow in the ipsilateral vertebral artery may be supplying the arm; during arm exercise, the diversion of blood from the contralateral vertebral artery through anastomotic channels may produce symptoms of brain stem ischemia. This condition has been aptly named the subclavian steal syndrome. Most instances of reversed vertebral artery flow with subclavian artery stenosis or occlusion are asymptomatic.[61]

Auscultation for bruit over the neck is helpful in identifying sites of extracranial stenosis. A bruit heard under the angle of the mandible suggests occlusive disease of the carotid artery, and a bruit heard medially in the supraclavicular fossa is associated with vertebral or subclavian artery stenosis. In more than 75% of patients, the presence of a loud and localized bruit is associated with atherosclerotic obstruction at that immediate side.[61]

Fundoscopy, although not specific for vertebrobasilar arterial problems, affords a general visual impression of the state of the vascular bed through a sampling of the retinal vessels. Other tests helpful in identifying the causes of pulse differences are Adson's, Allen's, Eden's, Wright's and the costoclavicular maneuver, which is useful when the practitioner suspects a thoracic outlet syndrome or occlusive disorder.[62]

Tests To Help Ensure the Safety of Manipulation

Manipulation should be considered only if joint dysfunction is present, as the purpose of manipulation is to increase the range of motion when limited, decrease pain, and reduce undesirable muscle tension. Unless the manipulation is skilled and well applied, however, harm may be the result.

Houle[63] advocated and applied the de Kleyn test as a premanipulative maneuver. The clinical evaluation of vertebral artery syndrome was further advanced in the chiropractic literature by Giles,[64] Henderson,[2] Kleynhans,[65] Jaskoviak,[30] Ladermann,[66] Gatterman,[67] George,[54] as well as Terrett[25,68,69] whose contributions are the most detailed work on this subject. European literature by medical authors experienced in manipulation have also provided much to the present understanding of vertebral artery syndrome.[26,27,70-75]

The positional tests of provocation preparatory to manipulation are helpful, but not infallible, diagnostic maneuvers. They fall short of simulating the position and effect of the manipulative adjustment. Notwithstanding the need to analyze their predictive value in the future,[76] positional tests are well accepted as the most sensitive screening tests available to detect vertebrobasilar compression or occlusion in the vulnerable patient. If, during the history taking, the patient reveals that a certain motion or neck position elicits dizziness, the practitioner should note this position and avoid it when providing manual treatment.

De Kleyn or Houle Test. In the de Kleyn or Houle test, the patient is supinely positioned, and the head and neck are passively rotated and extended first to one side and then the other for at least 30 seconds in the initial examination. On subsequent visits, a lesser period of 5 to 10 seconds is prudent, particularly if the patient has reported any lightheadedness or dizziness. A rest period of several seconds between the tests of the sides should allow some "catch-up" of latent or subtle signs or symptoms. The eyes should be observed not only because nystagmus or altered pupillary response may occur, but also because a patient who experiences vertigo nearly always closes the eyes. If any clinical manifestations (eg, dizziness, vertigo, nystagmus, nausea, faintness, or visual disturbances) develop, manipulation should not be performed. The side of provocation should be recorded.

Rotation of the head and neck normally diminishes contralateral vertebral artery flow by as much as 75%.[77] If the ipsilateral artery is diseased or is anomalous, symptoms will occur because the dominant healthy artery is under physiological compression, resulting in a loss of sufficient or compensatory blood flow to the hind brain. Vestibular mechanism impairment results in disorientation and vertigo.

In a patient with joint restriction, adequate vertebral artery challenge may not be possible until joint function is restored. Hence, subsequent provocation testing is necessary in order to reduce the risk of stroke at a later stage in the treatment. It is also hypothesized that the younger, more mobile cervical spine allows more vascular challenge at the end of active range of motion than does the degeneratively stiff neck.[31] In the latter instance, however, intrinsic conditions, such as atherosclerotic plaquing, are more likely to lead to transient ischemic attacks, whereas immediate or delayed mechanical injury to the vertebral artery may lead to vertebral artery syndrome in younger age groups. The premanipulative position should always be considered a test in itself and should be routinely held for a few seconds to check the patient's tolerance before the manipulation is performed.

Although the results are inconclusive, Houle's positional test of sustained cervical rotation and extension appears to be the best available test of vertebral artery involvement. The small number of patients in whom results are positive either do not undergo manipulation or are referred for further investigation; hence, documented evidence of test validity is difficult to establish. The predictive value of these tests has yet to be determined.

Standing Balance Test. A more sensitive test, the standing balance test may prompt an early, obvious response due to dependency of postural tone and balance. The components of the nervous system that play a major role in the maintenance of static equilibrium are visual cues, vestibular mechanisms, and proprioceptive and kinesthetic reflex activities. Vestibular function is dependent on vertebral artery flow. An increased contribution from the other two components must compensate for any impairment within one component if normal balance is to be maintained.

The standing balance test can be done with the eyes opened and then repeated with the eyes closed in order to eliminate visual cues. In the latter situation, some postural sway is normal, so the examiner should be nearby in the event of a loss of balance. Feet are placed approximately shoulder width apart. The patient is asked to flex the arms to 90 degrees with the palms up; then to extend the head and neck; and, while in this position, to rotate the neck first to one side and then the other, each for a period of approximately 20 seconds. A rest before performing the procedure on the second side allows for a catch-up of possible symptoms and/or the neutralization of sensitive balance receptors in the inner ear. Observation of loss of balance, fainting (drop attack), or nystagmus requires further investigation, as does any report of nausea, visual disturbance, extremity dysfunction, or difficulty with speech and swallowing. Referral to a neurologist or vascular specialist may be necessary, depending on the patient's response to testing. The test can be done sitting if the patient prefers more stability, but proprioceptive balance disturbances will be less apparent in this position.

Another variation of the balance test is marching in place while the neck is extended and rotated, requiring further postural reinforcement of righting reflexes in subclinical or suspicious cases.[59] Added to the cervical involvement, lower limb hyperemia and mechanical jolting of the extended neck may augment any sign of vertebrobasilar insufficiency.

Hautant Test. Performed while sitting or standing, the Hautant test indicates any deviation or stray of the arm during contralateral neck rotation that can be interpreted to result from labyrinthine or upper cervical joint dysfunction.[78,79] Impairment of vertebral artery flow to the labyrinth and vestibular nuclei is manifested as vertigo.

The amount of lateral arm stray through kymographlike recordings called cervicovertigograms can be registered.[79] While the patient holds a pencil against the moving graph paper and rotates the neck from one side to the other, lateral arm movement caused by the onset of dizziness is measured. The use of left and right quadrant weight scales, or stabilometry, also objectifies the degree of balance disturbance. Lewit considered a 5-kg difference in weight distribution during comparative neck rotation with or without extension to indicate disequilibrium.[79] The documentation of these slight arm stray and weight differences is academic, however, and more appropriate in the research of righting reflexes in association with upper cervical joint dysfunction. Disturbances in balance and involuntary arm movement are magnified where vertebral artery flow is impaired.

Barany Rotary Test. Designed to differentiate inner ear from cervicogenic triggers in the development of cephalic disturbances, such as vertigo and nystagmus, the Barany rotary test is best conducted in a multidisciplinary research or specialized clinical setting. The patient sits in a chair that can be easily rotated or swivelled and is quickly spun around; the head and torso remain in a constant position. The head is successively placed in various planes to test each of the semicircular canals horizontally.[2,64] When the chair is suddenly stopped, the endolymphatic momentum briefly continues, causing the cupola to bend in the direction of motion. This flow triggers a short-term nystagmus that lasts approximately 10 to 20 seconds. The slow component is the direction of rotation; the fast component, in the opposite direction. The patient has a sensation of vertigo in which he or she seems to be rotating in a direction opposite to the spin of the chair seconds before.

This test is designed to investigate the synchronous action of the semicircular canals on both sides, but it has been superseded by the specialist's use of the caloric water test. Its significance lies in the fact that, since the head is held constant and is rotated with the body, the vertebrogenic triggers that produce exaggerated reflex responses are not in operation. This test discounts cervical involvement in vertigo and nystagmus either through righting reflex disturbances or vertebrobasilar insufficiency.

Swinging Chair Test. A neurological disturbance arising from proprioceptive reflex effects on the brain stem and cerebellum may be demonstrated through the swinging chair test.[79] If the vertebral nerve surrounding the vertebral artery has more than a vestigial function reflex, vasospasm may represent another, albeit questionable, cause of vertigo and nystagmus.

Like the Barany rotary test, this test should be conducted in a specialized setting. During this test, the patient sits in a swivel chair while an assistant's hands fix the head position and the examiner rotates the chair to and fro. The head position can be successively changed, depending on cervical movement restriction. The magnitude of rotation depends on the patient's own range of left and right rotation. In this test, the positional triggers that incite endo-lymphatic motion are not in operation, excluding the possibility of a laby-rinthogenic origin of the patient's cephalic complaints. The test incorporates a rapid and rhythmic change too brief to challenge the vertebral arteries in a significant way, however.

Laboratory Examination

Like the positional tests of provocation previously described, laboratory tests do not necessarily unveil the cause of any vascular impairment in the susceptible patient. It is prudent, however, to reflect on any test result that provides insight into the patient's state of health, particularly into any hidden pathology of the cerebrovascular system.

Many laboratory tests do not fall within the domain of generalized medi-cal/chiropractic practice, but the results from procedures used to evaluate patients suspected to be at risk for stroke or transient ischemic attacks may be made available to the chiropractor.[80] In order to determine the cardiovascular and cerebrovascular status of the patient, the physician may call for blood tests, including a complete blood count and determinations of the erythrocyte sedimentation rate, serum cholesterol and lipid levels, postprandial glucose levels, and the blood urea nitrogen concentration. Skull and chest film studies and electrocardiograms may also be ordered. These test results may be of little value in the characteristic vertebral artery syndrome patient, however, unless arteriosclerotic problems coexist.

The most definitive diagnostic procedure for abnormalities in the structure and function of the vertebrobasilar vessels is angiography.[39] Valuable in differential diagnosis, angiography accurately demonstrates the site, extent, and incidence of arterial obstructions that may be surgically corrected. It has little practical value in screening because of the expense and risk of compli-cations with the procedure. Permanent worsening and death may follow angiography, although these occur in less than 1% of patients.[61]

Computed tomography scans are useful only in the investigation of the cervical and cranial area, where they make it possible to determine the eventual consequences of stroke in the vertebrobasilar territory. Magnetic resonance imaging has a higher sensitivity in exploring pathological fields in the central nervous system and may be helpful in cerebral blood flow measurements.[39] Similarly, cochleovestibular evoked potentials may be helpful where transient ischemic attacks and stroke have developed. Doppler scanning produces a good estimation of vertebral artery flow only when applied and interpreted by well-trained personnel, because the vessel has a small diameter and lies deep within the cervical bony canal.[39]

Because the predictive value of the clinical examination may be somewhat limited, any simple and cost-effective investigation that reduces patient risk by revealing any anomalous or acquired bony lesion is a tool worth considering. Plain film radiography falls into this category. It is used routinely following cervical trauma and is no less important when manipulative adjustments are being contemplated.[81-85] So long as the risk:benefit ratio of exposure to ionizing radiation is considered and attention is given to good radiographic detail, those experienced and qualified in spinal manipulation deem the radiograph to be an essential and readily available method of examination.[84,85] It reveals many anomalous or pathological processes that weaken or destabilize the supportive elements of bone and joint and, thus, may be associated with vertebral artery syndrome. Radiographic conditions that may be associated with vertebral artery insufficiency include:

- exuberant hypertrophic changes in the apophyseal and uncovertebral joint of Luschka
- congenital anomalies
  1. os odontoideum
  2. atlantal assimilation
  3. condylar hypoplasia
  4. increased atlantodental interval (ADI) spacing (Down syndrome)
  5. aplasia of the posterior atlantal arch (clefting anomalies)
  6. basilar impression (achondroplasia)
  7. Klippel-Feil syndrome
- acquired disorders
  1. occipitocervical dysplasia (Paget's disease, osteomalacia)
  2. infection (Grisel's syndrome, tuberculous involvement about the transverse ligament)
  3. rheumatoid-like involvement at the atlantodental joint (rheumatoid arthritis, systemic lupus erythematosus, psoriasis)

- trauma
  1. odontoid fracture
  2. rupture of the transverse ligament (widened ADI)
  3. hypermobility or instability at the craniocervical junction
  4. severe "whiplash" injuries
- tumors
  1. primary, benign and malignant
  2. secondary, leading to destructive instability

These are but a few of the conditions that a chiropractor should exclude in the assessment of a patient with neck complaints.

Clinical Impression (Working Diagnosis)

After analyzing the signs and symptoms to ascertain the pathophysiological processes involved, the practitioner may set down an interpretation of the causation(s) in a tentative conclusion called the clinical impression or working diagnosis. Before this is done, however, there must be a differential determination of the patient's signs and symptoms.[86] A painfully stiff neck may be

1. spinal or nonspinal in origin, requiring the differentiation of a nonspinal condition sufficient for an appropriate referral
2. related to a spinal disorder that is due to dysfunction or structural pathology, requiring the differentiation of vertebral conditions sufficient for an appropriate referral
3. related to a dysfunctional or mechanical problem sufficient for a clinical impression or diagnosis

More than one clinical impression may be recorded. One impression may relate to the functional disturbance of the cervical spine, while another may relate to the impact of this disturbance on a disorder or syndrome. For example, C2-3 dysfunctional hypomobility may be contributing to tension headaches and torticollis. If no mechanical disturbances are evident or the diagnosis is in doubt, the chiropractor should refer the patient to another health care provider who can investigate the patient's problem further. Although diagnostic and management variations occur in individual cases, the seed algorithm shown in Figure 6-2 is presented as a general guide in the decision-making process.

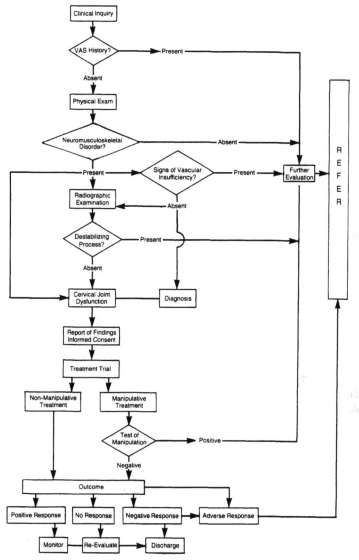

Figure 6-2 Decision-making flow chart for the chiropractic clinical evaluation and management of patients with upper cervical dysfunction.*

* Clinical guidelines are designed to assist clinicians by providing an analytical framework for the evaluation and treatment of common clinical problems. This seed algorithm, as proposed, is not intended to replace a clinician's clinical judgment or to establish a protocol for all patients with cervical joint dysfunction. All decision-making processes are subject to continuous review, and guidelines rarely establish the only appropriate approach to a clinical condition.

Doctrine of Informed Consent

After reviewing the case history, conducting physical and other specialized tests to rule out vertebrobasilar involvement, and establishing a clinical diagnosis of cervical joint dysfunction, the practitioner must discuss manipulative treatment with the patient. The discussion should include an explanation of the causative factors in the patient's problem and an outline of the possible outcomes, both with and without treatment.

Ethically, every attempt should be made to allow a patient to choose freely between available therapies. In order to make this choice, a patient must have information about the alternatives and consequences of care, as well as the expected benefits and risks. Such information should include[87]

1. the proposed regimen of treatment, including the manipulative adjustment, expected benefits, risks, pain or other obvious inconvenience, expected frequency, duration of care, and costs
2. alternatives, if the patient chooses either to do nothing or to pursue a different form of care; the benefits, risks, and inconveniences of such choices

If signs, symptoms, or tests of provocation suggest some risk, even if negligible, informed consent should be sought.[31] Some practitioners routinely inform their patients of the slight risk of stroke if cervical manipulation is contemplated (Exhibit 6-2).[88] Although the possibility of vertebral artery syndrome associated with manipulation is remote, disclosure of such material risk is legally mandated in many jurisdictions because of the syndrome's serious consequences.[89,90] Informed consent, however perceived, should not be an end, but a means for optimal patient care.

Practitioners and patients should strive for good communication to arrive at an agreement about a treatment to be undertaken. Just as a patient has an obligation to provide the practitioner with all relevant information about the condition, the practitioner has an obligation to provide all the information a patient needs to make adequately informed decisions regarding care. If there is a question of patient competency (eg, because the patient is a child, has a psychological difficulty, or is mentally handicapped), the practitioner should consult with family, guardians, or another health care provider before deciding on a course of treatment. If agreement cannot be reached, the practitioner should recommend that the patient seek a second opinion from another qualified practitioner. If the probable treatment outcome is in doubt, referral to a more qualified colleague is prudent. It is best to defer to the patient's informed and reasonable judgment if he or she chooses not to have treatment.

Exhibit 6-2 Informed Consent Form

INFORMED CONSENT FORM

Physicians, chiropractors, osteopaths and physiotherapists are required to advise their patients with neck problems such as yours of the following. In recent years there have been incidents of injury to the vertebral artery during the course of treatment. This has caused strokes or stroke-like occurrences, which are usually of a temporary nature. The chances of this happening are between one in one million and one in one and a half million. Tests with or without x-rays have been performed on you to minimize this risk to yourself. Chiropractic is considered to be one of the safest, most effective forms of therapy for your type of problem. If you have any questions about this, please ask your chiropractor.

I have read the above statement and consent to treatment.

Signed ....

Date ....

Source: Reprinted with permission from *Journal of the Canadian Chiropractic Association* (1988; 32[2]:91-94), Copyright © 1988, Canadian Chiropractic Association.

In circumstances involving apparently contentious issues of informed consent, the practitioner should record in the patient's clinical file all relevant information concerning the acquisition or, alternatively, the waiving of consent.[91] It is a wise practice to record in the patient's file the specific topics explained and discussed in connection with consent to treatment of the cervical spine.

Manipulative Treatment and Management

The controlled act of the manipulative adjustment may be defined as a passive manual maneuver—a sudden impulsion or thrust of controlled velocity and amplitude—applied to a joint at the end of its limited range of passive motion without exceeding the boundaries of anatomical integrity.[92,93] It is usually accompanied by a cracking noise. The aim of the adjustive thrust is to correct joint dysfunction. As in all procedures that carry material risk, the manipulation should be performed only by practitioners properly trained and experienced in its application.

Once the patient has consented to treatment for cervical joint dysfunction, the practitioner should review the manipulative procedure, especially if the patient has never consulted a chiropractor before. Although some patients perceive manipulation as a relatively gentle procedure, the adjustive thrust can be a traumatic event for the first-time chiropractic patient who is in pain. Explaining that the mobilizing or manipulative technique may result in a cavitating "crack" is essential.

Initial treatments should be light and never unduly forceful.[31] It is better to work up to the required adjustive thrust gradually over the first few treatments than to risk a painful muscle reaction. The thrust should be applied in the direction that accomplishes the therapeutic goal of mobility with the least pain possible. The practitioner should record the objective and subjective results of the manipulation, as these notes will be helpful in the selection of appropriate techniques in the future.

The practitioner should avoid any extension of the neck when manipulating a patient in the supine position; rather, it is important to keep the head rest up and the neck partially flexed. Rotational positions should be within the patient's comfort zone, with the motion segment to be adjusted just at the premanipulative passive movement barrier. At this point, "joint slack" is taken up and held for a few seconds, and the patient is asked if he or she is comfortable in this position; this test of manipulation ensures that no unusual symptoms arise before a short-lever, low-amplitude, high-velocity thrust is delivered to the segmental restriction.

If the patient is uncomfortable, the practitioner should consider using another nonthrust technique. For instance, joint mobilization, gentle muscle stretching maneuvers within the passive range of movement, or muscle energy techniques may prove effective in the early stages of an acute problem. Manipulative adjustments, in which the practitioner slowly works up to the desired thrust, can be given in subsequent treatments. The practitioner should instruct the patient on postures or tasks to avoid, as well as on the use of heat or cold at home, to help reduce muscle spasm and inflammation brought about by the initial injury. Mobilizing or strengthening exercises should be given as soon as conveniently possible.

The management of the patient's problem, rather than just the treatment of joint dysfunction, should be the practitioner's objective. Once the patient's joint function has been restored and pain or discomfort has disappeared, manipulative treatment can be phased out in favor of exercises. Preventive measures at home or work should be recommended if the problem is likely to recur.

A number of authors have questioned the wisdom of administering rotational upper cervical adjustments at all.[27,33,94] Controlled rotational thrust techniques have proved effective in the treatment of joint dysfunction, however. In the absence of contraindications, this procedure has remained within the reasonable and expected standard of chiropractic care.[95] A consensus approach that includes consideration of quality assurance and research that addresses technique utilization, risk management, and peer review are required to resolve such controversial issues.

Iatrogenic Causes of Complications and Adverse Reactions

Kleynhans reviewed the various factors in practitioner-related manipulative incidents and noted several causes.[65]

Lack of Knowledge. Formal training in the diagnosis and treatment of neuromusculoskeletal disorders ensures reasonable, acceptable clinical decisions and the provision of optimal patient care. Knowledge of the contraindications and indications for manipulative treatment comes from an academic review of the literature, specialized clinical training, and practical experience.

Lack of Skill. The performance of spinal manipulation can be dangerous in the hands of the unqualified. Because manipulation is proving to be a practical and cost-effective treatment for common complaints such as low back and neck pain, a new trend toward unqualified manipulation has emerged. Quality assurance of an acceptable standard of patient care can be provided only by those practitioners who are equipped by their education and training to carry out spinal diagnosis and therapy at a sophisticated and refined level on a continuing full-time basis. Livingston concluded that "medical and paramedical personnel would do well to either study spinal manipulation thoroughly or avoid it."[96] Other physicians with experience in the field of manipulative care agree.[97,98]

Lack of Rational Attitude and Technique. Among the problems that result from a lack of rational attitude and technique are a number of inappropriate practices.

- inadequate diagnostic habits; ambivalence toward diagnostic procedures and locating the mechanical source, if any, of the patient's problem prior to the application of the manipulation.
- inadequate radiographic evaluation. Failure to assess the structural integrity of the primary area requiring manipulative care objectively can result in misdiagnosis and injury. Radiographs should be of adequate quality and quantity to ensure that there are no contraindications to manipulation.
- delay in referral. Where manipulative treatment is inappropriate, ineffective, or not the treatment of choice, a delayed referral delays the correc-

tion of the patient's problem through alternative care. In the event of an adverse reaction to manipulation, time may be of the essence if more serious complications are to be avoided.

- delay in reevaluation. A patient's response to manipulative treatment should be assessed at various stages to determine if the therapeutic objective has been reached within a reasonable period of time. If the expected outcome has not been reached, the patient's problem should be reevaluated, as further treatment may not be warranted.

- lack of interprofessional cooperation. If the patient has a health problem for which manipulation may be of questionable value or states that he or she is receiving alternative care or therapy, failure to inquire further may result in harm to the patient.

- failure to take into account patient tolerances. The practitioner should be alert and sensitive to the patient who feels that the treatment may not be beneficial, reports a worsening of the condition, or describes the manipulation as unduly painful.

- poor technique selection or implementation. Unproved or inappropriate use of manipulation, like inadequate experience, training, and skill, invariably leads to injury. The application of excessive force in an unsafe direction or patient position at an inappropriate segmental level or in the presence of a contraindication for manipulation is, no doubt, the cause of many adverse reactions.

- excessive or unnecessary use of manipulation. Applying manipulation without regard to the need for it constitutes not only blatant disregard of the principles of cost containment, but also, more important, the worst form of abuse of the patient's best interest. Endless treatments with no added therapeutic gain also breach professional ethical behavior.

Practitioner Response to Vertebral Artery Syndrome

In the unlikely event that vertebral artery syndrome occurs, it is important that the practitioner *not* repeat the manipulative treatment in the hope that it will reverse the problem. The importance of cervical immobilization with a cervical collar and immediate arrangement for hospital transportation can not be overstressed. Anticoagulant therapy may be the only medical emergency measure that will reduce the complication of ischemia to vital central nervous system tissues.

It is essential to monitor the patient's vital signs. Blood pressure, pulses, respiratory rate, and pupillary response to light should be measured and recorded at timed intervals. Cardiopulmonary resuscitation must be performed in the event of an arrest. The practitioner should be prepared to take charge until the patient is under the care of emergency medical staff. Later, all precise details of the incident should be recorded and the appropriate protective association be notified as soon as possible.

CONCLUSION

All forms of treatment carry some risk of patient harm, and manipulation of the spine for dysfunctional disorders is no exception. The risk of harm is greatly reduced, however, when a profession's commitment to quality assurance is linked with research, risk management, and peer review programs. Standard of practice and care guidelines provide practitioners of manipulation with a structured approach to all aspects of improved patient care, facilitating the accurate assessment and manipulative treatment of dysfunction of the upper cervical spine.

REFERENCES

1. American Chiropractic Association, Department of Statistics. Department of statistics completes 1985 survey. *Journal of Chiropractic*. 1986;23:68–69.

2. Henderson DJ. Significance of vertebral dyskinesia in relation to the cervical syndrome. *Journal of Manipulative and Physiological Therapeutics*. 1979;2:3–15.

3. de Kleyn A, Nieuwenhuyse P. Schwindelanfalle and Nystagmas bei einer bestimmten Stellung des Kopfes. *Acta Oto-Laryngolica*. 1927;11;155–157.

4. Stopford JSB. The arteries of the pons and medulla oblongata. *J Anat Physiol*. 1916;50:131–164.

5. Sheehan D, Smyth GE. A study of the anatomy of vertebral thrombosis. *Lancet*. 1937;2:614–618.

6. Kubik C, Adams R. Occlusion of the basilar artery—A clinical and pathological study. *Brain*. 1946;69:73–121.

7. Tissington-Tatlow WF, Bammer HG. Syndrome of vertebral artery compression. *Neurology*. 1957;7:331–340.

8. Hutchinson E, Yates P. The cervical portion of the vertebral artery—A clinicopathological study. *Brain*. 1956;79:319–331.

9. Toole J, Tucker S. Influence of the head position upon cerebral circulation. *Arch Neurol*. 1960;2:616–623.

10. Selecki BR. The effect of rotation of the atlas on the axis: Experimental work. *Med J Aust*. 1969;56:1012–1015.

11. Sheehan S, Bauer RB, Meyer JS. Vertebral artery compression in cervical spondylosis. *Neurology*. 1960;10:968–986.

12. Bauer RB, Wechsler N, Meyer JS. Carotid compression and rotation of the head in occlusive vertebral artery disease. *Ann Intern Med*. 1961;55:283-291.

13. Powers S, Drislane T, Nevins S. Intermittent vertebral artery compression—a new syndrome. *Surgery*. 1961;49:257-264.

14. Bauer RB, Sheehan S, Meyer JS. Arteriographic study of cerebrovascular disease. *Arch Neurol*. 1961;4:119-131.

15. Chrast B, Korbicka J. Die Beeinflussung der stromungsverhaltnisse in der Arteria vertebralis durch verschiedene Kopt und Halshaltungen. *Deutsche Zeitschrift fur Nevenheilkunde*. 1962;183:426-448.

16. Faris A, Poser C, Wilmore D, Agnew C. Radiologic visualization of neck vessels in healthy men. *Neurology*. 1963;13:386-396.

17. Hardesty W, Whitacre W, Toole J, Randall P, Royster H. Studies on vertebral artery flow in man. *Surg Gynecol Obstet*. 1963;116:662-664.

18. Fields W, Ratinoy G, Weibel J, Campos R. Survival following basilar artery occlusion. *Arch Neurol*. 1966;15:463-471.

19. Husni E, Storer J. The syndrome of mechanical occlusion of the vertebral artery. *Angiology*. 1967;18:106-116.

20. Malpractice: Death resulting from chiropractic treatment for headache. *JAMA*. 1934;103:1260.

21. Pratt-Thomas HR, Berger KE. Cerebellar and spinal injuries after chiropractic manipulation. *JAMA*. 1947;133:600-603.

22. Terrett AGJ. Vascular accidents from cervical spine manipulation: Report of 107 cases. *Journal of the Australian Chiropractic Association*. 1987;17:15-24.

23. Opala G, Arkuszewski I. Rotation of the cervical spine and angiographic picture of the internal carotid artery. *Man Med*. 1989;4:47-48.

24. Lyness SS, Simeone FA. Vascular complications of upper cervical spine injuries. In: Sherk HH, Fielding JW, eds. Symposium on the upper cervical spine. *Orthop Clin North Am*. 1978;9(4):1029-1038.

25. Terrett AGJ. Vascular accidents from cervical spine manipulation. *Journal of the Australian Chiropractic Association*. 1987;17:131-144.

26. Gutmann G. Injuries to the vertebral artery caused by manual therapy. *Manuelle Medizin*. 1983;21:2-14.

27. Dvorak J. Orelli F. How dangerous is manipulation of the cervical spine? *Manuelle Medizin*. 1982;20:44-28.

28. Maigne R. Manipulations vertebralis et les thromboses vertebrobasilares. *Angeiologie*. 1969;21:287.

29. Cyriax J. *Textbook of Orthopaedic Medicine*. 7th ed. London: Balliere Tindall; 1978;1:165.

30. Jaskoviak PA. Complications arising from manipulation of the cervical spine. *Journal of Manipulative and Physiological Therapeutics*. 1980;3:213-219.

31. Henderson DJ. Vertebrobasilar vascular accidents associated with cervical manipulation. In: Vernon H, ed. *Upper Cervical Syndrome—Chiropractic Diagnosis and Treatment*. Baltimore: Williams & Wilkins; 1988:194-206.

32. Inglis BD. *Chiropractic in New Zealand: Report of the Commission of Inquiry*. Wellington: Government Printer; 1979;3:77-78.

33. Terrett AGJ. It is more important to know when not to adjust. *Chiropractic Technique*. 1990;2:1-9.

34. Gotlib A, Thiel H. A selected annotated bibliography of the core biomedical literature pertaining to stroke, cervical spine, manipulation and head/neck movement. *Journal of the Canadian Chiropractic Association.* 1985;29:80–89.

35. McGuire CH. Medical problem-solving: A critique of the literature. *J Med Educ.* 1965;60:587–595.

36. Riegelmann R, Hirsch R. *Studying a Study and Testing a Test: How To Read the Medical Literature.* 2nd ed. Boston: Little Brown & Co; 1981.

37. Holzer FJ. Verschlub der wirbelsaulenschlagader am kopfgelenk mit nachfolgender thrombose durch seitwartsdrehen des kopfes. Eine gefahr bei operationen am hals mit starker seitwartsdrehung. *Deutsch Z Ges Gerichtl Med.* 1955;44:422–426.

38. Schneider RC, Schemm GW. Vertebral artery insufficiency in acute and chronic spinal trauma. *J Neurosurg.* 1961;18:348–360.

39. George B, Laurian C. *The Vertebral Artery—Pathology and Surgery.* New York: Springer-Verlag; 1987:91–114.

40. Wolfson RJ, Schlosser WD, Winchester RA. *Vertigo.* Summit, NJ: Ciba Pharmaceutical Company; 1965:99–133.

41. Yates PO. Birth trauma to the vertebral arteries. *Arch Dis Child.* 1959;34:426–431.

42. Sharpe G. *The Law and Medicine in Canada.* 2nd ed. Toronto: Butterworths; 1987: 17–85.

43. Emson HE. *The Doctor and the Law—A Practical Guide for the Canadian Physician.* 2nd ed. Toronto: Butterworths; 1989:85–118.

44. Vear HJ. Standards of chiropractic practice. *Journal of Manipulative and Physiological Therapeutics.* 1985;8(1):33–43.

45. Council on Chiropractic Education (USA). *Educational Standards for Chiropractic Colleges.* Des Moines, IA: Council on Chiropractic Education; 1987.

46. Vear HJ. A study into the complaints of patients seeking chiropractic care. *Journal of the Canadian Chiropractic Association.* 1972;16(3):9–13.

47. Rose P. Statistical analysis of chiropractic patients. *Bulletin of the European Chiropractic Union.* 1973;22(1):21–24;22(3):12–13.

48. Sherman RA. A statistical investigation of 500 patients. *Bulletin of the European Chiropractic Union.* 1976;24:35–40.

49. Phillips RB. A survey of Utah chiropractic patients. *ACA Journal of Chiropractic.* 1981;18:113–123.

50. McNulty MJ, Ferguson AC. Patient response to chiropractic care. *Research Forum.* 1987;4(1):11–16.

51. Nyiendo J, Haldeman S. A prospective study of 2000 patients attending a chiropractic college teaching clinic. *Med Care.* 1987;25:516–527.

52. Nyiendo J, Olsen E. Visit characteristics of 217 children attending a chiropractic college clinic. *Journal of Manipulative and Physiological Therapeutics.* 1988;11(2):78–84.

53. West HG. Physical and spinal examination procedures utilized in the practice of chiropractic. In: Haldeman S, ed. *Modern Developments in the Principles and Practice of Chiropractic.* New York: Appleton-Century-Crofts; 1980:269–296.

54. George PE, Silverstein HT, Wallace H, Marshall M. Identification of the high risk pre-stroke patient. *ACA Journal of Chiropractic.* 1981;15:26–28.

55. Caronna JJ. Transient ischemic attacks—Pathophysiology and medical management. *Postgrad Med.* 1976;59(3):106–111.

56. Foreman SM, Hooper PD. Transient ischemic attacks and their significance in the chiropractic practice: Technical and clinical considerations. *Chiropractic Technique.* 1989;1(2):57–59.

57. Reinke TS, Jahn WT. Preventing legal suicide with medical records. *JMPT.* 1988;11(6):511–513.

58. Grice AS. A biomechanical approach to cervical and dorsal adjusting. In: Haldeman S, ed. *Modern Developments in the Principles and Practice of Chiropractic.* New York: Appleton-Century-Crofts; 1980:331–358.

59. Schafer RC, Faye LJ. Motion palpation and chiropractic technique. Huntington Beach, Calif: Motion Palpation Institute; 1989:43–139.

60. Fligg B. Motion palpation of the upper cervical spine. In: Vernon H, ed. *Upper Cervical Syndrome.* Baltimore: Williams & Wilkins; 1988:113–123.

61. McDowell FH. Cerebrovascular diseases. In: Beeson PB, McDermott W, eds. *Textbook of Medicine.* 13th ed. Baltimore: WB Saunders; 1971:189–216.

62. Lord JW, Rosati LM. *Thoracic-outlet Syndromes.* Summit, NJ: CIBA Pharmaceutical Company; 1971:1–32.

63. Houle JOE. Assessing hemodynamics of the vertebrobasilar complex through angiothlipsis. *Journal of the Canadian Chiropractic Association.* 1972; 41:35–36,41.

64. Giles LGF. Vertebro-basilar artery insufficiency. *Journal of the Canadian Chiropractic Association.* 1977;21:112–117.

65. Kleynhans AM. Complication and contraindications to spinal manipulative therapy. In: Haldeman S, ed. *Modern Developments in the Principles and Practice of Chiropractic.* New York: Appleton-Century-Crofts; 1980:133–141.

66. Ladermann SP. Accidents of spinal manipulation. *Annals of Swiss Chiropractic Association.* 1981;7:161–208.

67. Gatterman MI. Contraindications and complications of spinal manipulative therapy. *ACA Journal of Chiropractic.* 1981;15:75–86.

68. Terrett AGJ, Webb M. Vertebrobasilar accidents following cervical spine adjustment manipulation. *Journal of the Australian Chiropractic Association.* 1982;12:24–27.

69. Terrett AGJ. Importance and interpretation of tests designed to predict susceptibility to neurocirculatory accidents from manipulation. *Journal of the Australian Chiropractic Association.* 1983;13:29–34.

70. Gutmann G, Tiwisina T. *Zum problem der irritation der arteria vertebralis.* Stuttgart: Hippokrates-Verlag; 1957:15.

71. Gutmann G. Halswirbelsaule und durchblutungsstorrungen in der vertbralis-basilaris-strombahn. In: *Die Wirbelsaule in Forschung und Praxis.* Stuttgart: Hippokrates; 1962;25: 138–155.

72. Gutmann G. Durchbluntungsstorungen der arteria vertebralis im zusammenhang mit Halswirbelsauleenverletzungen. *Manuelle Medizin.* 1971;5:112–116.

73. Gutmann G, ed. *Arteria vertebralis—traumatologie und funtionelle pathologie.* Berlin/Heidelberg: Springer-Verlag; 1984.

74. Lewit K. Komplikationen nach chiropraktischen manipulationen. *Dtsch Med Wschr.* 1972;97:784.

75. Hulse M. *Die zervikalen gleichgewichtsstorungen.* Berlin: Springer-Verlag; 1983:4–9.

76. Jansen RD, Nansel DD. Diagnostic illusions: the reliability of random chance. *Journal of Manipulative and Physiological Therapeutics.* 1988;11(5):355–365.

77. Gutmann G. *Arteria Vertebralis—Tramatologie und Funktionelle Pathologie.* New York: Springer-Verlag; 1985:2–6.

78. Lewit K. *Manipulative Therapy in Rehabilitation of the Motor System.* Toronto: Butterworths; 1987:24,140–146,172, 326.

79. Lewit K. The contribution of clinical observation to neurobiological mechanisms in manipulative therapy. In: Korr IM, ed. *The Neurobiologic Mechanisms in Manipulative Therapy.* New York: Plenum Press; 1978:3–21.

80. Triano JJ. The use of instrumentation and laboratory examination procedures by the chiropractor. In: Haldeman S, ed. *Modern Developments in the Principles and Practice of Chiropractic.* New York: Appleton-Century-Crofts; 1980:231–267.

81. Phillips RB. The use of x-rays in spinal manipulative therapy. In: Haldeman S, ed. *Modern Developments in the Principles and Practice of Chiropractic.* New York: Appleton-Century-Crofts; 1980:189–208.

82. Yochum TR, Rowe LJ. *Essentials of Skeletal Radiology.* Baltimore: Williams & Wilkins; 1987.

83. Yochum TR, Rowe LJ. Arthritides of the upper cervical complex. In: Idczak RM, ed. *Aspects of Manipulative Therapy.* Victoria, Australia: Lincoln Institute of Health Sciences; 1980:22–32.

84. Henderson DJ. Radiographic evaluation of the upper cervical spine. In: Vernon H, ed. *Upper Cervical Syndrome.* Baltimore: Williams & Wilkins; 1988:18–47.

85. Sherman RA. Chiropractic x-ray rationale. *Journal of Canadian Chiropractic Association.* 1986;30:33–35.

86. Vear HJ. An approach to the chiropractic scope of practice. *Journal of Canadian Chiropractic Association.* 1977;21(1):20–30.

87. Burgess MM. Chiropractic informed consent. *Journal of Canadian Chiropractic Association.* 1990;34(1):24–26.

88. Carey P. Informed consent—The new reality. *Journal of Canadian Chiropractic Association.* 1988;32(2):91–94.

89. *Mason v Forgie* (1984) 31 C.C.L.T. 66 (N.B.Q.B.).

90. *Reibl v Hughes* (1980) 2 S.C.R. 880.

91. *Informed Consent—Ethical Consideration for Physicians and Surgeons.* Toronto: Biomedical Ethics Committee of the Royal College of Physicians and Surgeons of Canada; 1987.

92. Sandoz R. Some physical mechanisms and effects of spinal adjustments. *Annals of Swiss Chiropractic Association.* 1976;6:91–141.

93. Cassidy JD, Kirkaldy-Willis WH. Manipulation. In: Kirkaldy-Willis WH, ed. *Managing Low Back Pain.* 2nd ed. New York: Churchill Livingstone; 1988:287–296.

94. Martienssen J, Nilsson N. Cerebrovascular accidents following upper cervical manipulation: The importance of age, gender and technique. *American Journal of Chiropractic Medicine.* 1989;2(1):160–163.

95. Chapman-Smith DA. Report on the first international chiropractic conference, September 24–26, 1987. *Chiropractic Report.* 1987;2(1):7.

96. Livingston M. Spinal manipulation causing injury. *British Columbia Medical Journal.* 1971;14:78.

97. Dvorak J. Manual medicine in the United States and Europe in the year 1982. *Man Med.* 1983;1:3–9.

98. Kirkaldy-Willis WH, Cassidy JD. Spinal manipulation in the treatment of low back pain. *Canadian Family Physician.* 1985;31:535–540.

7

An Algorithm for the Analysis of Chiropractic Methods

Robert Boal, Mark Kaminski, David H. Peterson, and Richard G. Gillette

There are numerous ways to approach the difficult, controversial, and often emotional issue of standards for the diagnostic and therapeutic methods used in the practice of chiropractic.[1-7] One of the most common methods employed in health care today is to convene a panel of experts who review the relevant literature and then apply consensus methods to produce a statement on the appropriateness of a given diagnostic or therapeutic procedure.[1] Although the selection of experts and the determination of consensus rules may be difficult tasks, the paramount difficulty in using this approach is to develop appropriate criteria for acceptability.

For a health care discipline, the most rigorous solution to the development of clinical standards is the requirement for full validation of clinical effectiveness,[8-11] using accepted standards for validation of diagnostic measures and clinical treatment trials.[12-14] Full validation should be the goal for any profession; however, in the practice of health care, full validation is not always possible. New information, theories, and practices are continually emerging; a method that balances the ongoing validation process with continued practice is needed.

The antithesis of full validation by clinical research is the acceptance of any method used by any practitioner as part of the standards of practice. In the chiropractic profession, for example, anything that a chiropractor does would become a chiropractic standard. In its first 95 years, the chiropractic profession approached the entire area of standards in much this manner.[15] Although there have been calls for formalized standards,[16-20] few standards for the practice of chiropractic have been widely adopted. In particular, no criteria for the acceptability of chiropractic clinical methods have been set forth and accepted by the profession. At the present time, rulings by state licensing boards and the testimony of expert witnesses in court cases appear

The authors would like to thank the members of the Western States Chiropractic College Standards Committee, in particular Mitch Haas and Fred Colley, for their comments and ideas with respect to the diagnostic and therapeutic questions presented in this chapter.

to be the only routine methods by which chiropractic standards are established.[21]

Given the demands of accountability in today's health care environment, it seems prudent for the chiropractic profession to adopt a formalized, consensus-based approach to develop standards of practice. The first step in setting any standard of practice is to establish the status of a particular procedure. The procedure should then be assessed by means of a model that requires clinical validation for full acceptability. Furthermore, a useful scheme allows provisional acceptance for some methods before their clinical effectiveness has been systematically investigated. These methods must be well defined, measurable, and consistent with present scientific knowledge, however. This approach best addresses the continued use and the current state of understanding of diagnostic and therapeutic methods employed by the chiropractic profession.

DEVELOPMENT OF THE WSCC MODEL

Teaching institutions such as the Western States Chiropractic College (WSCC) are continually analyzing new information and methodologies in order to incorporate these new concepts into their curricula. Struggling with this issue and also justifying elements already taught within a college curriculum is an ongoing problem at all institutions of higher education.[22] In chiropractic, these dilemmas are further compounded by the limited research that has been conducted in the past to establish the effectiveness of chiropractic clinical methods,[9,23] as well as by the lack of a mechanism to establish professional standards for these methods.[20] The only guidelines have been the generally diffuse statements of state statutes that define the scope of chiropractic practice[24,25] (but do not address specific clinical methodologies) and those standards that legal precedent establishes.[20] It was within this climate that WSCC, under the direction of then president Herbert J. Vear, created a standards committee in the spring of 1983. Their charge was to develop a method to evaluate the elements within a chiropractic curriculum.

After struggling with numerous attempts to develop evaluation guidelines, Kaminski suggested an algorithm based on the scientific method. The resultant scheme (the WSCC model) is a useful tool to determine systematically the current state of understanding of diagnostic procedures and therapeutic methods.[26]

OVERVIEW OF THE WSCC MODEL

Designed as an algorithm, the WSCC model represents a logical progression of questions that should be considered when any procedure is under evaluation. Throughout this scheme, various elements of the scientific method are incorporated. The analysis focuses on such principal issues as the identification of parameters, their relation to known information, and published research.

The flowchart in Figure 7-1, which depicts the WSCC model, is punctuated by the following four important headings: (1) definition and description, (2) measurable observations, (3) science knowledge, and (4) experimentation and testing. At each of the four steps, guidelines are given as criteria for a major evaluation, and it must be decided whether a procedure meets these criteria. From this process, a status of *provisional acceptance, acceptance,* or *unsubstantiated* is assigned.

No matter how elaborate, however, a decision-making flowchart cannot answer questions; this must be done by appropriate experts. Any group that uses the model must resolve how they will specifically determine when a procedure passes or fails at each stage in the flowchart. An evaluative panel must weigh responses and come to final decisions based on their own protocols, but the alogrithm should begin to objectify and delineate many of the relevant questions and important issues that must be considered in systematic validation.

Definition and Description

Inquiries or evaluations initially require a definition that includes a detailed description of the procedure or practice, a comprehensive list of unique terminology, a history, and a basic statement of rationale. A procedure or practice that is indefinite or indescribable lacks the characteristics necessary to analyze it further.

Measurable Observations

It is essential to describe and catalog observations. Although literature citations are not necessary, a detailed description of observations is required. Important questions that must be answered include what parameters are measured, how they are measured, and how the measurement relates to the procedure.

A science must establish whether there is a consistent and meaningful relationship between two or more observed events. For example, does a specific manipulation predictably result in a specific outcome? Claims of relationship can be based on many types of observation (eg, coincidence, consensus, or intuition). Unless a collection of observations and their relationships are measurable, however, the resultant conclusion is unsupportable.

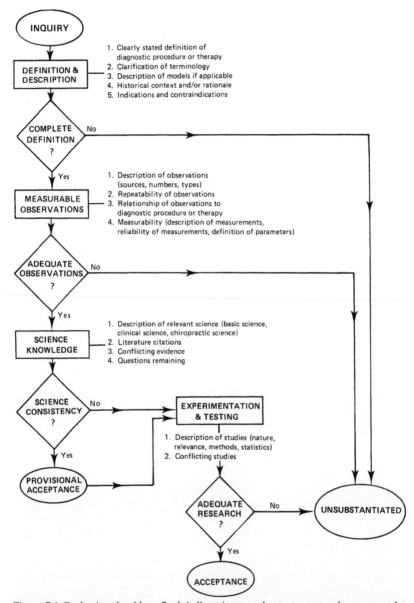

Figure 7-1 Evaluation algorithm. *Ovals* indicate inputs and outputs, *rectangles* represent data entry steps (with key questions), *diamonds* involve a decision based upon information previously gathered and *arrows* delineate the flow of thought. *Source:* Reprinted with permission from M Kaminski, R Boal, RG Gillette, DH Peterson, TJ Villnave, "A Model for the Evaluation of Chiropractic Methods" in *Journal of Manipulative and Physiological Therapeutics,* (1987;10:61–64), Copyright © 1987, National College of Chiropractic.

The measurable observations step is the most flexible in the WSCC model. The spirit of this component lies in its call for quantifiable assessment. The suggested criteria allow many procedures to qualify before they have been clinically validated. Reliability questions are asked at this point in the algorithm in order to gather general information, not to eliminate further analysis of a procedure. Any panel of evaluators has the option of modifying the measurable observations criteria to increase the demands of this section of the model. As the chiropractic profession matures, it seems likely that a procedure will have to meet increasingly higher criteria at this point in the path to a provisionally acceptable status.

Science Knowledge

Because science is both knowledge and a process, new knowledge must be analyzed in the context of current understandings. Proved mechanisms are not necessarily expected, but a consistency with current scientific models is sought. A procedure or practice should possess a rationale that is both reasonable and logical. Even a new concept or piece of evidence that radically alters the understanding of a scientific discipline must first be evaluated in the environment of previously analyzed and accepted "truths." If such new ideas do ultimately change the state of scientific understanding, they will do so subsequent to experimental verification.[27,28]

When a procedure or practice meets the test of scientific consistency and appears to be biologically plausible, it receives provisional acceptance. This status identifies emerging ideas and does not imply validation or tested efficacy. This unique, intermediate stage represents an allowance for procedures that, although not fully acceptable, may be considered for temporary inclusion within the methods of the profession. Provisionally accepted concepts are expected to move toward acceptance through traditional experimentation and testing.

Experimentation and Testing

Most of the clinical procedures in chiropractic and many of the clinical procedures in medicine have not yet passed the rigors of clinical testing and validation. This situation leaves health care providers facing clinical decisions in an environment of some uncertainty.

Experimentation and testing require the evaluation of pertinent research to substantiate all procedures with clinical studies and, ideally, the delineation of basic mechanisms; procedures that pass this extensive inquiry are given *acceptance*. The evaluation of clinical methods that have undergone limited testing should emphasize the procedure's consistency with scientific knowledge and its biological plausibility; as discussed earlier, these methods may be given provisional acceptance. Without passing a test of scientific consistency and being clinically validated, a method should be considered unsubstantiated.

Procedures or practices that are inconsistent with current scientific knowledge may still gain acceptance by demonstrating appropriate experimental validation. This divergent path has been included in the WSCC model to create the necessary latitude for a radically different idea to gain acceptance. Although a procedure may lack a mechanism, model, or explanation, it deserves an avenue for possible validation (albeit one that lacks a provisional state).

Comments

Some methods used under the umbrella of chiropractic are "self-contained," for lack of a better term. In these treatment procedures, a unique diagnostic finding serves as an indicator for treatment. After treatment, the practitioner uses the same diagnostic procedure to monitor the effectiveness of therapy. For example, muscle testing as an indicator of the need to supplement nutrients is a self-contained method. If the unique diagnostic finding has no relationship to other established clinical measurements and lacks biological plausibility, the procedure will probably have failed at the level of measurable observations or scientific consistency and will not have received provisional acceptance. Furthermore, if the procedure does not satisfy the criteria for experimentation and testing, it will have been labeled as unsubstantiated by the WSCC model. In these cases, however, the diagnosis and treatment come as a package. Both elements must be considered for their individual merits, as well as for the known relationship of the diagnostic indicator/clinical outcome measure to the disorder being treated.

Regardless of the path employed subsequent to the issue of scientific consistency, the goal of any procedure or practice is to gain acceptance. The idea of acceptance is often an elusive one, frequently only tacitly understood,[27-29] but most authorities insist on numerous and meaningful clinical trials.[8-11] Ultimately, acceptance is not what makes the model fundamentally useful. The evaluative scheme best addresses new ideas that may be provisional in nature or presently unsubstantiated.

Failure to receive provisional acceptance or acceptance results in a status best labeled as "unsubstantiated." It is necessary to use a form of rejection that provides the failed procedure with a neutral status rather than a negative one. A negative status would unduly discourage further investigation in the area of question. One of the inherent values of the WSCC model is that *it identifies the strengths and weaknesses of an unsubstantiated procedure*; this should prove useful for further exploration of its promising aspects.

IMPLEMENTATION OF THE WSCC MODEL

Since the original publication of the WSCC model,[26] the WSCC Standards Committee has applied the model to a limited number of specific procedures. From these analyses, a generic set of detailed questions has been created. As part of a general protocol, these questions would generally be sent to an advocate of the clinical method to be evaluated. An analysis of the advocate's replies would serve as the basis for a consensus opinion by a panel of experts. With many commonly used clinical procedures, the panel may be able to answer the model's questions even without an advocate. It should be noted, however, that a fair application of this assessment device to any clinical procedure has proved to be an arduous and time-consuming activity.

The instrument was designed basically to provide an evaluation structure for panel or committee members involved in the assessment of chiropractic procedures. It does not address the issues that surround the development of a consensus, but focuses on the important questions that must be asked about procedures. Time limitations, procedural rules, and specific methods for responding to questions vary according to the size and resources of the evaluating body. Each group must determine its own response times, ability to review pertinent literature, methods for finalizing a decision on the status of a procedure, and a means for publicizing its consensus opinions. All deliberations should be governed "in spirit" by the consensus guidelines recommended for health science professions in a number of recent publications.[1,7]

Diagnostic Procedures

Several questions should be addressed by the advocate of a diagnostic procedure. The evaluation of the advocate's answers to these questions is the basis of a determination of that procedure's status.

Definitions and Descriptions

1. What is the operational definition of the diagnostic procedure? Is the description of the procedure adequate for others to duplicate results independently? If not, explain.

2. What are the specific definitions of any special terminology associated with this procedure?

Descriptive terms that are unique to this procedure should be defined. Also, common clinical terms should be clarified if there is wide variation in their use. For example, how is a *joint challenge* performed? Do practitioners push on the joint to assess pain, or is muscle testing or leg length testing used in conjunction? What is being tested? Is it joint pain, joint alignment, joint mobility?

3. What is the clinical condition being identified by this diagnostic procedure? Provide a rigorous description of this condition, including the associated pathophysiological and/or pathomechanical changes. Relevant references must be included.

For example, is joint dysfunction theorized to be a mechanical derangement with disturbances in the periarticular soft tissues or an internal derangement of the joint or intervertebral disk? Are there assumed physiological changes producing inflammation or local dysfunction in the nervous system? Does the advocate suggest pathophysiological effects beyond the joint and its periarticular tissues? If so, what are they?

4. How is the diagnostic procedure used? For example, is it a screening device, diagnostic indicator, or test for achievement of a treatment goal?[30]
5. Define a "normal" population[14,31] and an "abnormal" population with respect to the condition in question. What is the typical variation for this diagnostic finding in the "normal" population?
6. Are there additional diagnostic procedures that are routinely used to supplement this method? If so, explain their use.
7. What are the possible benefits and risks of this diagnostic method in comparison to the benefits and risks of other diagnostic tools used to identify this clinical condition?
8. What is the historical context of the development and use of this diagnostic procedure?

Measurable Observations

1. How are the clinical findings quantified? Are they nominal, ordinal, interval, or ratio scale measurements?[31,32]
2. What is the relationship between the diagnostic procedure and the clinical condition that is being evaluated? Is this procedure relevant?

3. What constitutes an abnormal finding, and how is this measured? Is the determination of an abnormal finding clearly outside the normal range? Is there a threshold between normal and abnormal clinical findings? Explain.
4. Can the same observer obtain similar assessments on different occasions (ie, intra-observer reliability)?[12-14]

At this point, questions on reliability (see also Question 5), correlations to other clinical observations (see Question 7), and preliminary empirical measurements (see Question 8) are asked in order to obtain general information. Methods for which these issues have not been addressed may pass to the next step (scientific knowledge) without rejection, but with a label of unsubstantiated. If the method is consistent with science knowledge, it may receive *provisional acceptance*. Questions of reliability and correlation to other procedures must be critically addressed under the umbrella of experimentation and testing before the method receives *acceptance*, however.

5. Can different observers independently obtain similar assessments using this method (interobserver reliability)?[12-14]
6. Is the diagnostic finding graded to the severity of the clinical condition? Explain.
7. Does the diagnostic finding correlate with some other relevant clinical observation (eg, mobility, pain, x-ray films, blood chemistry, laboratory findings)? Explain.
8. What preliminary empirical observations or measurements have been collected?

Science Knowledge

1. Is there literature to support any special terminology used in the context of this procedure? Explain.

For example, how is the term *nerve pressure* defined, and is this particular use of the term valid? The advocate may submit literature citations where the term is used representatively.

2. Are statements of fact supported by relevant literature citations? Explain.

In some cases, a statement of fact may be so basic that no reference is required (eg, there are 12 thoracic vertebrae). A statement such as "functional disease of the spine causes a functional short leg" should be supported by literature citations, however.

3. Do the basic premises of this procedure have biological plausibility (ie, are they consistent with established scientific thought), or do they represent a new or alternative theory? Explain.

For example, does a basic understanding of human physiology support a claim that muscle testing can identify a specific endocrine disorder or nutritional deficiency? Is there an established knowledge of physical phenomena to suggest that rubbing a plastic instrument over a body site would detect pathology?

4. Are there conflicting pieces of evidence and/or remaining questions with respect to the basic premises behind this diagnostic procedure? Explain.

Experimentation and Testing

1. Has the evaluation of this procedure met standards for validity testing? Explain. If yes, include references.

A diagnostic procedure should be evaluated with respect to a number of criteria (eg, comparison to a "gold standard," blinded investigation, determination of reliability, determination of specificity and sensitivity, randomized trials, broad cross-section of patients, clear definition of patients).[12-14]

2. Compared to other diagnostic tests, how well does this diagnostic method measure the given specific clinical condition?

Comparisons should be made on the basis of published work in indexed, peer-reviewed journals and valid, relevant statistical analyses.[33]

3. Has the effectiveness of this diagnostic procedure been investigated over the course of the condition in question?
4. Does the diagnostic finding correlate with relief or abatement of signs and symptoms? Explain.

Treatment Methods

The advocate of a treatment method should also address several types of questions. An evaluation of the answers forms the basis of a determination of that treatment method's status.

Definitions and Descriptions

1. What is the operational definition of the treatment method? Is the description of the procedure adequate for others to duplicate results independently? If not, explain.
2. What are the therapeutic goals for this treatment method? Are they curative, palliative, or preventive?[12,34]
3. What are the specific definitions of any special terminology associated with the procedure?

As for a diagnostic procedure, the advocate of a treatment method should define descriptive terms that are unique to this treatment method, particularly if there is wide variation in their use.

4. What is the clinical entity being treated? Provide a rigorous description of this condition, including the associated pathophysiological and/or pathomechanical changes. Relevant references must be included.
5. Define a "normal" population[14,31] and an "abnormal" population with respect to the condition in question. How was this established?
6. What diagnostic procedures are used to identify the treatment group? What is the status of these diagnostic procedures according to the WSCC model?

Appropriate diagnostic procedures should at least be provisionally accepted by the criteria set forth in the WSCC model (see Figure 7-1).

7. Are there specific contraindications for the treatment? Explain. Are there certain conditions or situations in which the problem is more appropriately treated by other, conventional forms of therapy? Explain.
8. What are the clinical outcome measures for determining that the condition has been effectively treated?

If this is a clinical test, it should meet the same standard as a diagnostic indicator; that is, it should have provisional or full acceptance according to the WSCC model. If the outcome measure represents a quality-of-life issue, the measure should be quantifiable and relevant to the treated condition.

9. Are there additional therapeutic methods that are routinely used to supplement this procedure? If so, explain their use.

10. What are the expected or hypothesized benefits and risks of this treatment in comparison to the benefits and risks of other therapeutic methods used to treat this condition?
11. What is the hypothesis that explains how this treatment changes the pathophysiological and/or pathomechanical states associated with the condition being treated?

If the therapy is theorized to affect dysfunctional joints, for example, an explanation of the mechanisms is in order. Does the treatment stretch post-traumatically shortened fibrotic tissue, repositioning a displaced joint, or does it have a purely analgesic effect?

12. What is the historical context of the development and use of this therapeutic method?

Measurable Observations

1. How is the given clinical entity measured?

When it is being claimed that a treatment is effective for a disorder, the disorder in question should be measurable. For example, in some idiopathic conditions, pain may be the measure of a treatment's effectiveness; by using subjective patient assessment of pain, the effectiveness of treatment can be quantified. Similarly, if it is claimed that the treatment in question normalizes something such as "neurolymphatic points," these structures should be measurable and the treatment effects quantifiable.

2. How does the clinical outcome measurement relate to the condition in question? Is it relevant?
3. What preliminary empirical observations or measurements have been collected?

Questions on reliability, correlations to other clinical observations, and preliminary empirical measurements are asked at this point for the purpose of general information—just as they are in the evaluation of diagnostic procedures. Although treatment methods may be provisionally accepted without validation, questions of reliability and correlation to other methods must be critically addressed under the umbrella of experimentation and testing before these treatment methods are fully accepted.

Science Knowledge

1. Is there literature to support any special terminology used in the context of this procedure? Explain.

   How is each term defined, and is each use of the term valid? The advocate may submit literature citations where the term is used representatively.

2. Are statements of fact supported by relevant literature citations? Explain.

3. Do the basic premises of this method have biological plausibility (ie, are they consistent with established scientific thought), or do they represent a new or alternative theory? Explain.

4. Are there conflicting pieces of evidence and/or remaining questions with respect to the basic premises behind this therapeutic method? Explain.

Experimentation and Testing

1. What is the clinical effectiveness of this therapeutic method as reported in the literature?

   The advocate can simply list the relevant literature citations.

2. Has the evaluation of this method met standards for clinical design and analysis? Explain.

   The evaluation of the treatment method should meet basic standards for clinical research design, such as a clearly stated hypothesis; a complete description of the patient population; randomized sampling and allocation of patients; blinding of patients, assessors, and treating physicians; study sample size sufficient to establish significance; valid and reliable outcomes; and minimal attrition.[9,12–14]

3. How does the treatment effectiveness vary with the severity of the clinical complaint?

   The advocate should describe any change in treatment frequency, methodology, or effectiveness that may occur when there is a variation in the severity of the described condition.

4. How does the effectiveness of this method compare to that of other treatment approaches for the clinical condition in question?

Comparisons should be made using published work in indexed, peer-reviewed journals and valid, relevant statistical analyses.[34]

5. Has the effectiveness of this therapy been investigated over the course of the condition being treated? Explain.

APPLICATIONS AND IMPLICATIONS

Through the use of the WSCC model for their evaluation, topics within a college curriculum receive labels of *acceptance*, *provisional acceptance*, and *unsubstantiated*. A particular label should not exclude a procedure from the curriculum, but a status of unsubstantiated should never be lost in the presentation of such a procedure. Unsubstantiated procedures may be extremely interesting, but they should be discussed as ancillary to those topics that are considered provisionally accepted or accepted.

The WSCC model will be useful for the further investigation of unsubstantiated diagnostic procedures and treatment methods. One of the most noteworthy aspects of the scheme is that it is ultimately heuristic. Specifically, the determination of a "status of understanding" for any chiropractic technique or procedure through the application of the model should naturally lead to relevant, testable research questions or hypotheses. Once formalized, such questions can be examined by the proponents of a technique or by the profession at large through the application of rigorous research programs.

Using this model in the larger context of profession-wide standards for chiropractic practice would be a more complicated issue than is using it in the consideration of curriculum offerings in a college's instructional program. The economic and social issues that must be considered when making decisions on the standards of care are multifaceted and complex.

- Is society and its health care organizations willing to expend the energy and money necessary to evaluate health care procedures?
- How can cost-effectiveness be included in decisions on standards of care?
- Will the public be willing to accept a slower introduction of new technology in an environment of greater scrutiny?
- What alternative procedures are available to a given therapy?
- How will these procedures affect the patient's psychological well-being and quality of life?

Notwithstanding these additional issues, the WSCC model will prove useful to those delegated to make decisions on standards of care. The model itself may be modified; for example, a different set of labels may be selected (eg, orthodox, provisional, experimental, mainstream, anecdotal, investigational, unacceptable), or additional questions may be required in evaluating methods under the umbrella of standards of care. The way in which the process of evaluation should begin and the procedures that should be evaluated first are difficult decisions that face all health care professions.

Perhaps the most fertile area for expansion of the algorithm lies in the establishment of formal rules to achieve a consensus at the decision-making junctures. Although the reliability of consensus methods is unresolved, collective expert opinion can be satisfactorily derived. Of critical importance are objective criteria; without them, a consensus of opinion becomes subjective and arbitrary. Educational institutions, professional societies, entrepreneurs, government regulatory and research organizations, and insurance carriers all have vested interests and roles to play in making these decisions.

CONCLUSION

The algorithm and its questions will not solve any of the problems of standards of practice, clinical validity, or curricular design. The chiropractic profession itself will have to resolve these problems. Although the WSCC model can establish a status for the current understanding of clinical procedures, its real importance is that it represents a formalized process for the evaluation of chiropractic methods. As the chiropractic profession matures, it will need to move beyond its current failings at self-evaluation. The identification and description of the state of understanding of chiropractic procedures and practices must involve objective criteria that are based on the tools of science and a process of agreement that facilitates the application of these criteria.

REFERENCES

1. Fink A, Kosecoff J, Chassin M, Brook RH. Consensus methods: Characteristics and guidelines for use. *Am J Public Health*. 1984;74:979–983.

2. Sacks HS, Berrier J, Reitman D, Ancona-Berk VA, Chalmers T. Meta-analysis of randomized controlled trials. *N Engl J Med*. 1987;316:450–455.

3. Kent DL, Larson EB. Diagnostic technology assessments: Problems and prospects. *Ann Intern Med*. 1988;108:759–761.

4. Lawler FH, Hosokawa MC. Evaluation of standards of practice for primary care physicians using 12 hypothetical cases. *J Fam Pract*. 1987;24:377–383.

5. Kelly JT. Practice guidelines: A view from organized medicine. *Internist.* 1989;30(5):9–11,15.

6. Guyatt G, Drummond M, Feeny D, Tugwell P, Stoddart G, Haynes RB, Bennett K, Labelle R. Guidelines for the clinical and economic evaluation of health care technologies. *Soc Sci Med.* 1986;22:393–408.

7. Chassin MR. Standards of care in medicine. *Inquiry.* 1988;25:437–453.

8. Deyo RA. Conservative therapy for low back pain. Distinguishing useful from useless therapy. *JAMA.* 1983;250:1057–1062.

9. Brunarski DJ. Clinical trials of spinal manipulation: A critical appraisal and review of literature. *J Manipulative Physiol Ther.* 1984;7:243–249.

10. Basmajian JV, ed. *Manipulation, Traction and Massage.* 3rd ed. Baltimore: Williams & Wilkins; 1985.

11. Buerger AA, Tobis JS, eds. *Approaches to the Validation of Manipulation Therapy.* Springfield, Ill: Charles C Thomas; 1977.

12. Sackett DL, Haynes RB, Tugwell P. Clinical epidemiology: A basic science for clinical medicine. Boston: Little, Brown; 1985.

13. Fletcher RH, Fletcher SW, Wagner EH. *Clinical Epidemiology: The essentials.* 2nd ed. Baltimore: Williams & Wilkins; 1988.

14. Feinstein AR. *Clinical Epidemiology: The Architecture of Clinical Research.* Philadelphia: WB Saunders Co; 1985.

15. Keating JC. Philosophical barriers to technique research in chiropractic. *Chiropractic Technique.* 1989;1(1)23–29.

16. Haldeman S. The importance of research in the principles and practice of chiropractic. *J Can Chiropractic Assoc.* 1976;20(3):7–10.

17. Vear HJ. Standards for chiropractic practice. *J Manipulative Physiol Ther.* 1985;8:33–43.

18. DeBoer KF. Eine kleine nacht musing. *American Journal of Chiropractic Medicine.* 1988;1:41–43.

19. Bergmann T. Proceedings of consensus conference on validation of chiropractic methods. *Chiropractic Technique.* 1991;2(3):71–161.

20. Sutherland DC. Validation: Chiropractic's next challenge. *Am Chiropractic Assoc J Chiropractic.* 1990;27(4):50–56.

21. Jahn WT. Malpractice in chiropractic. *Am Chiropractic Assoc J Chiropractic.* 1980;17(9):64–67.

22. Rudolph F. *Curriculum: A History of the American Undergraduate Course of Study since 1636.* San Francisco: Jossey–Bass; 1977.

23. Leboef C. A review of data reports published in the *J Manipulative Physiol Ther* from 1986–1988. *J Manipulative Physiol Ther.* 1990;13:89–95.

24. Lamm LC, Wegner E. Chiropractic scope of practice: What the law allows. *American Journal of Chiropractic Medicine.* 1989; 2:155–159.

25. Official Directory of the Federation of Chiropractic Licensing Boards, Chicago. Kremmling, Col; 1990.

26. Kaminski M, Boal R, Gillette RG, Peterson DH, Villnave TJ. A model for the evaluation of chiropractic methods. *J Manipulative Physiol Ther.* 1987;10:61–64.

27. Chalmers AF. *What Is This Thing Called Science.* St Lucia, Australia: University of Queensland Press; 1978.

28. Kuhn T. *The Structure of Scientific Revolutions*. 2nd ed. Chicago: University of Chicago Press; 1970.

29. Polyani M. *The Tacit Dimension*. New York: Doubleday; 1966.

30. Haynes RB. How to read clinical journals: II. To learn about a diagnostic test. *Can Med Assoc J*. 1981;124:703–710.

31. Phillips DS. Basic statistics for health science students. San Francisco: WH Freeman; 1978.

32. Siegel S. *Nonparametric Tests for the Behavioral Sciences*. New York: McGraw-Hill Book Co; 1956.

33. Haas M. Statistical methodology for reliability studies. *J Manipulative Physiol Ther*. 1991;14:119–132.

34. Sackett DL. How to read clinical journals: V. To distinguish useful from useless or even harmful therapy. *Can Med Assoc J*. 1981;124:1156–1162.

8

Standards for Interprofessional Relations

Robert Anderson

Health care in the United States cannot and should not function as a monopoly of any one health care profession. Certainly, the various professions concerned in one way or another with the diagnosis, prevention, and treatment of musculoskeletal disorders need to interact as collegial disciplines that share common goals. White stated this position in emphatic terms.

> Who are we, the specialists in spine care, to whom patients turn? We are skilled. We are confident. But we are unorganized, with inadequate means of interprofessional communication. We know too little about the expertise of those outside of our own practice. We tend to feel competitive, even jealous, of one another. Patients do not benefit from these attitudes. Society does not benefit. It is clear that we as practitioners also do not benefit.[1(p5)]

In today's world, the chiropractor or any other clinician requires a mastery of appropriate modes of communication to foster interprofessional collaboration and to interact with the public. This mastery needs to include personal skills that can smooth the way for successful involvement in scientific and professional encounters. No kind of encounter is more important or more sensitive for any practitioner than referral to or collaboration with another type of provider. Confidence and ease in communicating appropriately with colleagues, both intraprofessionally and interprofessionally, are essential qualities—not only for the chiropractor who has a solo practice, but also for the chiropractor who works in an interdisciplinary group practice, in a health maintenance organization, or in a hospital.

I drew on the professional expertise and experience of those who read a first draft of this chapter: Scott Anderson, MD; Gerald P. Keane, MD; William C. Meeker, DC, MPH; Robert D. Mootz, DC; and Jerome Schoferman, MD. I am truly grateful for their contributions. Of course, I alone am responsible for any shortcomings that may persist.

REFERRAL TO OTHER PROVIDERS

A chiropractor should refer a patient to another professional provider of health care solely for the purpose of obtaining additional expertise, treatment, or counsel. The referring physician should neither directly nor indirectly receive payment from the other health care provider for making the referral. To send a patient to any apparently independent and separate entity in which the referring physician, a close associate, or a family member has an ownership interest is unethical and improper.[2]

When making a referral, a chiropractor should never forget that the ultimate goal is to achieve effective interaction by communicating successfully across professional or specialist boundaries. The watchwords are clarity and brevity.[3] The first task is to explain clearly and carefully to the patient the reason for the referral and the expected benefits.[4]

It is also necessary to explain the reason for the referral to the clinician whom the patient will see. A chiropractor who is sending a patient to a physician known only through colleagues or by reputation, for example, should call the physician personally to ensure that the referral will be welcome and appropriate.[5] This call is also useful when the chiropractor has worked with the physician before, as a succinct explanation of the purpose of the referral is beneficial to all who are involved.[4] It should not be left to the patient to make the initial call, although the patient may subsequently need to telephone to set the exact time of the appointment.

The referring chiropractor should also send a brief letter that describes in mutually understood language the reason for the referral. A short letter, concise and to the point, is more impressive than a long, drawn out essay full of inappropriate detail and negative findings.[6] The letter should include a short summary of the history, physical findings, laboratory test results, x-ray reports, chiropractic diagnosis, treatment to date, and treatment response. Above all, it is important to state clearly whether the referral is solely for diagnostic purposes or whether it is for treatment either to supplement or to replace the care that the referring practitioner has been providing.[4] Clarity on the purpose will ensure a good referral relationship, because it is unethical not to respect the referring doctor's intent. It is also important to keep track of what happens to the referred patient. If a written acknowledgment and report is not forthcoming, the referring practitioner should take the initiative to ask for follow-up information.

Straightforward, unambiguous communication is equally important for the practitioner to whom a patient has been referred. The practitioner should write a follow-up letter that summarizes his or her findings on the history, physical examination, and special studies. This statement of findings should be followed by the diagnosis, analysis, or clinical impression, along with treatment recommendations if the patient was sent for evaluation only. If the patient was sent for chiropractic treatment, which is the more common scenario, the chiropractor should indicate not only what treatment is planned, but how long or how many times the chiropractor expects to see the patient and what the prognosis is for a good outcome. When treatment has been completed, the chiropractor should send a brief report to the referring practitioner, describing the patient's current status and indicating that the patient has been either discharged as cured or referred back to the original provider.[4] It is a quaint, but welcome, custom to include a brief sentence of thanks for the opportunity to see the patient.

Just as important as following the appropriate formalities when making a referral is knowing when circumstances require a referral. Although chiropractors may find it necessary or advisable at times to refer to any kind of care provider, including ministers, priests, rabbis, and social workers (for whom the formalities are greatly truncated), they are especially likely to refer patients to specialists in radiology, neurology, neurosurgery and orthopedic surgery, physical medicine and rehabilitation (physiatry), rheumatology, internal medicine, psychiatry or psychology, and multidisciplinary evaluation.

Radiology

As part of the initial evaluation of a new patient, plain radiographic studies may be undertaken. Like many orthopedic surgeons and other physicians, chiropractors often use office x-ray equipment and evaluate their own radiographs. The practitioner who uses in-office x-ray imaging in this manner is responsible for identifying any visible pathology, including soft tissue or osseous lesions that are not directly implicated in the complaint or illness that motivated the patient to seek treatment. This is a heavy responsibility, as the radiograph may show extremely subtle, easy-to-miss indications of an early stage in an infection or malignancy. Chiropractors and other physicians must be completely certain that their training and experience are adequate. Whenever they encounter uncertain or unclear findings, it is essential that they send the films involved to a board-certified chiropractic or medical radiologist for full evaluation or refer the patient to another health care provider for more extensive imaging. Many physicians and chiropractors routinely send all films to a specialist for a second reading or refer all patients who require imaging studies to radiologists.

Most patients with acute back pain can be treated in a chiropractic protocol that does not require spinal radiographs. The chiropractic literature provides ample justification for eliminating this expense and the exposure to ionizing radiation for these patients.[7] Current standards require x-ray analysis in acute back pain patients only if the patient is more than 50 years old; has recently experienced severe trauma, pain at rest, or unexplained weight loss; is undergoing treatment with corticosteroids; has a temperature above 101°F, a neuromotor deficit, or a history of cancer; or may have a rheumatoid disorder. [8-10] In the absence of these factors, the risks of missing serious pathology by not using x-ray evaluation are minimal.

The need for imaging studies must be reassessed in patients whose acute back pain does not improve after 2 to 3 weeks of chiropractic care (eight to ten spinal adjustments). These treatment failures require a more thorough diagnostic workup. In order to rule out more serious pathology, the treating chiropractor should order laboratory studies (minimally a complete blood cell count (CBC), chemistry panel, urinalysis, and erythrocyte sedimentation rate (ESR)) and should undertake or arrange for plain radiographs, if they were not obtained initially. Additional options must be considered in these instances. The chiropractor may use a different therapeutic approach for another trial of treatment or may refer the patient to another chiropractor or to a medical practitioner who can provide a different kind of therapy as a trial of treatment. Clinical judgment may require referral to a radiologist for more extensive imaging in order to identify the refractory disease process.

Neurology

A chiropractor should determine whether a patient's signs and symptoms relating to muscular strength, skin sensation, patterns of pain perception, and deep tendon reflexes are consistent with a lesion that is treatable by chiropractic adjustment or with injuries that are suitable for chiropractic management. [11] Post-treatment reexamination should confirm that the patient remains an appropriate patient for chiropractic care. Inconsistent or additional neurological findings mandate a more extensive diagnostic evaluation. When competent chiropractic or medical judgment suggests that the patient may have a serious neurological disorder, the chiropractor should refer the patient to a neurologist for definitive evaluation. Signs of ataxia (including a positive Romberg's test), upper motor neuron defects, paradoxical changes in neurological status, and indications of peripheral neuropathy are among the findings that require a complete neurological evaluation by a specialist. Symptoms of speech impairment, unexplained disturbances of vision, pain independent of movement, or patterns of pain that suggest the presence of space-occupying lesions also require this type of investigation.

In some patients, electrodiagnostic studies can be helpful in determining the extent of the disease, including whether the neuromuscular dysfunction is acute or chronic and whether it is treatable or permanent. The chiropractor may request an electromyographic (EMG) evaluation in order to finalize the diagnosis and treatment plan. Such a referral may be to a practitioner in any of several specialties in which EMG studies are performed. Usually, but not always, the referral is made to a specialist in neurology or physical medicine and rehabilitation (physiatry).

Neurosurgery and Orthopedic Surgery

With rare exceptions, no patient should undergo surgery without a prior trial of conservative treatment. If an adequate trial of conservative care, including spinal adjusting, fails to result in improvement, a chiropractor should consult with a chiropractic, medical, or surgical specialist who may be able to suggest or to offer a new approach.

In the uncommon cases in which a patient suddenly loses all power in the distribution of a single nerve root or a minor neurological deficit, such as a slight dorsiflexor weakness, increases during the period of chiropractic treatment, a neurosurgical or orthopedic opinion is mandatory. These are conditions in which there is a threat of permanent nerve damage, and surgery may be necessary. Consultation with a surgeon, of course, does not automatically indicate that the patient will be best served by a surgical intervention.[12]

Radiculopathy patients sent for a surgical consultation should report back to their primary chiropractic or medical physician, whose advice for or against surgery should weigh heavily in the decision. The final decision must be based on an evaluation of all opinions, including those of the patient and the patient's significant others. The patient should be aware that surgery is not a sure cure. Indeed, on the basis of the literature, as well as his experience as a spine surgeon, White concluded that surgery is not beneficial for most people with back and leg pain.[12]

Conservative care can be at least as effective as surgery in selected cases. Saal and Saal, both physiatrists, demonstrated in one observational study that, in the absence of significant stenosis, herniated lumbar intervertebral disk syndromes with radiculopathy may improve dramatically if treated through an aggressive, nonsurgical, patient-active program—even though the condition had failed to improve with earlier conservative care in every patient in the study.[13] The decision on a treatment plan must take into account the fact that not everyone is a good candidate for aggressive, patient-active conservative care, however, just as not everyone does well after surgery. The chiropractor assumes a heavy responsibility when orchestrating the decision between surgery and additional conservative care. The patient manager and other involved parties should not feel pressured into making a rapid decision; they need time to observe, study, and evaluate the options.

The only surgical emergency in the treatment of low back pain is the sudden onset of a cauda equina syndrome, characterized by saddle anesthesia, urinary incontinence, and/or loss of anal sphincter tone (or possibly urinary or bowel retention). When this rare condition occurs, the practitioner who made the findings should arrange a surgical consult on the same day. This patient should be monitored by an orthopedic surgeon or a neurosurgeon. Often, surgery is required within 24 hours of detection. Failure to recognize the seriousness of this condition and failure to refer the patient to an appropriate health care provider immediately can have extremely serious consequences, including permanent nerve damage and disability.

Physical Medicine and Rehabilitation

Physicians who specialize in physical medicine and rehabilitation are natural collaborators for chiropractors. Because they work with people who suffer from severe physical disabilities, including chronic pain syndromes, they are experienced in the diagnosis and treatment of severe musculoskeletal disorders. Historically, their specialty evolved from physical therapy, so they understand the role of physiotherapeutic modalities, proprioceptive and muscular retraining, and related medical and psychiatric problems. In addition to EMG studies, they can provide a complete medical workup. Thus, their help is especially valuable in working with patients who suffer from multiple disorders, such as the diabetic with both peripheral neuropathy and mechanical back pain or, a common kind of patient for them, the older person who has suffered a stroke.

Physiatrists can be helpful in providing medical expertise in diagnosis, treatment recommendations, and rehabilitative programs that are useful adjuncts to chiropractic management. Furthermore, they are excellent candidates for mutual referrals. All too often, chiropractors find that medical and surgical referrals tend to be in one direction only. Physiatrists, however, may realize that their patients can often benefit from spinal adjusting.

Rheumatology

The patients who seek care from chiropractors usually suffer from mechanical joint disorders or osteoarthritis.[14] Some, however, have rheumatoid arthritis, and the chiropractor should explore for signs and symptoms of this disease in the initial examination of any patient. In 1987, the American Rheumatism Association revised its criteria for the classification of rheumatoid arthritis, and every chiropractor should be thoroughly familiar with the association's criteria and recommendations.[15]

Patients with rheumatoid arthritis should be treated in collaboration with a rheumatologist or other appropriate medical doctor, because they will respond better to chiropractic care that is coordinated with an appropriate anti-inflammatory and analgesic medical regimen.[16] The chiropractor must exercise extreme caution on approaching the upper cervical spine in these patients; vertebral erosion and ligamentous instability puts them at risk for spinal cord compression, as well as for vertebrobasilar insufficiency.[17]

Other inflammatory and connective tissue disorders are also manifested by articular pain and dysfunction, at least in part. These include ankylosing spondylitis, Reiter's disease, inflammatory bowel disease, psoriatic arthritis, and lupus erythematosus, all of which are systemic diseases involving multiple organ systems.[17] They require medical management, although they may respond well to chiropractic care as ancillary treatment for pain and dysfunction.

Internal Medicine

Most of the clinical trials and laboratory experiments that relate to the efficacy of chiropractic have been limited to musculoskeletal disorders, and the resultant body of published research provides justification for chiropractic adjustments in the treatment of pain and dysfunction of spinal origin.[18,19] Many chiropractors treat nonmusculoskeletal disorders at times, however. Indeed, a minority practice with an emphasis on internal disorders.[20] The justification for the chiropractic treatment of nonmusculoskeletal disorders is almost entirely anecdotal.[21] Chiropractors who treat patients under these circumstances must rigorously follow appropriate standards of practice.

Above all, internal disorders under chiropractic treatment should be clearly and unequivocally benign to ensure that a period of nonmedical or nonsurgical treatment will do no harm. In certain more problematic disorders, cooperation and communication between the providers of chiropractic and medical care may be appropriate. Because a patient's complaint may be merely the most obvious symptom of a serious disease, a complete medical examination is essential to rule out dangerous or treatable pathology; this must never be omitted.

Not every patient requires a medical referral. On the contrary, most patients who seek chiropractic treatment of internal disorders have already tried medical treatment. They seek chiropractic treatment because medical treatment has failed. In taking the history of these patients, the chiropractor must document past medical evaluation and care. It is also essential to document a plan and expected outcomes. Progress should be closely monitored. It is appropriate to provide written progress reports to the patient's primary care physician as well.

Disorders that are commonly treated under chiropractic management include allergies, chronic sinusitis, acne, asthma, chronic constipation, and premenstrual syndrome. The chiropractor must identify and avoid treating potentially sinister presentations, such as acute appendicitis, peritonitis, osteomyelitis, septic joint disease, headache due to tumor, uncontrolled diabetes, medically unsupervised cardiac insufficiency, and medically unsupervised angina. Any patients who have these conditions and are attended by a chiropractor as their primary care provider should be promptly referred for appropriate medical care.

A chiropractor should never assume the medical and legal risk of providing treatment for a life-threatening condition. Occasionally, a patient refuses to accept a medical referral for a non–life-threatening disease. In such cases, the chiropractor should obtain a written informed consent form in the patient's own handwriting for the chart. If a short trial of conservative care then proves ineffective, the patient should again be offered a referral. If the patient again refuses to comply, the chiropractor should discharge the patient as suffering from a condition unsuitable for chiropractic care.

Psychiatry or Psychology

Referring especially to back injuries and chronic pain, Becker, who is board-certified in both orthopedic surgery and psychiatry, emphasized the importance of differentiating functional from organic back pain. "Of equal importance to the history of the present illness or condition is the parallel history."[22] Becker continued,

> The parallel history has two parts, analogous to the history of the present illness and past medical history: (a) concurrent events and circumstance, usually, but not always, in the domestic arena, and (b) the past personal history which forms the backdrop against which an individual's physical complaints are best viewed and understood.[22]

In short, a practitioner must be on the alert for the presence of a psychological component of distress that is distinguishable from pathophysiology as such. Personal, family, and job stressors may contribute to the illness. Chronic pain patients are characteristically downhearted, often manifesting the signs and symptoms of clinical depression. A chiropractor who suspects that psychosocial issues are confounding and impairing treatment progress should refer the patient for appropriate evaluation and possible concurrent treatment by specialists in psychosocial management.[23,24]

Multidisciplinary Evaluations

Most back and neck patients recover their health after undergoing chiropractic care, but a small number do not. Patients with pain of spinal origin may be unresponsive to conservative care. Some may have undergone multiple surgical procedures and yet continue to experience incapacitating pain. Although patients for whom treatment has been ineffective constitute only a small proportion of all back pain patients, the aggregate number in the United States and other industrialized nations is quite large.

Because these chronic pain patients require the best possible diagnosis, they should be referred to a tertiary medical center that specializes in spinal diagnosis. In order to obtain an accurate diagnosis, the condition of these patients should be evaluated by a team of experts, including chiropractic experts, who specialize in spinal disorders and who use forms of diagnostic training, experience, and technology that cannot be found in less well equipped and less broadly staffed centers. Based on such a multidisciplinary evaluation and the best possible diagnosis, the patient should then be scheduled for a course of conservative care (including chiropractic adjustment), surgery, a chronic pain program, vocational rehabilitation, or training for return to work as is appropriate in each case.[15]

The practitioner must always keep in mind the fact that patients with acute pain require different management from those with chronic pain. Although the acute pain patient usually responds well to chiropractic adjustment and/or other conservative care, an episode of back pain is the single most predictive risk factor for future pain. Thus, the acute pain patient will profit from instruction in spinal pathophysiology, basic biomechanics, ergonomics, and training in proper practices in posture and movement in order to prevent recurrence. A program of physical conditioning may also be advisable. Many patients, perhaps most, want only to be adjusted and thereby relieved of pain, but every acute pain patient nonetheless should be given the opportunity to learn these preventive measures. It is incumbent on the chiropractor either to provide education and conditioning for acute pain patients or to recommend programs in which these patients may participate. At the very least, every acute pain patient should be informed of the advisability of preventive measures.

Chronic pain patients often respond very well to chiropractic adjustment.[19,25] Nonetheless, like acute pain patients, they should be encouraged to enroll in an ancillary preventive program.[26] In order to break the cycle of re-injury through repetitive microtrauma, they need education and conditioning. For example, they may benefit from stabilization training in which they can learn posture and movement practices that protect the spine from stress and trauma. Chiropractors often supervise and administer these programs in their own facilities; when they do not, they should refer these patients to chiropractors, physical therapists, or other health care providers who do. The chiropractor is qualified to function as patient manager when a patient requires the ministrations of multiple health care providers. Proper care is best ensured if a single individual functions as coordinator of the total program of treatment and rehabilitation.[27]

PROTOCOL IN HOSPITALS

In the coming decade, more and more chiropractors will find themselves collaborating with medical practitioners, both in private practice and in hospitals or health maintenance organizations (HMOs).[28] Chiropractors who are interested in obtaining appointments to hospital staffs need to familiarize themselves with the laws that regulate hospital practice in their states to determine how they may qualify. They also need to determine exactly what privileges they want as members of a hospital staff. Are they interested only in the privilege of ordering laboratory or imaging studies? Do they want to examine and treat patients exclusively in the outpatient department, or do they want to see inpatients? Kranz summarized the issues well by advising chiropractors to

> Make sure you determine how you would fit into the scheme of a particular hospital's care plan. Be ready to emphasize the unique contribution chiropractic can make to the care given to the hospital's patients; that is, be clear about what you can provide that the patients are not now getting from other practitioners.[29(p112)]

In order to obtain hospital privileges, a practitioner must apply formally and in writing to the chief hospital administrator. It is best to precede the formal application with an informal meeting or telephone conversation. It is helpful to work through a medical colleague who is already on staff, if possible.

When a hospital opens its doors to one chiropractor, it will usually then admit several. Under these circumstances, an effort should be made to persuade the hospital to establish a department of chiropractic services with a chiropractor as department head. This arrangement ensures that chiropractic staff members are represented on the executive committee by one of their number who is fully qualified to speak for them. The chief of chiropractic services should also develop an orientation program to help chiropractors who are new to the staff learn proper hospital protocol.[30] Chiropractors should not hesitate, however, to turn to sympathetic physicians and nurses for initial guidance on procedures to order laboratory analyses, request imaging studies, schedule patient appointments, or make entries in a patient's chart. As students and residents, every medical physician was indoctrinated according to the aphorism, "watch one, do one, teach one." Although no longer a student or intern, the chiropractor in a new setting should take full advantage of this philosophy in order to learn to conform to administrative regulations.

One way to become comfortable with the hospital environment is to attend grand rounds, morbidity and mortality rounds, and departmental presentations. An important benefit of having hospital privileges is that it facilitates involvement in these learning situations. Conversely, chiropractors on staff should energetically seek opportunities to conduct in-service educational presentations of their own in order to explain chiropractic and respond to questions. Openness and learning are necessary in both directions if interprofessional collaboration is to succeed.

Chiropractors usually function in two ways in hospitals. First, they may see patients in the emergency department or outpatient clinic. In these circumstances, patients apply to a chiropractor through hospital administrative channels, but their interaction with the chiropractor is no different from that in a private office. Consultations and referrals, often to medical colleagues within the hospital setting, can be arranged as in any practice. The staff privileges of chiropractors who function in this way are very real, but limited. They are considered to have guest privileges, but not the full staff rights that authorize them to admit patients entirely on their own.

Second, chiropractors may provide inpatient care. Although admitting patients to the hospital requires a higher level of staff privilege than is granted to chiropractors, occasionally a chiropractor may feel that a patient needs hospitalization for a spinal disorder or, more frequently, that a patient who needs hospitalization for a medical disorder should continue to receive chiropractic care for a spinal disorder. Always, admitting a patient to a hospital requires a co-admission procedure in which a medical physician does a history, performs a physical examination, and provides a diagnosis that justifies admission. Again, full staff privileges are not accorded to the chiropractor, but within the scope of hospital practice, the chiropractor is entitled to provide full spinal manipulative evaluation and care. The co-admission procedure has advantages for the admitting chiropractor, as it leaves to another practitioner the time-consuming task of the patient's medical workup. This frees the chiropractor for specialty work in spinal treatment.[31] In addition, co-admission relieves the chiropractor of responsibility for oversight in the case of the rare patient who is treated chiropractically when the true condition is a medical or surgical problem.

COMMUNICATION AMONG PROFESSIONALS

A shared spoken language, an awareness of body language, and a sensitivity to the symbolism of dress and deportment facilitate communication.

The profession of medicine is distinguished by a specialized jargon that, along with subtleties of expression, serves both as a code for discussing health care issues and as a way to identify professional in-group membership.[32] Chiropractors have their own code, which is only partially congruent with that of medicine. For this reason, not only do chiropractic and medical physicians confront each other as competitors in the economic and political arena—a reality that must always be acknowledged—but also they speak different languages and act in different ways, which can affect the success of interaction.[33]

The divisive and counterproductive potentiality of interprofessional miscommunication is most apparent in the matter of professional vocabulary. Medical doctors enjoy the benefits of high status in the contemporary health care world. They can survive by being professionally "monolingual." None need learn to speak the "dialect" of chiropractic. Therefore, chiropractors who want a better kind of interprofessional interaction must become comfortable with the use of medical terms and phrases. Younger chiropractors were taught both "languages" in chiropractic colleges, so they can be "bilingual" with simple practice.

It has been argued that chiropractors with hospital privileges should persuade hospitals to amend their bylaws to permit the use of chiropractic terminology to describe the chiropractic approach to health care. As Gregg noted, "If we were to remain a chiropractic program and not just a specialty of medicine, I felt strongly that terms such as subluxation and adjustment be used in our bylaws, versus spinal manipulation and non-pathogenic lesion."[30] This raises an issue that is both difficult and contentious. When only a chiropractic term is precise and accurate, it seems that chiropractic wording should be permitted and encouraged. It should not be forgotten, however, that medical charting is not a place for cabalistic mysteries. Although chiropractic terminology contributes to a unique professional identity, the success of chiropractic does not rest on a distinctive terminology alone. On the contrary, the use of such a terminology can contribute to a failure of interprofessional communication and collaboration.

All the providers who must review a patient's progress should readily understand the chart. No reader will have trouble with the essentially synonymous terms *adjustment* or *manipulation*, even though subtle differences important to some chiropractors may be missed. Most readers in a hospital will be stymied, however, when attempting to decipher either the term *subluxation* or the term *nonpathogenic lesion* as used chiropractically. There are alternatives, and they should be used if they improve communication across disciplines. In the case of the subluxation, for example, terms such as *joint fixation, hypomobile vertebral segment, facet syndrome,* and *somatic dysfunction* (a codable diagnosis for the manipulable lesion) are all more comprehensible to nonchiropractors than is the term *nonpathogenic lesion* and less confusing than is the chiropractic term *subluxation*, which in medicine and surgery implies a partial dislocation. Careful review of the pros and cons of proposed terminology is essential before insisting on a vocabulary that may leave nonchiropractic colleagues uninformed and bewildered.

Because interprofessional societies can be especially influential in sharing information across disciplines,[34] chiropractors need to participate in professional associations that bring diverse health care providers together. They need to contribute to the meetings and to a growing clinical and scientific literature. In this way, medical personnel have the opportunity to learn about chiropractic. Simultaneously, chiropractors, in common with medical physicians in their many specialties, are continually updated on the rapidly changing fields of medicine that are relevant to their work. They keep informed about changing medical practices in prescribing medications, in performing surgery, and in interpreting laboratory and imaging findings.[35]

Interprofessional meetings provide important opportunities to facilitate understandings across disciplinary boundaries. They help to bring better unity to the universe of health care. The ultimate beneficiaries of interprofessional communication and understanding will be patients, who, in the past, have frequently found themselves neglected and confused by interprofessional rivalries.[35]

COMMUNICATION WITH THE PUBLIC

Every health care provider, including the chiropractor, must observe professional standards in advertising and in other public involvements. The well-dressed, well-spoken chiropractic physician builds valuable allies among ordinary people in this way, and they serve as good will ambassadors to other opinion leaders in health care and in the society at large.

The chiropractor, like all other health care providers, must avoid nonscientific statements, exaggeration, and hyperbole. Every provider must always speak with careful accuracy about health conditions, even if lay terms are used. It is unfair to the patient, for example, to speak of nerve pressure as though sciatic pain were the equivalent of stepping on a garden hose. The patient is entitled to an accurate statement, even if it is simple. This philosophy is not only a matter of proper relations with patients. It also influences relations with other health care providers, as patients frequently tell a provider what another said. Statements made to an uneducated working person in a private office must bear repeating by that patient to a medical physician in another private office.

Finally, professionals should not criticize one another publicly except under unusual circumstances and in rigorously circumscribed ways. It is inappropriate to accuse other physicians publicly of poor judgment, wrong treatment, or questionable motives. Because the prestige of anyone known as "doctor" is great and many people accept whatever a doctor says as authoritative, third parties tend to use such accusations wrongly by misplacing their trust in the accuracy of the statement, by misinterpreting it, or by denying authority to any professional when it appears that certain professionals are in disagreement. The place for confrontations is in professional meetings before audiences of peers. Accusations of malpractice belong in the courtroom or at the board of inquiry.

CONCLUSION

Most patients respond well to the ministrations of a single provider. In the present day, however, no clinician can know enough to take complete responsibility for every patient, even a clinician whose specialty is appropriate to that patient's diagnosis. Health care has become so complex that all practitioners must work in a context of specialization and subspecialization. Professional lives are more complex as a result, but they can also be more stimulating and productive.

Interprofessional collaboration can be a source of confusion, frustration, and disappointment if it is not done well, but it can also be a source of great satisfaction, personal growth, and successful practice. It has to happen, so let us make it happen in the best possible way.

REFERENCES

1. White AH. Introduction to conservative care. In: White AH, Anderson R, eds. *The Conservative Care of Low Back Pain*. Baltimore: Williams & Wilkins; 1991: 3-7.

2. Cole HM, ed. Law and medicine: Conflicts of interest. *N Engl J Med*. 1989;262(3):390-397.

3. Chapman-Smith D. The chiropractor on paper: The writing of reports, professional correspondence, consultations and journal articles. Workshop, The American Back Society Spring Symposium on Back Pain; May 3-6, 1990; Chicago, Ill.

4. Mootz RD. Interprofessional referral protocol. *Today's Chiropractic*. 1987;16:37-39.

5. Egerton JM. Is a referring chiropractor a colleague? *Medical Economics*. 1989;66:55.

6. Cassidy JD, Mierau DR, Nykoliation JW, Arthur B. Medical-chiropractic correspondence. *Journal of the Canadian Chiropractic Association*. 1985;29:29-31.

7. Mootz RD, Meeker WC. Minimizing radiation exposure to patients in chiropractic practice. *ACA Journal of Chiropractic*. 1989;26(4):65-70.

8. Deyo RA, Diel AK. Lumbar spine films in primary care: Current use and effects of selective ordering criteria. *Journal of General Internal Medicine*. 1986;1:20–25.

9. Frymoyer JW. Back pain and sciatica. *N Engl J Med*. 1988;318(5):291–300.

10. Liang M, Komaroff AL. Roentgenograms in primary care patients with acute low back pain: A cost-effectiveness analysis. *Arch Intern Med*. 1982;142:1108–1112.

11. Haldeman S. The neurophysiology of spinal pain syndromes. In: Haldeman S, ed. *Modern Developments in the Principles and Practice of Chiropractic*. 2nd ed. New York: Appleton-Century-Crofts; 1991.

12. White AH, Rothman RH, Ray CD, eds. *Lumbar Spine Surgery: Techniques & Complications*. St Louis: CV Mosby.

13. Saal JA, Saal JS. Nonoperative treatment of herniated lumbar intervertebral disc with radiculopathy: An outcome study. *Spine*. 1989;14(4):431–437.

14. Nyiendo J, Phillips RB, Meeker WC, Konsler G, Jansen R, Menon M. A comparison of patients and patient complaints at six chiropractic college teaching clinics. *Journal of Manipulative and Physiological Therapeutics*. 1989;12(2):79–85.

15. Arnett FC, Edworthy SM, Block DA, et al. The American Rheumatism Association 1987 revised criteria for the classification of rheumatoid arthritis. *Arthritis Rheum*. 1988;31(3):315–325.

16. Evans T, Hess EV. When to treat and when to refer your rheumatoid arthritis patient. *Journal of Musculoskeletal Medicine*. 1989;6(4):17–34.

17. Schumacher HR, ed. *Primer on the Rheumatic Diseases*. 9th ed. Atlanta: Arthritis Foundation; 1988.

18. Anderson R, Meeker WC, Wirick BE, Mootz RD, Kirk DH. A meta-analysis of clinical trials of spinal manipulation. Unpublished manuscript.

19. Meade TW, Dyer S, Browne W, Townsend J, Frank AO. Low back pain of mechanical origin: Randomised comparison of chiropractic and hospital outpatient treatment. *Br Med J*. 1990;300:1431–1437.

20. Anderson R. Chiropractors for and against vaccines. *Medical Anthropology*. 1990;12(2):169–186.

21. Leach RA. *The Chiropractic Theories: a Synopsis of Scientific Research*. 2nd ed. Baltimore: Williams & Wilkins; 1986.

22. Becker GE. Some historical reflections. *American Back Society Newsletter*. 1990;6(1):3–4.

23. Anderson DJ, Moskowitz MH. Psychiatric aspects of spine disease. In: White AH, Anderson R, eds. *The Conservative Care of Low Back Pain*. Baltimore: Williams & Wilkins; 1991:274–288.

24. Hunt RE, Goldstein RE. The psychologist's contribution to spine care. In: White AH, Anderson R, eds. *The Conservative Care of Low Back Pain*. Baltimore: Williams & Wilkins; 1991:288–296.

25. Cassidy JD, Kirkaldy-Willis WH. Manipulation. In: Kirkaldy-Willis WH, ed. *Managing Low Back Pain*. 2nd ed. New York: Churchill Livingstone; 1988:287–296.

26. Triano JJ. Standards of care: Manipulative procedures. In: White AH, Anderson R, eds. *The Conservative Care of Low Back Pain*. Baltimore: Williams & Wilkins; 1991:157–166.

27. White AH, Anderson R. The challenge of conservative care. In: White AH, Anderson R, eds. *The Conservative Care of Low Back Pain*. Baltimore: Williams & Wilkins; 1991:159–168.

28. Kranz KC, Hendrickson RM. *Chiropractic and the HMO-PPO Challenge*. Washington, DC: The International Chiropractors Association; 1988.

29. Kranz KC. *Chiropractic and Hospital Privileges Protocol*. Washington, DC: The International Chiropractors Association; 1987.

30. Gregg RJ. New Center Hospital: A successful model for the future. *Dynamic Chiropractic*. 1990;8(10):1, 44.

31. Sather T. Interprofessional relations: How to implement a multi-disciplinary approach to patient care. Workshop presentation, American Back Society, Fall Symposium on Back Pain; December 3–5, 1987: San Francisco, Calif.

32. Goffman E. *The Presentation of Self in Everyday Life*. New York: Doubleday; 1959.

33. Kuipers JC. "Medical discourse" in anthropological context: Views of language and power. *Medical Anthropology Quarterly*. 1989;3(2):99–122.

34. Haldeman S. Learned spine societies and meetings. In: White AH, Anderson R, eds. *The Conservative Care of Low Back Pain*. Baltimore: Williams & Wilkins; 1991:423–426.

35. Swartz AA. Editorial. *American Back Society Newsletter*. 1990;6(2):3.

9

Standards for Diagnostic Imaging

Cynthia Peterson

The health and welfare of every patient should be the prime concern of all physicians. The correct treatment can commence only after a thorough history has been taken, a diagnostic evaluation performed, and a working diagnosis developed. Radiography is one of the principal diagnostic tools used by most chiropractic physicians to confirm or rule out clinical suspicions of pathology, obtain additional information regarding the presence of anomalies, and to evaluate biomechanical disorders. Even the "normal" radiographic series offers vital information to the treating physician.

With rising malpractice costs, and heightened fears of litigation, an increasing number of chiropractors are becoming aware of the advantages of having a specialist analyze their patients' radiographs and provide a professional opinion for the protection of both patient and practitioner. Radiographic evaluations can be obtained from either medical or chiropractic radiologists. The chiropractic radiologists are able not only to interpret the pathological processes evident on the films, but also to evaluate any biomechanical aberrations.

Special imaging procedures, particularly computed tomography (CT) and magnetic resonance imaging (MRI), are becoming increasingly available for chiropractic referral, and a growing number of chiropractic radiologists are becoming involved in imaging centers. Although the examination procedures and interpretations of special imaging should be left to the radiological specialists, all chiropractors should have a basic understanding of these imaging modalities. Computed tomography, which involves ionizing radiation, provides axial images of very thin body sections. The computer is able not only to reformat the information that it receives in virtually any plane, but also to produce the images in a much greater variety of tissue densities than conventional x-ray techniques can. Spinal conditions that are well visualized on CT

179

include, but are not limited to, disc protrusions/herniations, spinal stenosis, lateral recess entrapments, neoplastic and infectious processes, and fractures.

With MRI, images are produced by means of a strong magnetic field and a radiofrequency to influence the orientation of tissue protons. Removal of the original radiofrequency causes the protons to relax and align themselves to the magnetic field. During this process the protons emit specific radiofrequencies that are detected and the information fed into a computer. No ionizing radiation is necessary. The body is imaged in the axial plane, as well as in the coronal and sagittal planes without reformatting. The area of the body imaged by MRI is usually larger than that imaged by CT. Furthermore, MRI gives exquisite soft tissue detail. Spinal conditions that are well visualized on MRI include, but are not limited to, disc protrusions/herniations, pathological processes involving the spinal cord and adjacent structures, disc degeneration, and spinal stenosis. Currently, MRI is considered more sensitive than CT for soft tissue visualization, while CT is more sensitive for osseous visualization.

LEGAL IMPLICATIONS RELATED TO DIAGNOSTIC IMAGING

Standard #1: The chiropractic physician is legally responsible to recognize all pathological processes, both osseous and soft tissue, visualized on each radiographic series.[1,2]

According to the claims department of the National Chiropractic Mutual Insurance Corporation,

The courts do not take into consideration what you were looking for. The courts will hold you responsible for the content of that x-ray in its entirety. You must realize, the standard you will be held to by your peers, the court and other experts, is that of someone who is qualified to read what is on the x-ray.[1]

Those patients with conditions that are not amenable to chiropractic treatment should be referred to the appropriate health care provider.

Standard #2: Radiographs must be of sufficient diagnostic quality that the presence or absence of pathological processes can be determined.

Many malpractice cases are settled simply because the poor quality of the radiographs cannot be defended.[1]

Standard #3:   Repeat radiographic evaluation of the patient should not be undertaken without significant observable clinical indication, as determined by the treating chiropractic physician. [3]

ADVANTAGES AND DISADVANTAGES OF OWNING AN X-RAY UNIT

Historically, chiropractic physicians had no other option but to purchase x-ray equipment and read all of their own films. This practice was so common that, until recently, no one questioned its continued feasibility. Today, advocates of owning x-ray equipment continue to cite convenience and control over the management of the patient as important reasons to purchase an x-ray machine. Many practice management and x-ray companies advise chiropractors to purchase x-ray equipment for the financial benefits to be gained from radiographing their own patients. This encourages the use of ionizing radiation for the wrong reasons, however, and may lead to abuse; the x-ray machine must be viewed as an important diagnostic tool, not a revenue generator.

Standard #4: Medical necessity is the only acceptable standard for exposing the patient to ionizing radiation.

Owning an x-ray machine is necessary for chiropractors in many regions of the United States. At present, the chiropractic profession does not have enough radiology specialists in strategically located x-ray laboratories to service a majority of practitioners. Although more and more medical facilities accept chiropractic radiological referrals and will provide spinal films taken with the patient in the upright position, medical radiologists in many areas still refuse to cooperate with chiropractors. Under these circumstances, there is no alternative to the purchase of an x-ray unit.

Many new chiropractic graduates are choosing to enter practice without purchasing x-ray equipment. Three factors contribute to this decision. First, most new graduates are extremely cognizant of the complexity of the field of radiology and the medicolegal implications of doing their own radiological evaluations. Second, many students have been able to complete chiropractic college only by obtaining large student loans, and they are looking for ways to lower their initial practice overhead costs; forgoing the purchase of radiological equipment can save the new practitioner at least $20,000. Third, some practitioners find that they make more money by using the space allocated for the x-ray room as a treatment room; the x-ray room in most clinics stands empty much of the time.

Chiropractic physicians who have decided not to purchase an x-ray unit should take this factor into consideration when choosing a location for their practices. The ideal location is one where chiropractic radiologists are nearby or where medical facilities accept chiropractic referrals. Often overlooked, but important, benefits of using a specialized radiographic center include

- consistent high-quality radiographic images. X-ray laboratories are in business to perform x-ray examinations. They have state-of-the-art equipment that is serviced regularly and physicians or technologists who are highly trained in radiography.
- a professional interpretation with every radiographic series, if desired.
- avoidance of the "hidden" costs of owning an x-ray unit. The costs of x-ray film, periodic machine calibration, chemicals, and preventive or reparative maintenance, for example, can become substantial if used equipment is purchased or if the screens, films, chemicals, and x-ray generator are not properly matched.

Most chiropractors who have practiced for a number of years without x-ray units in their offices state that the lack of an x-ray unit does not cause problems in patient management. Patients accept the idea of "specialization" within health care; many expect it. Advising a chiropractic patient that the radiologists are experts who assist the treating practitioner in providing the best possible diagnostic workup is very effective in obtaining the patient's cooperation and enhancing the patient's confidence in the treating doctor.

Obviously, many factors affect a chiropractor's decision regarding the purchase of x-ray equipment. Practitioners must assess their priorities and their individual practice situations before they can make a sound decision. It is important to remember that, unlike chiropractors in the past, many practitioners today have a real choice in this matter.

EQUIPMENT

Once a chiropractic physician has decided to include x-ray facilities within his or her office, a variety of decisions must be made, as an x-ray unit is a large financial investment in the chiropractic practice. Well-coordinated equipment that is properly maintained will not only produce better quality diagnostic images, but also will save the treating practitioner time, energy, and money in trouble-shooting problems arising from poor maintenance or substandard equipment (Table 9-1). Properly calibrated equipment, combined with standardized processing, filters, shields, and collimation, will provide the best quality images with the least risk to the patient.

Table 9-1 Minimum X-Ray Equipment Standards

Machine	Single phase 325 with aluminum equivalent filtration of 2.0 to 2.5mm in front of the tube.
Table	Upright table (patients 28 cm AP measurement should be referred for recumbent studies).
Grids	Fine line 10:1 or 12:1 focused grids. (Bucky system is not necessary).
Intensifying Screens and Cassettes	Rare earth intensifying screens. Film/screen combination: 200 or 400. No gradient screens. 4–14×17s, 4–10×12s, 4–8×10s.
Processing	Hand tanks or automatic processor.
Markers and Identification	Right/left markers. Patient identification to include: name, age, sex. Examination date, name, and address of doctor or clinic should be included on each radiograph.
Radiation Protection	Gonad and breast shields. Collimation at least to film size. Compensating filters.

Location of the X-Ray Room

The practitioner first must choose the location of the x-ray room and dark room within the office space. Because office settings vary dramatically, a radiation physicist should help the practitioner select the most appropriate location for the x-ray room and determine the proper amount of lead shielding for each wall.

Standard #5: The x-ray room must have the proper amount of lead (or lead equivalent) barriers and must be inspected by the local radiation protection office.

New vs Used Equipment

Choosing between new or used x-ray equipment is the next major decision. The financial burden of purchasing x-ray equipment encourages the new chiropractor to buy used equipment, which has a limited additional life span, may have limited technical capabilities, and often produces less than desirable images.[4] Older machines may not be adequately calibrated and may have inaccurate mechanical timers, resulting in an inconsistent radiation output. Older mechanical timers often lack the range of time settings that the new electronic timers offer and may not be compatible with the new rare earth film/screen combinations.[4,5] In addition, older machines may not have the option of the higher mA (milliamperage) settings. Low mA settings[5] require longer time settings to obtain the appropriate mAs. This increases the likelihood of motion artifact. Thus, many older x-ray machines not only deliver higher radiation exposures than is currently deemed necessary, but also produce images of inconsistent radiographic quality.

If purchasing an older piece of equipment, the practitioner should avoid buying into "package deals" (ie, generator, tube, cassettes, film, processing and dark room supplies) unless assured that all of the equipment is compatible. It is necessary also to check the type of service available from the dealer and the warranties offered.[6]

Modern machines have electronic timers that ensure more accuracy and consistency in the radiation exposure. These machines also offer higher mA settings and a wider range of time options, which make them compatible with rare earth intensifying screens. Some newer and more expensive models have a photo-timer option that automatically shuts off the exposure when the correct penetration has been achieved. Although photo-timers are theoretically ideal, they require exquisite patient positioning for good image quality and sacrifice operator control of the latitude for film quality.

The practitioner has the option of a single-phase or a three-phase x-ray generator. The single-phase generator is the most widely used within the chiropractic profession, because it is substantially less expensive than is the three-phase generator and is usually more than adequate for the typical chiropractic practice. Busy hospital radiology departments favor three-phase generators. Because the single-phase x-ray generator has significantly more fluctuation in the kVp (kilovolt peak) than does the three-phase generator, the most efficient three-phase machines can cut exposure times in half without changing the kVp or mA settings.[6] This decreases the likelihood of motion artifact. Three-phase generators also reduce the heat load on the x-ray tube and, therefore, prolong the tube life. For heavily used equipment, this is an important consideration. Several manufacturers are currently producing high-frequency single-phase generators that simulate three-phase generators, but cost significantly less.

An x-ray unit that will meet the radiological needs of the vast majority of treating chiropractors should be rated at a minimum of 300 mA and 125 kV.[4] This type of machine is often referred to as a "325." Small and large focal spot size options are also helpful features, as the small focal spot adds clarity to small body parts.[4] Federal performance standards for certified equipment require intrinsic aluminum equivalent filtration of 2 to 2.5 mm permanently installed in front of the primary x-ray beam.[7] This filration does not affect the radiographic quality, but it reduces the radiation dosage to the patient.[7]

Grids

Reciprocating grids (the Bucky system) are no longer considered essential if fine line stationary grids (100 to 110 lines/inch) are used.[8,9] The grid ratios typically employed are either 10:1 or 12:1 and should be focused for the FFD (focal film distance) used.[8,9] Higher grid ratios require an increased radiation dosage and are used with higher kVp techniques. The use of stationary grids rather than reciprocating grids reduces the radiation exposure by approximately 15%.[9]

X-Ray Tables

Most chiropractors take all their radiographs with the patient in the upright position. Many practitioners feel that, because the number of patients who need to be radiographed in the recumbent position is so low, they cannot justify the expense of purchasing an x-ray table. An advantage of the x-ray table is the ease of radiographing extremities, however. All practitioners should consider the practicality of purchasing an x-ray table for radiographing patients in both upright and recumbent positions.

> *Standard #6:* It is difficult to obtain adequate diagnostic studies of patients who measure more than 28 cm in the frontal dimension while they are in the weight-bearing position; consequently, these patients should be radiographed in recumbency.[9]

Taking films on large patients in the upright, weight-bearing position sacrifices significant diagnostic detail, gives higher than necessary radiation exposure, and taxes the x-ray tube. Furthermore, a fracture or other pathological process that may be missed if the obese patient is radiographed in the upright position is not worth the risk. If the chiropractor can radiograph patients only when they are upright, larger patients should be referred to a facility capable of taking radiographs of recumbent patients.

Intensifying Screens

> *Standard #7:* All physicians should use rare earth intensifying screens.[4,6]

New practitioners should start out with new screens and cassettes. Practitioners seeking to upgrade their equipment and improve their radiographic quality should begin by obtaining rare earth screens and new cassettes. Old screens and cassettes may have artifacts or may be warped, resulting in poor film-screen contact.

Rare earth intensifying screens have undergone dramatic improvement in the last decade. When combined with the proper film, they provide better diagnostic detail than do the older calcium tungstate screens.[4,10] In addition, because the phosphors in the rare earth screens are very efficient at emitting light when struck by x-rays transmitted through the patient, the radiation dose to the patient is reduced.[4,10]

Speeds of x-ray systems vary from 60 to 800 (based on the par speed of 100), depending on the film-screen combination selected. Slower speeds offer better diagnostic detail, but higher radiation dosages; the reverse is true for faster speed systems.[10] For convenience and simplicity, chiropractic physicians generally use only one speed, most often a 200 or 400 speed system. (The 400 speed system offers half as much radiation exposure as does the 200 speed system, but less detail.) To achieve particularly good detail, many reserve a 100 speed system for extremity studies. Thus, the option is available to use lower speeds to obtain exquisite detail or higher speeds to reduce radiation exposure and protect the x-ray tube in examinations of obese patients.

Practitioners must remember that both the intensifying screens and the radiographic films are assigned a speed. It is the combination of the speed of the screen with the speed of the film that gives the total speed of the system (Table 9-2). Furthermore, practitioners must use only those films for which the screens are designed.[6,10] "Split" or gradient intensifying screens result in a more even exposure of the radiograph, but they unnecessarily increase radiation exposure to the patient.

Standard #8: Gradient intensifying screens are outdated technology and must be abandoned.[3,11]

Some practitioners expect intensifying screens to last indefinitely. This is an unrealistic expectation; the average life of intensifying screens is approxi-

Table 9-2 Commonly Used Dupont Films and Screens, and the Resultant System Speed

Quanta III Screens (800 speed)	Cronox 4 Film (full speed)	800 Speed System
Cronex 7 or 10 Film (1/2 speed)	Quanta Fast Detail Screens. (400 speed)	200 Speed System
400 Speed System	400 Speed System	

mately 7 years.[6] The use of rare earth intensifying screens can prolong the life of the x-ray tube (tube replacement cost > $5,000), however, and are worth the cost.[6]

Practitioners should purchase sufficient screens and cassettes to permit an efficient examination (Exhibit 9-1). It is at best inconvenient to stop in the middle of an x-ray examination to process films and reload cassettes in order to finish the examination. Those who have too few cassettes may be tempted to perform an incomplete diagnostic series of the areas of complaint because of this inconvenience.

Markers

Standard #9: The patient's right or left side must be labeled on each anteroposterior, posteroanterior, and oblique view. The general rule for lateral and oblique views is to label the side closest to the film.[12]

Film Processing

Standard #10: Specific patient identification information must appear on every radiograph.

The patient's name, date of exposure, and the name of the facility where the x-ray examination was performed should appear on every radiograph.[12] Identification information is easily imprinted on the radiograph by using the film identification printer in the dark room prior to film processing.

The debate continues concerning the cost-effectiveness of hand tank development vs automatic processing. Recent chiropractic graduates tend to

---

Exhibit 9-1 Recommended Number of Cassettes

Minimal Number and Sizes	*Additional Recommendations for Quality Service*
4 14 × 17's	2 7 × 17's
4 10 × 12's	2 11 × 14's
3 8 × 10's	3 8 × 10's (for a total number of 7 for a complete cervical series.)
1 14 × 36 (if full spine X-ray is required)	2 extremity cassettes (single screens for exquisite detail)

use hand tanks because the initial cost is less. Some chiropractic radiologists are convinced that the operating costs of a 3-minute table top automatic processor are no higher than are those associated with hand tank development, however, and the results of automatic processing are certainly more consistent.[6,10] Hand tanking is a very lengthy and messy procedure that requires time away from the patient. Practitioners who use hand tanks often do not properly monitor, replace, or stir the chemicals, nor do they keep the chemicals at the proper temperature. This results in wide fluctuations of image quality. Automatic processors are more efficient and produce better quality images.[10]

Most problems concerning image quality can be traced directly to processing. Practitioners must remember that processing chemistry and processing conditions must match the intensifying screens and film.[8] Even in automatic processors, temperature is important, as are the replenishment rates of the chemicals.[9] Many automatic processors are designed so that they must process a minimum number of films per day to replenish the chemicals adequately. If a processor is underutilized and the chemicals are not being replenished at a sufficient rate, problems may arise concerning image quality and consistency. Cleared films may be passed through the processor at periodic intervals to alleviate this problem until utilization increases.

Many practitioners try to save money by not purchasing service contracts for their x-ray equipment. Without a service contract, however, technical problems and equipment failures may not be properly addressed, and the x-ray machine may not be calibrated every 18 months as it should be. The automatic processor may not be cleaned regularly nor the processing chemistry monitored. Attention to these and other details of maintenance can save more money by extending the life of the equipment than is saved by not purchasing service contracts.

Radiation Protection Standards

Compensating aluminum filters are important devices that not only reduce radiation exposure to the patient, but also significantly improve radiographic quality.[11,12] These "wedge" filters, which come under a variety of brand names, are designed so that the thicker part of the filter is placed over less dense areas of the patient's body. Their original purpose was to improve the quality of the diagnostic image. The emphasis has shifted more recently from image consistency to patient safety, however, because they increase the protection for radiosensitive areas of the body. The effects of compensating filters are best appreciated on anteroposterior or posteroanterior full spine radiographs, but they also enhance the radiographic image of anteroposterior thoracic spine films and lateral lumbar films if the patient has a marked difference in the anatomic measurement from the waist to the hip region.

> *Standard #11:* In addition to aluminum wedge filters, lead shielding must be used to protect the radiosensitive areas of the body in the path of the primary beam.[8,10,12-14]

The exposure field for spinal radiography includes many radiosensitive organs, such as the thyroid gland, lungs, spleen, ovaries, testes, and breasts. Shields are made of lead and, therefore, prohibit penetration by the primary x-ray beam. Gonad shielding should be a routine procedure for males. Unfortunately, the position of the ovaries within the female pelvis varies, and small round shields may not protect them. In females who are small to medium in size, the posteroanterior projection offers significantly less radiation to both breast and ovarian tissue while minimally reducing osseous detail.[8,12,13]

> *Standard #12:* The posteroanterior position should be used for both full spine and lumbar spine radiographs in small- to average-sized patients.

The incidence of breast cancer is rising. Those who perform radiographic examinations cannot neglect their responsibility to make every effort to protect the breast tissues from ionizing radiation. Both lead shields and the posteroanterior projection substantially reduce the radiation exposure to this radiosensitive tissue and should be used whenever possible.[13,14] Shields are also available under a variety of trade names to protect the eyes and thyroid gland.

> *Standard #13:* Collimation should be used to reduce exposure to nonessential areas of the body.

Collimation decreases the amount of scatter radiation, which reduces the exposure of the patient and improves diagnostic detail. Scatter radiation degrades image quality by superimposing an overall exposure on the useful image, thereby reducing contrast.[8-10] The primary x-ray beam should be collimated to include only the area of interest.

CLINICAL JUSTIFICATION FOR X-RAY EXAMINATIONS

The following list was developed by Western States Chiropractic College to assist new chiropractors in determining whether radiographic examinations should be included in the diagnostic workup:

1. trauma
2. acute nontraumatic symptoms
3. prolonged chronic symptoms
4. scoliosis or deformity
5. possible presence of a foreign body
6. differentiation of infectious, metabolic, congenital, and tumorous disease
7. abnormal clinical findings
    a. abnormal orthopedic tests/signs: Soto Hall; neurovascular compression; SLR; Patrick Fabre; Valsalva/jugular compression; cervical compression
    b. abnormal neurological tests/signs: muscle atrophy, hyperesthesia, hypesthesia along specific dermatomes
    c. physical tests/signs: abnormal heart sounds, blood pressure; chest pain, cough, sputum production, vascular changes/atherosclerosis, aneurysm, intermittent claudication
    d. unusual palpatory findings: masses (either hard or soft tissue), unusual spinal curvatures (eg, kyphoscoliosis or "Gibbus")
    e. abnormal limitation in ranges of motion: flexion, extension, lateral flexion, rotation

Standard #14: Standards of practice require that a minimal diagnostic series be performed for each area radiographed.[12,15]

A minimal diagnostic series is necessary to ensure adequate visualization of the entire area in order to rule in or out pathological processes or determine necessary follow-up views (Table 9-3).

There are only two legal reasons to expose a patient to ionizing radiation. The first is to apply radiation therapy, as in the treatment of some cancers.

Standard #15: Radiation therapy is beyond the scope of practice of the chiropractic profession.

The second reason to use ionizing radiation is to diagnose pathology.

Standard #16: Radiographing patients simply to determine the presence of subluxations is not, in and of itself, sufficient justification for the use of radiation.

Certain chiropractic techniques promote nonstandard radiographic views to determine subluxations. A classic example of this is the anteroposterior nasium view.

Table 9-3 Minimal Diagnostic Series and Common Supplementary Views

Body Part	Minimal Series	Supplementary Views
Cervical spine	AP, AP-open mouth, odontoid, lateral	Swimmer's lateral, lateral right and left oblique, flexion-extension
Thoracic spine	AP, lateral	Swimmer's lateral
Lumbar spine	PA or AP, lateral (angled AP or PA lumbosacral spot)	Right and left oblique, flexion/extension, lateral bending, spot lateral lumbosacral
Pelvis	AP	
Full spine	AP or PA with lateral cervical, thoracic and lumbar, AP odontoid	Angled AP or PA, lumbosacral
Shoulder	AP internal, AP external rotation	
Acrom/clav	AP-weight- and nonweight-bearing bilaterally	
Elbow	AP and lateral	
Wrist	PA, medial oblique, lateral	PA with ulnar deviation (navicular view), dorsal oblique
Hand/finger	PA, medial oblique, lateral	
Hip	AP hip or AP pelvis, frog leg	
Knee	AP and lateral	Tunnel
Ankle	AP, medial oblique, lateral	
Foot	Dorsoplantar, medial oblique, lateral	
Chest	Upright PA	Lateral
Ribs	AP or PA—above/below diaphragm, Ant/Post oblique −45 degrees	
Abdomen	Recumbent AP or PA—upper/lower separately if necessary	
Skull	PA or Caldwell, Towne, right/left lateral	

Note: AP, anteroposterior; PA, posteroanterior.

Standard #17: Nonstandard radiographs cannot substitute for films taken in the minimal diagnostic series and must be viewed as supplementary.

THE CHIROPRACTIC RADIOLOGIST: A SPECIALIST

What is a "chiropractic radiologist"? The chiropractic radiologist is a specialist who has become a diplomate of the American Chiropractic Board of Radiology (ACBR). In the past, chiropractors have had two traditional options to earn this credential. One option, which is now a declining one, is to complete a 300-hour, nonresident postgraduate program in radiology. This route involves one weekend per month for 3 years. Recent advances in special imaging technologies, coupled with the vast amounts of experience and knowledge necessary to pass the ACBR examinations, have left most of the candidates who chose this route ill-prepared to sit for board examinations, however, and this route is no longer a realistic one to diplomate status. The second route to eligibility for the ACBR examinations is to complete a formal residency program at a chiropractic college accredited by the Council on Chiropractic Education. This is a 2- to 3-year program of intensive training in all aspects of diagnostic imaging, including skeletal radiology, biomechanics, soft tissue diagnosis, and special imaging.[16] With successful completion of a residency program, the candidate is eligible to take the ACBR examination. All 10 parts of the examination must be passed with a score of 80% or higher before the credential of diplomate is granted to the practitioner. Diplomates are recognized as experts by the chiropractic profession, the legal profession, and third-party payers.

There are several clinical indications for using a chiropractic radiologist. Some practitioners send every film of every patient to chiropractic radiologists for consultation. Doing so assures them of a thorough evaluation of each radiograph and greatly diminishes the chance of missing a potentially significant problem. It provides peace of mind to treating practitioners and gives them more time to focus on other aspects of patient care. To have a radiologist's report on file is also a major asset in any subsequent litigation. Furthermore, the diplomate's credentials add strength and credibility to the case.

Practitioners also consult a chiropractic radiologist for assistance with difficult cases. One of the most common consultations with a radiologist involves a practitioner's specific questions on a particular film. For example, "What is causing the unusual density/lucency seen over the right transverse process of L4?" The answer to this type of question is often as simple as a variation in normal anatomy, summation shadows, or artifacts. There may be a pathological process, however.

The field practitioner should consider sending the patient to the radiologist's office to have radiographs taken and interpreted.

Standard #18: The referring practitioner should provide a brief history, in addition to a description of the patient's chief complaint.

A knowledge of the history will enhance the reading and provide a more accurate impression of the patient's diagnosis through a correlation of clinical and radiographic findings. One major advantage to this approach is that the radiologist can immediately take any additional views necessary for maximal visualization of an abnormality; this saves time and expense for both the patient and the treating chiropractor. The radiologist can also obtain additional pertinent history related to the complaint or the abnormalities observed. Because the diplomate is considered an expert in the field of radiology, good quality films should be assured.

The chiropractic radiologist can provide a specialist's opinion on the need to refer a patient for special imaging procedures, such as a bone scan, ultrasonography, CT, MRI, angiography, or intravenous pyelography. It is imperative that chiropractors be able to make wise and appropriate referrals for these sophisticated diagnostic procedures. These technologies can be abused easily, with unnecessary risk and cost to the patient. When indicated, however, special imaging is invaluable in the diagnostic workup.

An often overlooked expertise possessed by the chiropractic radiologist is in the area of film quality control. The diplomate is able to assist the chiropractic physician in improving film quality, selecting and trouble-shooting x-ray equipment, and choosing appropriate supplementary views to clarify problem areas.

As more chiropractic radiologists enter practice and become known to the profession, treating practitioners will appreciate the variety of services available. The ultimate goal is to serve the patient and, thus, the profession in the best way possible.

The names and addresses of chiropractic radiologists can be obtained from:

The American Chiropractic Association
1701 Clarendon Boulevard
Arlington, VA 22209 (703) 276-8800

REFERENCES

1. National Chiropractic Mutual Insurance Corporation Claims Department. Comments. *NCMIC Informer.* 1987; 87-1.

2. Rosenfeld HN. Straight chiropractic and the duty to diagnose: A New Jersey case. *Beacon.* 1985; 13.

3. Sowby FD. New radiographic guidelines for use in chiropractic. *Journal of Manipulative and Physiological Therapeutics.* 1985; 8(1):47.

4. Chiropractic radiologists stress benefits of updated equipment. *ACA Journal of Chiropractic.* 1988; 25(7):26–28.

5. Howe J, Leverone R, Winterstein J. Guidelines for radiographic equipment and procedure. *Journal of the American Chiropractic Association.* 1975; 12(7):66–72.

6. Getting the most for your x-ray dollar. *ACA Journal of Chiropractic.* 1988; 25(8): 56–59.

7. Picker Corporation. *The Production of X-Rays: A Matter of Energy Conversion.* PG 369S/872B316. Cleveland: Picker Corporation Medical Marketing Division; 1988.

8. *Fundamentals of Radiography.* 12th ed. Rochester, NY: Eastman Kodak Company; 1980.

9. Better radiographic quality within reach, experts say. *ACA Journal of Chiropractic.* 1988, 25(11):55–58.

10. Bushong SC. *Radiologic Science for Technologists.* 3rd ed. St. Louis: CV Mosby; 1984.

11. Field TJ, Buehler MT. Improvements in chiropractic full spine radiography. *Journal of Manipulative and Physiological Therapeutics.* 1981; 4(1):21–25.

12. Yochum TR, Rowe LJ. *Essentials of Skeletal Radiology.* Baltimore: Williams & Wilkins; 1987.

13. Gray JE, Hoffman AD, Peterson HA. Reduction of radiation exposure during radiography for scoliosis. *J Bone Joint Surg.* 1983; 65-A(1):5–12.

14. Protecting the breast during scoliosis radiography. *FDA Drug Bulletin.* 1985; 15(1).

15. Bontrager KL, Anthony BT: *Textbook of Radiographic Positioning and Related Anatomy.* 2nd ed. St. Louis; CV Mosby; 1987.

16. Howe J. Roentgenology in chiropractic: State of the art—1974. *ACA Journal of Chiropractic.* 1974; 11(5):VIII, S66–72.

10

Standards for Thermography in Chiropractic Practice

Susan L. Vlasuk

Thermography is a neurodiagnostic imaging system that has great applicability to chiropractic practice. The image is a photograph of the spontaneous heat emission arising from the body's immediate subcutaneous microcirculation. The volume of subcutaneous circulation, being under local chemical and autonomic nervous system control, provides *physiological* or functional data. Thus, while the other diagnostic imaging systems provide *anatomical* data, a thermogram can provide significantly different clinical information. Certainly, various localized inflammatory conditions manifest themselves via local circulatory changes, but these conditions are visible to inspection. It is the physiological data less superficially visible that are of particular interest to the clinician—the superficial circulatory changes that can occur secondary to deeper neuromusculoskeletal abnormalities, mediated by neurotransmitters, sympathetic nerve fibers, and autonomic end organ receptors.

Information supplied by a thermogram cannot be equated to or replaced by information obtained through any other diagnostic imaging procedure. The nervous system has sensory, motor, and autonomic components. There are other diagnostic tests used to evaluate the sensory and motor functions. In a routine physical examination, the physician performs a sensory evaluation via pinprick and light touch evaluation, and examines motor function via deep tendon reflexes and muscle strength assessment. Furthermore, the physician can order Somato-Sensory Evoked Potentials (SSEPs) or needle electromyographs. There is no readily available test other than thermography, however, that monitors autonomic function.

One important advantage of thermography is that it is completely noninvasive, risk-free, and painless. It involves no radiation dose to the patient, being simply a photograph of the normal heat that is spontaneously emitted from the surface of the body.

Skin thermal images can be acquired via two new methods. Liquid crystal contact thermography (LCT) involves the use of framelike structures, called detector screens or cassettes, each of which holds a flexible sheet that contains cholesteric liquid crystals. These crystals change color in response to various levels of heat directly conducted from the skin, as in the popular contact strip body temperature measuring devices. At least six different screens, calibrated to measure various ranges of temperatures, are available in each liquid crystal contact thermography set. This process requires the physical touching of the patient. Once the liquid crystal screen has completed its color change, the resulting image is photographed, usually with instant prints, for permanent archiving. The use of liquid crystal thermography has gradually been de-emphasized over recent years.

In infrared electronic telethermography (IR), an infrared scanner measures spontaneously radiated heat emission without touching the subject. The infrared radiation from the patient's body strikes the detector crystal within the scanner, producing an electronic signal that is processed in an accompanying control unit. The control unit can regulate the window of temperature ranges desired (generally 5°C or 10°C) and the level of temperature being measured; usually it can also provide a white-on-black, black-on-white (inverted), or color image. Modern IR units measure real temperature referenced to an internal calibrated standard; and they have sophisticated software programs for image display and analysis, often with color printers. If a printer is not available, the images are photographed, either with 35-mm print or slide film, for later analysis and archiving.

Whereas research during the 1980s showed comparable findings from thermal data obtained either by liquid crystal or by infrared electronic methods, the lesser proclivity to operator error in electronic studies, along with greater precision in temperature measurement, have now caused virtually all major thermographic organizations to consider high-resolution infrared electronic thermography the state-of-the-art procedure for thermal imaging.

HISTORICAL PERSPECTIVE

The science of heat detection and measurement was still quite primitive when modern chiropractic was developed in 1895.[1-3] The participation of chiropractors in the investigation of heat detection and its significance has been documented from the very origin of the profession.[4] The first reference to superficial heat emanation came from D. D. Palmer himself, who felt subtle paraspinal skin temperature differences with the sensitive dorsum of his hand, referring to abnormal areas as "hot boxes."[5] Numerous thermometry instruments were devised and used throughout early chiropractic history,[6-14] some of which are still used at the present time. As early papers on neuromuscular thermography began to appear in the medical literature, the chiropractic colleges were showing a parallel interest as early as 1968.[15-18]

In 1987, the House of Delegates of the American Chiropractic Association (ACA) approved bylaws for the formation of the American Chiropractic College of Thermology (ACCT), which functions under the direction of the ACA Council on Diagnostic Imaging. The American Chiropractic College of Thermology maintains an examining board known as the American Chiropractic Board of Thermography.[4] On June 23, 1988, the ACA House of Delegates approved a policy statement on thermography issued by the American Chiropractic College of Thermology, in cooperation with the ACA Council on Diagnostic Imaging. It stated

> The American Chiropractic College of Thermology and the Council on Diagnostic Imaging of the American Chiropractic Association accept . . . "that thermography is a legitimate diagnostic methodology which may be germane to chiropractic practice and which may also be a potential source for chiropractic research."
>
> Currently there are two recognized methods of thermographic imaging, Infrared Electronic Telethermography (IR) and Liquid Crystal Contact Thermography (LCT). Both methods require a high level of operator competency and an adherence to established and consistent protocol.
>
> Thermography, as a diagnostic aid, may be indicated when a physiological imaging test is needed for differential diagnosis. It is a procedure which objectively records evidence of skin temperature differences. Such test results must be properly correlated with a thorough history, an appropriate clinical examination, and other diagnostic studies/tests as may be indicated by clinical necessity. In this setting, diagnostic thermography may be an aid in establishing a differentiated diagnosis and in determining a prognosis.
>
> Thermography may also be utilized as objective documentary evidence of skin temperature differentials which may or may not be causally related to neuromuscular injury or abnormality. Such objective evidence is sometimes used for litigation and/or research related purposes. The utilization of thermography in this context is not intended to relate to, or affect, case management.[19]

On June 13, 1991, the ACA House of Delegates again considered its policy on thermography and voted without dissension to approve the revised policy statement jointly submitted by the ACA Council on Diagnostic Imaging and its College of Thermology. The new policy statement, designed to utilize the contemporary terminology of "High Resolution Infrared (HRI) Imaging" and to delete Liquid Crystal Thermography as an approved procedure, states:

> High Resolution Infrared (HRI) Imaging (electronic infrared thermography) is a diagnostic procedure which measures skin surface temperature. It is germane to chiropractic practice in cases where a physiologic test is required for the diagnosis of selected neurological and musculoskeletal conditions.
>
> High Resolution Infrared Imaging requires a high level of operator and interpreter competency and an adherence to established and consistent protocol.
>
> The results of High Resolution Infrared Imaging must be properly correlated with a thorough history, an appropriate clinical examination, and other diagnostic studies/tests as may be indicated by clinical necessity. In this setting, High Resolution Infrared Imaging may be an aid in establishing a differentiated diagnosis and in determining a prognosis.[20]

The study of thermography is included in the core curriculum of many chiropractic colleges, and most of these colleges are also offering postdoctoral seminar work in thermography.

At this time, no state prohibits the practice of thermography by chiropractors. Because of the historical interest in paraspinal heat detection, modern thermography is considered a usual and customary analytical procedure, although the current method of skin surface temperature evaluation is more technologically advanced than were previously available methods.

EDUCATIONAL GUIDELINES

It is generally accepted that doctors of any specialty who interpret thermograms should have completed a minimum of 60 hours of instruction in thermography in their college core curriculum, in the college clinic during internship, or through postdoctoral symposia. This is usually sufficient to ensure minimal competency. Expert credentials generally require board certification.

The specialty certification board of the American Chiropractic College of Thermology is known as the American Chiropractic Board of Thermography (ACBT). It grants certification in a two-stage process. Stage 1 requires

Part I:

1. 60 hours postgraduate thermography classroom instruction presented by a chiropractic college and pre-approved by the board
2. completion of a minimum of 50 thermographic studies
3. submission of two of the doctor's own thermography studies (one cervical with upper extremities and one lumbar with lower extremities, *or* one full body), with a written report to the board
4. application to the board

If these prerequisites are met, the applicant then takes a written examination. Stage 2 requires

Part II:

1. successful completion of the written examination in Stage 1
2. completion of an additional 40 hours (total of 100 hours) of postgraduate thermography classroom instruction presented by a chiropractic college and pre-approved by the board
3. completion of an additional 200 (total 250) thermographic studies
4. personal use of thermography in practice for 2 years
5. submission of five of the doctor's own thermographic studies (at least two cervical and two lumbar), with written reports
6. completion of a second examination that is both written and practical/oral

The stage 1 and 2 examinations may not be completed at the same sitting. These examinations are offered on a semiannual basis.

The ACBT is an ACA-affiliated organization, but an applicant need not be an ACA member to be a candidate for examination and to hold "board-certified" status from the ACBT. Even though board-certified in thermography, however, a practitioner who is not an ACA member is not eligible to become a member of the professional specialty organization, the American Chiropractic College of Thermology. In order to be a member of the college, the applicant not only must be board-certified by the ACBT, but also must be a licensed chiropractor, a member of the ACA, and a member of its Council on Diagnostic Imaging.

Members of the American Chiropractic College of Thermology must demonstrate evidence of continuing education each year in order to continue to qualify for membership. Acceptable methods are any one of the following:

1. attending an approved seminar or symposium on thermology, such as would be credited toward certified status, for 12 or more credit hours

2. teaching an approved seminar on thermology, such as would be credited toward certified status, for 12 or more credit hours for those attending the seminar
3. writing and submitting a paper that is accepted by the college

Educational guidelines for technicians who perform thermographic studies can be far less, perhaps 24 hours, because a technician can produce a good study by careful adherence to a predetermined procedure. Adequately trained practitioners can usually provide acceptable training for a technician in their own offices, making it unnecessary for a technician to attend college courses. The technical component of performing a thermogram is little more complicated than taking visible light photographs, and there is, of course, no component of risk for the patient; the technician should be conscientious and careful to observe proper protocol, however. It is ultimately the practitioner's responsibility to provide a good quality study, no matter who performs the study.

GUIDELINES FOR THERMOGRAPHY IN CHIROPRACTIC PRACTICE

Although the majority of physicians in all specialties are dedicated to ethical and scientific practice procedures, they tend to become uneasy or sometimes even belligerent when a set of practice guidelines or standards is proposed. A cut-and-dried or "average case" approach to patient care violates the patient's right to be treated according to his or her individual signs, symptoms, and history, as decided by his or her own doctor, who is intimately familiar with his or her condition. Traditionally, the doctor's burden in carrying this responsibility has been accompanied by his or her sole authority to make independent decisions and to take appropriate action. The responsibility remains, but various administrators within government and payor agencies, who are not licensed to practice the healing arts, are eroding the authority for decision-making and action.

Doctors may be wary of participating in standard setting, but they are even more reluctant to have standards imposed by others. As a result, as in many other specialty fields, proposals for guidelines/standards for thermography are currently developing at a decidedly measured and methodical pace. Until 1991, there was no national organization, chiropractic or medical, that had any detailed guidelines for thermography; only technical protocols had been developed. The thorny utilization questions of medical necessity and appropriate timing had not been officially addressed. It is virtually impossible for a professional association to address the issue of fees because of serious legal implications caused by antitrust and restraint-of-trade considerations. Even amid this confusion, however, it is clear that guidelines are best designed to advance quality patient care.

Medical Necessity

If a thermogram is to be considered "medically necessary," the chiropractic physician who orders the thermogram must document in the patient's chart notes the clinical question that, in his or her opinion as treating practitioner, would best be answered by a thermogram; it is also necessary to note that the thermogram, even if the findings are normal, will help the practitioner reach any of the following decisions:

1. formulating or confirming a diagnosis
2. determining the most effective site(s), type(s), frequency, duration, or end of treatment
3. determining the presence and/or extent of residual impairment
4. determining the prognosis

Indications

Thermography is highly germane to chiropractic practice because it is known chiefly for its effectiveness in demonstrating spinal radiculopathy[21-32] and peripheral neuropathy.[33-39] In addition, it is now considered the test of choice for the demonstration of reflex sympathetic dysfunction.[32,40-49] It is also useful in the evaluation of thoracic outlet syndrome[35,50-64] and many generalized neuromusculoskeletal conditions, such as facet syndrome,[55-61] strains/sprains, myofascial pain syndromes, trigger points and scleratomal referred pain syndromes,[32,62-81] peripheral compartment entrapment syndromes,[34,35,37,39] and the inflammation associated with joint injury, arthritis, and bursitis.[82-90] Thermography can be useful, as well, for the differential diagnosis of headache.[91-100] Normal findings on a thermogram play an important role in determining the need for further diagnostic testing.[28,101-115] Because of the significantly small percentage of false-negative results of thermograms (0.05%), [106] thermography is helpful in eliminating the need for further invasive diagnostic testing such as myelography, which involves hospitalization, pain, risk, and exposure to radiation; electromyography, which is often painful; computed tomography (CT), which requires the use of ionizing radiation; and magnetic resonance imaging (MRI), which is very costly.

Thermography is particularly useful for evaluating chronic pain.[28,108,112,116–123] Although not a "picture of pain," thermography does document the autonomic disturbances that frequently accompany pain. In addition to its low incidence of false-negative test results, thermography has a greater degree of sensitivity in documenting neuromuscular abnormality than do any of the other imaging systems,[28,101–115] again because it is a test of physiology rather than a test of anatomy. Its results compare very favorably with the results of other imaging tests, and it poses no danger or discomfort to the patient. In certain circumstances, thermography may have a lesser degree of specificity than does CT or MRI. On the other hand, it has a far greater degree of specificity than does a radionuclide bone scan. There are no physiological contraindications to thermography.

Common indications for thermographic imaging in chiropractic practice include

- evaluation for reflex sympathetic (autonomic) dysfunction
- differentiation between neurological and myofascial causation of persistent pain
- differentiation between neurological and vascular involvement
- differentiation between radicular, compartment, and peripheral neuropathy
- evaluation for myofascial trigger points
- evaluation for thoracic outlet syndrome (neurovascular compression)
- evaluation for physiological significance of minor anatomical findings noted on CT or MRI, or for further evaluation in cases of clinically suspicious radiculopathy when results of prior CT or MRI are normal
- chronic pain of undetermined origin, particularly when strong symptomatic picture is accompanied by few or no positive orthopedic or neurological findings
- evaluation for subclinical findings that preclude patient release or return to work
- evaluation for chronic and/or severe headache
- differentiation between primary joint dysfunction (sprain, capsulitis, arthritis) and neurological or myofascial disorders
- evaluation of somatic dysfunction not responding to treatment as expected by the treating chiropractor
- evaluation of the autonomic component of neuropathy (rather than limiting examination to the motor and sensory components, which are commonly examined).

- evaluation for multiple levels (sites) of neurological involvement that may not be apparent upon physical examination
- evaluation for possible fabrication, malingering, or symptom magnification
- other proposed uses justified "by report"

Procedures

The following procedural guidelines are necessary for diagnostic thermography:

1. Thermographic study should be ordered by a state-licensed doctor, who may be either the treating doctor or a chiropractic consultant who is retained to offer a second opinion.
2. Thermographic study should be ordered *following* the history taking and physical examination, the results of which indicate that a clinical question is best answered, in the opinion of the treating chiropractor, by a thermogram.
3. The area of thermographic study should be related to the patient's complaint or to findings discovered by the practitioner during the physical examination.
4. "Medical necessity" and "indication" should be documented in the patient's chart.
5. Pre-examination, facility, and study protocol should be accomplished according to the protocols published by the American Chiropractic College of Thermology, Academy of Neuromuscular Thermography,[124] or American Academy of Thermology.[125]
6. The interpreter should have appropriate training through courses and seminars offered by accredited chiropractic or medical colleges and universities.

Timing for Thermographic Evaluation

Thermographic imaging may frequently be required immediately or shortly after injury when there is a clinical suspicion of

- reflex sympathetic dysfunction, also known as causalgia, dysautonomia, or sympathetically maintained pain, because thermography is the test of choice for this condition and rapid initiation of specific appropriate treatment is vital

- vascular injury, as expeditious referral to a vascular specialist may be necessary

Thermographic imaging may be required shortly after injury for the evaluation of clinically suspicious segmental or peripheral neuropathy, if the treating chiropractor determines that the case management would be affected by the findings.

Full-protocol thermographic imaging is not routinely required shortly after injury when the appropriate mode of initial treatment is apparent to the treating chiropractor after the history and physical examination; however, scout or limited thermograms may be used to assist in the physical examination. A full-protocol diagnostic thermogram may be required at a later time during the course of the same condition if the patient fails to respond according to the treating chiropractor's expectations. Any follow-up thermographic studies are subject to the same requirements (eg, establishment of medical necessity and adequate indication, adherence to proper procedures) that apply to initial studies.

Stress (Provocative) Testing

Mechanical or thermal stress testing may be required for adequate interpretation of thermal findings, and such testing should be conducted according to established protocols.[124–127] In mechanical stress testing, the patient is asked to perform the normal body movements that cause or aggravate pain; images are then collected. For thermal stress testing, applications of cold or heat (usually by water immersion) are used to stimulate a vascular response; the examiner then determines if a symptomatic part reacts in the same manner and at the same rate as does an asymptomatic control part similarly challenged. Such provocative testing is performed *after* neutral baseline images have been collected; for example, between the second and third replications of a triplicate study.

Other Uses of Thermography

Documentary Thermography

A thermogram that is performed solely to acquire objective evidence of neuromuscular injury or other abnormality and is not expected to affect case management is considered a documentary procedure. Whereas producing a documentary thermogram is analogous to, and as acceptable as, producing photographs of a patient's contusions and abrasions, such a thermogram does not qualify as a "medically necessary" diagnostic test.

Screening Thermography

Abbreviated thermographic testing, because it is noninvasive, may be useful for screening asymptomatic populations. For example, it may be appropriate for scoliosis screening and pre-employment screening of candidates for heavy industrial activities. These abbreviated screening tests are not "medically necessary," as they are performed on asymptomatic individuals; however, they may reveal an abnormality that would require another form of diagnostic testing, which may include a full-protocol thermogram. In that case, that justified follow-up thermogram or other type of diagnostic test would be considered "medically necessary."

Breast Thermography

The production and interpretation of a thermogram by a chiropractic physician solely for the purpose of evaluating breast disease is not an established procedure. Chiropractic physicians should, however, make a notation of abnormal breast findings visualized incidentally on a neuromusculoskeletal thermogram and refer the patient for mammographic evaluation and appropriate management.

On June 13, 1991, the ACA House of Delegates approved "Guidelines for Thermography in Chiropractic Practice," which essentially summarized, in an abbreviated fashion, the discussion included above. These Guidelines are as follows:[128]

Thermographic Description:
Thermography is a diagnostic procedure which measures skin surface temperature distribution.

Thermographic Policy:
This diagnostic imaging procedure is germane to chiropractic practice in cases where a physiologic test is required. High Resolution Infrared (HRI) Imaging* is a useful procedure for the diagnosis of selected neurological and musculoskeletal conditions.
*Electronic Infrared Thermography

Guidelines for Determining Medical Necessity:
The treating doctor shall certify as to the medical necessity of the thermographic study based upon a diagnostic clinical question and

the effect of the results on case management decisions. The referring doctor shall certify to the medical necessity by prescription.

HRI Imaging is of value in the diagnostic evaluation of patients when the clinical history suggests the presence of one of the following situations:

1. Early diagnosis and monitoring of reflex sympathetic dystrophy syndromes.
2. Evaluation of spinal nerve root/fiber irritation and distal peripheral nerve fiber pathology for detection of sensory/autonomic dysfunction.
3. To evaluate and monitor soft tissue injuries, including segmental dysfunction/subluxation, sprain, and myofascial conditions (strains and myofascial pain syndromes) not responding to clinical treatment.
4. To evaluate for the physiological significance of equivocal or minor anatomical findings seen on myelogram, CT and/or MRI.
5. To evaluate for feigned disorders.

Utilization Review:
Because of the detailed knowledge, training, and skill level required, thermographic studies ordered, produced, or interpreted by chiropractic physicians must be reviewed only by a licensed chiropractor who holds appropriate** credentials with regards to knowledge, skill, and experience in thermography. Only licensed chiropractors holding such credentials can claim sufficient competence to make valid judgments or comments regarding appropriateness, necessity, or accuracy of thermographic studies, and their relevance to chiropractic case management.

**Board Certified status with the American Chiropractic Board of Thermography or other national thermographic certifying board which restricts its examination to candidates who have completed a prescribed postgraduate syllabus program offered by a chiropractic college having status with a national chiropractic accrediting agency approved by the United States Department of Education (USDE).[128]

PROTOCOL

In March of 1988, the American Chiropractic College of Thermology issued the following statement on neuromusculoskeletal thermographic protocol.[127]

Rules of Protocol:

1. Any of the rules of protocol can be altered by a physician if more than one study is performed, providing he can give a plausible reason for the alteration not having a significant effect on the results of the studies, show that the results of the studies are consistent, show that the thermographic diagnostic impressions correlate well with other physical, orthopedic, myofascial, neurological examination or laboratory findings, and show that the diagnostic impressions are consistent with the patient's history and his presenting complaints.

Number of Studies:

2. A thermographic evaluation consisting of three studies is preferred for diagnostic criteria. Studies are usually performed consecutively on the same day. However, this is not a fixed rule. Two studies could be done on one day, and the third study could be done days or weeks later.
3. Two studies can be adequate for routine office diagnosis. If the results of the studies are consistent, this is sufficient for a diagnostic impression.
4. One study is adequate for a *screening* type of evaluation. Based on positive results, one or more additional studies could be ordered by a physician, if a diagnostic impression were required.

Stress Studies:

5. If three studies are performed on the same day, the patient may be asked, by a physician, to move in such a way as to exacerbate the symptoms (in between the second and third study). This permits an evaluation of the effects of stress on the patient's condition. These movements must be performed bilaterally.
6. It may be necessary for a physician to have the patient stressed by an autonomic challenge. This should be done as the last part of the thermographic examination.
7. If a part of the body is to be cooled utilizing an alcohol spray, a water mist, or a blow dryer set on cool, followed by an equilibration period, and this is to be followed by thermographic views being taken of that region, then this should be performed as the final procedure after all other studies are complete.

Examining Room:

Temperature:

8. The temperature of the room should be such that the patient is not perspiring and not shivering. However, under arm perspiration might be present with some nervous patients and could be blotted by the technician. 20° Celsius to 29° Celsius is acceptable.
9. Room temperature changes during the course of an examination must be very gradual so that all parts of the patient's body can adjust uniformly. A rule of thumb is for the room temperature to not change by more than one degree Celsius over the course of a single study.
10. The examining room must have at least one thermometer to record the room temperature during the examination.
11. The temperature gradient between the surfaces to the right and the left sides of the patient must be less than 1° Celsius. This must also be true for the temperature gradient between the surface immediately either in front or behind the patient and an equal distance in the opposite direction.
12. The thermographic examination room should be carpeted. If this is not the case, then the patient area should be covered with heavy matting.

Room Size:

13. The room size should be of sufficient size for the patient and technical personnel to have enough freedom of movement to properly use the thermographic equipment.

Windows and Doors:

14. Windows should be covered to prevent infrared radiation from entering or escaping from the room. Shades and blinds are adequate for this purpose. Windows should be sealed to prevent drafts in the area around the patient. Doors should not allow drafts in the area around the patient.

Lighting:

15. Standard fluorescent or diffused incandescent lights are adequate.

Drafts:

  16. The area where the patient stands must be relatively free of air
      currents.

Ventilation:

  17. Room ventilation should be such that the above specifications
      for drafts and temperature stability are maintained.
  18. Heat sources should be minimized in the room and must be
      kept well away from the patient. Heat sources must also be
      directed away from the patient.

Humidity:

  19. Humidity needs only the same control that would be normally
      expected in a professional office. It must be low enough that
      the patient is not perspiring.

Views:

  20. The views taken should encompass the symptomatic region of
      the body and all neurovascular components appropriate for
      the test.
  21. Local spot studies are appropriate when the physician has
      justification, such as a patient history indicating a local
      trauma or possibly a tentative diagnosis of a local problem.
  22. Once an initial thermographic evaluation has been performed
      and a patient is to be re-evaluated at a later date, in order to
      monitor the patient's condition and/or the effectiveness of
      treatment, a physician has the discretion to restrict the ther-
      mographic studies to the views which were positive in the
      original thermographic evaluation.
  23. Areas capable of being viewed should be appropriate for the
      equipment.

Equilibration and Disrobing:

  24. It is necessary for each region of the body to be studied to
      have been uncovered (completely exposed to the room air)
      and to not have touched anything, for at least 15 minutes
      before a thermographic study of that area is made. The soles

of the feet are an exception. However, specialized gowning techniques may be appropriate under certain conditions.

Time between Studies:

25. When one study is finished, the next one can be started immediately, provided the parts of the body to be studied have been uncovered and have not touched anything for the previous 15 minutes. The soles of the feet are an exception. However, there must be at least 15 minutes of elapsed time between the beginning of one study and the start of the next study.

Equipment:

26. Contact thermographic equipment utilizing a range of interchangeable screens is appropriate for neuromusculoskeletal thermographic studies.
27. Electronic thermographic equipment utilizing an infrared scanner, which scans in two directions is appropriate for neuromusculoskeletal thermographic studies.
28. Temperature repeatability and accuracy of 0.1° Celsius is adequate for electronic equipment. (This gives a signal to noise ratio of 5:1 for 0.5 degree temperature differentials.) Absolute temperature measurements are not required, only relative temperatures and temperature differentials are important.
29. When multiple views are used for bilaterally equivalent areas, the equipment settings and technique are recommended to be identical.
30. For electronic studies, the scanner must be aimed perpendicular to the surface to be viewed.

Patient Identification:

31. The thermographic composite, captured on archival media, should have the following minimum information:
    a. Patient's name or identification code
    b. Either the name or identification code of the clinical facility or the name or identification code of the doctor rendering the service
    c. Date the service was rendered
    d. An indication to which study the view pertains, if not obvious

32. The following instructions or something similar will be given to the patient prior to coming for the examination. Many of these instructions may exceed the minimum requirements. However, due to lack of research documentation, and given a patient's propensity to ignore instructions, a considerable buffer has been provided. Should these instructions not be adhered to, then it is the physician's judgment as to whether the test should be performed, canceled, or rescheduled.

   a. Shower or bathe the night before your scheduled test. Do not shower, bathe, or use a sauna, whirlpool, etc. within four (4) hours of your scheduled test.

   b. For 24 hours prior to your test, take *only* those medications which a physician has told you are required.

   c. Avoid sunburn.

   d. Do not do heavy exercise for four (4) hours before the test, or undergo any kind of physical therapy, chiropractic care, or use a Transcutaneous Electrical Nerve Stimulator (TENS unit) for 24 hours prior to the test.

   e. Wear loose-fitting clothing, and remove all rings, jewelry, watches, etc., if possible, prior to entering our facility. Girdles and support hosiery should not be worn to the test. Hair should be bound up on the top of the head.

   f. Do not consume any food or beverages for two (2) hours prior to the test.

   g. Do not smoke for at least two (2) hours prior to your test.

   h. Do not use liniment or skin irritants for 24 hours prior to your test.

The foregoing technical protocols, approved in 1988, encompass liquid crystal thermography. It is likely, in view of the 1991 decision to delete liquid crystal thermography as an approved procedure, that relevant sections of the technical protocols will be changed.

TYPES OF STUDIES

The Current Procedural Terminology (CPT) categorization for thermography is clearly insufficient.[129] The two categories currently included in CPT-4 are a "cephalic" study, which is coded 93760, and a "peripheral" study, which is coded 93762. These codes are categorized under vascular procedures, and they would be adequate for a thermogram ordered to evaluate the venous or arterial systems. They are not adequate for neuromuscular examination, however.

Ultimately, it will be more appropriate to devise new CPT codes under the diagnostic imaging section 7xxxx. The following categorization is adequate for the thermography purposes usually undertaken within the chiropractic profession:

1. upper body (currently being informally coded as 93762WC)
2. lower body (currently being informally coded as 93762WD)
3. limited thoracic (currently being informally coded as 93760WA)
4. full body (currently being informally coded as 93762WC and 93762WD)
5. special limited study (currently being informally coded as 93762)
6. facial (currently being informally coded as 93760)

The number of images necessary to comprise a complete study varies, depending on the equipment used. There are two separate circumstances: (1) typical resolution infrared equipment and (2) high-resolution infrared equipment. Typical resolution electronic infrared equipment ($30,000 to $65,000 equipment cost) requires the following views:

1. upper body: posterior cervicothoracic, including posterior arms; close-up posterior cervical; anterior cervicothoracic, including anterior arms; left lateral neck, shoulder, arm; right lateral neck, shoulder, arm; anterior (palmar) forearms and hands; posterior (dorsal) forearms and hands; additional optional views to visualize further anything not well demonstrated in the aforementioned standard views; for example, separate views of the hands, radial forearms and hands, ulnar forearms and hands. Many facilities also include an anterior face, anterior and lateral thoracic, and/or superior shoulder views.
2. lower body: posterior thoracolumbar/gluteal; close-up posterior lumbar qualitative (black and white); posterior thighs; anterior thighs; left lateral thigh; right lateral thigh; anterior legs; posterior legs; dorsal feet; plantar feet; additional optional views to visualize further anything not well demonstrated on the aforementioned standard views; for example, oblique gluteals, lateral hip and flank, medial and lateral legs, qualitative (black and white) views of vascular abnormalities.
3. limited thoracic: anterior, posterior, left lateral, right lateral.
4. special limited study: anterior, posterior, medial, and lateral views of limited comparable parts, such as hands or feet, for the evaluation of a specific localized condition such as reflex sympathetic dysfunction or local inflammation.
5. Facial: anterior, left lateral, right lateral.

The newest wide-field high-resolution electronic infrared systems ($80,000 + equipment cost) provide such spectacular image clarity that the entire body can be imaged in one field. Thus, only a front view, a back view, and left and right lateral views are necessary. These images can then be segmented and enlarged by means of the software computer programs that are a part of this equipment, providing data fully comparable to the data produced by spot views with less sophisticated equipment.

In the final analysis, the number of views is not nearly as important as ensuring that the entire region being studied is included in the fields presented. As an example, some electronic scanners may be able to image forearms and hands on the same view and other types of equipment may necessitate separate views in order to adequately visualize all parts.

Furthermore, all views must be repeated three times, with a minimum 15-minute equilibration period between like views, in order for the study to be considered a full-protocol thermogram. Practitioners may decide on a case-by-case basis when a full-protocol thermogram is not necessary.

COSTS

In determining the costs of thermography, it is important to take into account the frequent necessity of producing the required views in triplicate. This considerably increases the tie-up of the operator, equipment, and examination room. It is not appropriate, therefore, to equate the cost of thermography to the cost of diagnostic ultrasound or electromyography. The cost of a full-protocol upper body *or* lower body thermogram more closely corresponds to that of CT, but it is not as expensive as MRI. This comparison applies to *regional* thermography, that is, a lumbar thermogram compared to a lumbar CT scan. A *full-body* thermogram is performed much more frequently than are full-body CT studies, and such a thermogram would, of course, result in greater costs. A full-body thermogram may be ordered not only because thermography is completely risk-free, but also because, being a physiological rather than an anatomical test, it frequently provides vital data on the effect of one region on another region. For example, chiropractors have traditionally recognized that cervical spine symptoms frequently arise from lumbopelvic biomechanical disorders. With thermography, this information relative to somatic dysfunction and physiology can be discerned at no risk to the patient.

Whereas the equipment costs for CT and MRI are substantially higher than are equipment costs for thermography, the unusual length of time required to produce a full-protocol thermogram must be emphasized. A facility could produce three unenhanced lumbar CT studies (performed by technicians) in the length of time that it would take to produce one full-protocol lumbar thermogram.

Making a comparison to plain film x-ray, we find that the time required for a lumbar thermogram is approximately six times greater than the time required for a typical lumbar plain film x-ray study, and the equipment cost for infrared thermography is two to three times higher than the cost for plain film x-ray equipment. Good x-ray equipment for producing plain film skeletal x-ray studies may cost roughly $25,000 to $30,000; a typical lumbar x-ray study, which may consist of five views, takes an operator approximately 15 minutes to perform. The average electronic infrared thermography euqipment would cost roughly $50,000; a typical electronic lumbar thermographic study which may consist of 10 to 12 views, all of which are generally repeated three times (30 to 36 views total), requires 75 to 90 minutes to perform.

It is necessary only to determine the fees per study, thus computing the amount of revenue that can be generated in a comparable length of time by a diagnostic imaging center, to recognize the profound impact of patient through-put in any reckoning of costs involved. It does not take long to begin to negate the effect of the high initial equipment cost, particularly when considering the related tax implications of purchasing and maintaining that equipment, as well as staff costs.

Scout views or single or duplicate studies are sometimes performed in order to answer less formal clinical questions, resulting in lower costs than are encountered in full-protocol triplicate studies. A "single" study (the production of only one view of each surface in the region being studied) requires the same amount of patient and facility preparation as does a triplicate study, however. The effort required to perform a single set of views is, therefore, greater than one-third of the full-protocol triplicate study; rather, it requires approximately one-half of the effort required for a triplicate study. A duplicate study would require two-thirds to three-fourths of the effort required of a triplicate study.

CONCLUSION

In its present state, thermography is a highly sensitive and very effective imaging method that has three distinct advantages over other diagnostic methods: it is risk-free, it is painless, and it provides physiological information. Properly correlated with the finding of the history and physical examination, a thermogram may provide diagnostic assistance not otherwise available and may help to avoid more costly or dangerous testing. Furthermore, it is becoming increasingly apparent that the availability of physiological information may refine surgical decisions to the point of improving results.[130]

Indeed, modern thermal imaging equipment simply adds sophistication to an analytical process that has traditionally been employed within the chiropractic profession. As of 1987, thermography has been brought under the guidance and direction of chiropractic political and educational institutions, and its further development and utilization will be dictated by continued research and by reliance on the protocols and guidelines that have been discussed.

REFERENCES

1. Bar-Sella H. Infrared thermography—An historical perspective. In: *Academy of Neuro-Muscular Thermography Clinical Proceedings*. Dallas: Postgraduate Medicine Custom Communications; 1985:104–106.

2. Mueller J, Christiansen J. *Historical Aspects of Medical and Chiropractic Thermology*. Lombard, Ill: National College of Chiropractic; 1988. Monograph.

3. Gershon-Cohen J. A short history of medical thermometry. *Ann NY Acad Sci.* 1965;122:4–11.

4. Vlasuk SL. Chiropractic and thermography: A historic perspective. *ACA Journal of Chiropractic.* 1989:42–52.

5. Christiansen J. Thermography boon or bust for chiropractic. *ACA Journal of Chiropractic.* 1985;19:60–62.

6. Dye AA. *The Evolution of Chiropractic.* Richmond Hall; 1939.

7. Eddy HC, Taylor HP. Experiences with the dermatherm (tycos) in relation to peripheral vascular disease. *Am Heart J.* 1931:683–689.

8. Palmer BJ. Precise posture spinograph comparative graphs. Davenport, Iowa; Palmer School of Chiropractic Press; 1938;20.

9. Biron WA, Wells BJ, Houser RH. *Chiropractic Principles and Technic.* Chicago: National College of Chiropractic; 1939.

10. Kimmel EH. The dermathermograph. *Journal of Clinical Chiropractic.* 1969;1:78–86.

11. Novick ND. The VNT photo-electric instrument. *Journal of Clinical Chiropractic.* 1969;2:78–83.

12. Sherman LW. Neurocalometer, neurocalograph, neurotempometer research. Davenport, Iowa: Palmer School of Chiropractic Press; 1946.

13. Haldeman S. First impressions of the synchro-therme as a skin temperature reading instrument. *J CA Chir Assn.* 1970:7–8.

14. Haldeman S. Observations made under test conditions with the synchro-therme. *J CA Chiro Assn.* 1970:9–12.

15. Janse J. Personal communication to Maurer EL. Lombard, Ill, October 4, 1968.

16. Dudley WN. Thermography and the body. *ACA Journal of Chiropractic.* 1973;7:530–532,

17. Dudley WN. Personal communication to Vlasuk SL. Howell, Mich, October 20, 1986.

18. Jenness M. The role of thermography and postural measurement in structural diagnosis. In: Goldstein M, ed. *The Research Status of Spinal Manipulative Therapy.* Bethesda, Md: US Department of Health, Education and Welfare; 1975:255–263. DHEW Pub No (NIH) 76-998, NINCDS.

19. Policy statement on thermography, American Chiropractic College of Thermology and ACA Council on Diagnostic Imaging, ratified by ACA House of Delegates, June 23, 1988.

20. Policy statement on thermography, American Chiropractic College of Thermology and ACA Council on Diagnostic Imaging, ratified by ACA House of Delegates, June 13, 1991.

21. Deunsing F, Becker P, Rittmeyer K. Thermographic findings in lumbar disc protrusions. *Arch Psychiatr Nervenkr.* 1973;217:53-70.

22. Raskin MM, Martinez-Lopez M, Sheldon JJ. Lumbar thermography in discogenic disease. *Radiology.* 1976;119:149-152.

23. Ching C, Wexler CE. Peripheral thermographic manifestations of lumbar disk diseases. *Applied Radiology.* 1978;100:53-58.

24. Wexler CE. Lumbar, thoracic, and cervical thermography. *Journal of Neurol and Orthop Surg.* 1980;1(2).

25. Pochaczevsky R, Wexler CE, Meyers PH, Epstein JA, Marc JA. Liquid crystal thermography of the spine and extremities. *J Neurosurg.* 1982;56:386-395.

26. Fischer AA, Chang CH, Kuo JC. Value of thermography in diagnosis of radiculopathy as compared with electrodiagnosis. *Arch Phys Med Rehabil.* 1983;64:526.

27. Green J, Noran WH, Coyle MC, Gildemeister RG. Infrared electronic thermography (ET): A non-invasive diagnostic neuroimaging tool. *Contemporary Orthopedics.* 1985;11:39-48.

28. Hubbard JE. Statistical review of thermography in a neurology practice: Pain evaluation. In: *Academy of Neuromuscular Thermography Clinical Proceedings.* Dallas: Postgraduate Medicine Custom Communications; 1985:65-72.

29. Adatto KN, Phillips SI, Manale BL, Watermeier JJ, King AG, Bartholomew PM. Thermography and computed tomography in evaluation of lumbar disc disease. In: Abernathy M, Uematsu S, eds. *Medical Thermology.* Washington, DC: American Academy of Thermology; 1986:170-174.

30. Hubbard JE. Thermal imaging of radiculopathy: A review. In: *Academy of Neuromuscular Thermography Clinical Proceedings.* Orlando, Fla: Modern Medicine Public; 1986:65-71.

31. Hubbard JE, Maultsby J, Wexler CE. Lumbar and cervical thermography for nerve fiber impingement; A critical review. *Clinical Journal of Pain.* 1986;2:131-137.

32. Council on Scientific Affairs. *Thermography in Neurological and Musculoskeletal Conditions.* Chicago: American Medical Association; 1987.

33. Pulst SM, Haller P. Thermographic assessment of impaired sympathetic function in peripheral nerve injuries. *J Neurol.* 1981;226:35-42.

34. Herrick RT, Herrick SK. Thermography in the detection of carpal tunnel syndrome and other compressive neuropathies. *J Hand Surgery.* 1981;12A:943-949.

35. Nakano KK. Liquid crystal contact thermography (LCT) in the evaluation of patients with upper limb entrapment neuropathies. *J Neurol Orthop Surg.* 1984;5:97-102.

36. Brelsford KL, Uematsu S. Thermographic presentation of cutaneous sensory and vasomotor activity in the injured peripheral nerve. *J Neurosurg.* 1985;62:711-715.

37. Uematsu S. Thermographic imaging of cutaneous sensory segment in patients with peripheral nerve injury. *J Neurosurg.* 1985;62:716-720.

38. Jablecki CH. Thermography in carpal tunnel syndrome. In: Abernathy M, Uematsu S, eds. *Medical Thermology.* Washington, DC: American Academy of Thermology; 1986:153-157.

39. Gateless D, Gilroy J, Nefcy P. Thermographic evaluation of carpal tunnel syndrome during pregnancy. *Thermology.* 1988;3:21-25.

40. Ecker A. Contact thermography in diagnosis of reflex sympathetic dystrophy: A new look at pathogenesis. *Thermology.* 1985;1:106-109.

41. Adatto KN, Phillips SI, Manale BL, Watermeier JJ, Brickmann I, Dudek JK. Thermography: A useful tool in the diagnosis of post-traumatic sympathetic dystrophy. In: *Academy of Neuromuscular Thermography Clinical Proceedings.* Orlando, Fla: Modern Medicine Public; 1986:30-34.

42. Green J, Reilly A, Hazelwood C, Becker C. Sympathetic skin response abnormalities correlated with abnormal infrared thermography in patients with low back pain and radiculopathy. In: *Academy of Neuromuscular Thermography Clinical Proceedings.* Orlando, Fla: Modern Medicine Public; 1986:89–92.

43. Perelman RB, Adler D, Humphreys M. Reflex sympathetic dystrophy: A thermographic evaluation. In: *Academy of Neuromuscular Thermography Clinical Proceedings.* Orlando, Fla: Modern Medicine Public; 1986:21–29.

44. Uricchio JV. Reflex sympathetic dystrophy and causalgia. In: *Academy of Neuromuscular Thermography Clinical Proceedings.* Orlando, Fla: Modern Medicine Public; 1986:13–20.

45. Ignacio D, Azer RN, Shibuya J, Pavot AP. Thermographic monitoring of sympathetic nerve block. *Thermology.* 1986;2:21–24.

46. Ochoa J. The newly recognized painful ABC syndrome: Thermograhic aspects. *Thermology.* 1986;2:65–107.

47. Kobrossi T, Steimann I. Reflex sympathetic dystrophy of the upper extremity. *Journal of the Canadian Chiropractic Association.* 1986;30(1):29–32.

48. Edwards BE. Reflex sympathetic dystrophy since Livingston. *Thermology.* 1988;3:59–61.

49. BenEliyahu DJ. Thermography in the diagnosis of sympathetic maintained pain. *American Journal of Chiropractic Medicine.* 1989;2(2):55–60.

50. Nakano KK. Neurogenic thoracic outlet syndromes. *J Neurol Orthop Surg.* 1983;4:323–326.

51. Richardson RR, Torres H, Analitis S, Downie J. Traumatic thoracic outlet syndrome. *J Neurol Orthop Surg.* 1983;4(4):327–337.

52. Pavot AP, Ignacio DR. Value of infrared imaging in the diagnosis of thoracic outlet syndrome. *Thermology.* 1986;1:142–145.

53. Nakano KK. Liquid crystal contact thermography in the evaluation of patients with neurogenic thoracic outlet syndrome. In: Abernathy M, Uematsu S, eds. *Medical Thermology.* Washington, DC: American Academy of Thermology; 1986;92–98.

54. Conwell TD. Thoracic outlet syndrome: Current diagnostic concepts and case management. Brooklandville, Md.: DC Tracts, Data Trace Chiropractic Publishers, 1990;2(3):165–180.

55. Mooney V, Robertson J. The facet syndrome. *Clin Orthop.* 1976;115:149–156.

56. McFadden JW. Thermography used to diagnose the facet syndrome. *J Neurol Orthop Surg.* 1983;4:353–357.

57. Wexler CE. *Atlas of Lumbar Thermographic Patterns.* Tarzana, Calif: Thermographic Services; 1983.

58. Chapman G, Britt BA. *Clinical Thermography: II and III.* Chula Vista, Calif: CTA Publications; 1984.

59. Leroy P, Christian CR, Filasky R. Diagnostic thermography in low back pain syndromes. *Clinical Journal of Pain.* 1985;1:4–13.

60. McFadden JW. Liquid crystal thermography and the facet syndrome. In: Abernathy M, Uematsu S, eds. *Medical Thermology.* Washington, DC: American Academy of Thermology; 1986:799–782.

61. Hobbins WB. Initial, private publ. *Thermal Image Analysis.* Madison, Wis: Author; 1987;8(2):8–9.

62. Head H. On disturbances of sensation with special reference to the pain of visceral disease. *Brain.* 1893;4:1–158.

63. Kellgren JH. Observations on referred pain arising from muscle. *Clinical Sci.* 1938;3:175–190.

64. Kellgren JH. The anatomical source of back pain. *Rheumatol Rehabil.* 16;1:3–9.

65. Pedersen HE, Blunck CFJ, Gardner E. The anatomy of lumbosacral posterior rami and meningeal branches of spinal nerves (sinuvertebral nerve). *J Bone Joint Surg.* 1956;38A(2):377–391.

66. Karpman HL, Knebel A, Semel CJ, Cooper J. Clinical studies in thermography: II. Application of thermography in evaluating musculoligamentous injuries of the spine. *Arch Environ Health.* 1970;20:412-417.

67. Hobbins WB. Thermography and pain. In: Gautherie M, Albert E, eds. *Biomedical Thermology.* New York: Alan R. Liss; 1982:361-375.

68. Travell JG, Simons DG. *Myofascial Pain and Dysfunction: The Trigger Point Manual.* Baltimore; Williams & Wilkins; 1983.

69. Simons DG, Travell JR. Myofascial origins of low back pain. *Postgrad Med.* 1983;73(2):66-108.

70. Kobrossi T. Clinical use of thermography in the diagnosis of soft tissue lesions. *Journal of the Canadian Chiropractic Association.* 1984;28(3):319-327.

71. Fischer AA. Correlation between site of pain and "hot spots" on thermogram in lower body. In: *Academy of Neuromuscular Thermography Clinical Proceedings.* Dallas: Postgraduate Medicine Custom Communications; 1985:99.

72. Weinstein G. The diagnosis of trigger points by thermography. In: *Academy of Neuromuscular Thermography Clinical Proceedings.* Dallas: Postgraduate Medicine Custom Communications; 1985:96-98.

73. Fischer AA, Chang CH. Temperature and pressure threshold measurements in trigger points. *Thermology.* 1986;1:212-215.

74. Fischer AA. Pressure threshold measurement for diagnosis of myofascial pain and evaluation of treatment results. *Clinical Journal of Pain.* 1987;2:207-214.

75. Diakow PRP. Thermographic imaging of myofascial trigger points. *Journal of Manipulative and Physiological Therapeutics.* 1988;11:114-117.

76. Simons DG. Myofascial pain syndromes: Where are we? Where are we going? *Arch Phys Med Rehabil.* 1988; 69:207-212.

77. Fischer AA. Documentation of myofascial trigger points. *Arch Phys Med Rehabil.* 1988;69:286-291.

78. Conwell TD. Musculoskeletal thermography. *Colorado Chiropractor.* 1989; 2:32-37; 3:24-30.

79. Kent C, Gentempo P. Objective documentation of soft tissue lesions with thermography and electromyography. *Am Chiropractor.* 1989:22-25.

80. Jinkins JR, Whittemore AR, Bradley WG. The anatomic basis of vertebrogenic pain and the autonomic syndrome associated with lumbar disc extrusion. *Am J Roentgenol.* 1989;152:1277-1289.

81. BenEliyahu D. Thermography in clinical chiropractic practice. *ACA Journal of Chiropractic.* 1989;26:59-72.

82. Ring EFJ, Collins AJ, Bacon PA, Cosh JA. Quantification of thermography in arthritis using multi-isothermal analysis. *Am Rheum Dis.* 1974;33:353-356.

83. Binder A. A clinical and thermographic study of lateral epicondylitis. *British Journal of Rheumatol.* 1983;22:77-81.

84. Lobenko AA. Use of liquid crystal thermography for diagnosis of trauma of the extremities. *Ortho Tramatol I Protez.* 1983;6:26.

85. Devereaux MD, Parr GR, Lachmann SM, et al. The diagnosis of stress fractures in athletes. *JAMA.* 1984;252:531-533.

86. Hazelman BL. An improved method for using thermography to assess activity in rheumatoid arthritis. *Int Med.* 1985;5:63-67.

87. Goodman PH, Heaslet NW, Pagliano JR, Rubin BD. Stress fracture diagnosis by computer-assisted thermography. *Physician and Sportsmedicine.* 1985;13(4):114-132.

88. Devereaux MD, Parr GR, Lachmann SM, Page-Thomas DP, Hazleman BL. Thermographic diagnosis in athletes with patellofemoral arthralgia. *J Bone Joint Surg.* 1986;68:42-44.

89. Ignacio DR, Pavot A, Azer RN, Jackson H. Thermography and decompensated shoulder syndrome. In: Abernathy M, Uematsu S, eds. *Medical Thermology.* Washington, DC: American Academy of Thermology; 1986:120-123.

90. Hobbins WB. Thermography in sports medicine. In: Appenzeller O, ed. *Sports Medicine.* Urban and Schwarzenberg; 1988:chap 22.

91. Lance JW, Anthony M. Thermographic studies in vascular headache. *Med J Aust.* 1971:240–243.

92. Kudrow L. Thermographic and doppler flow asymmetry in cluster headache. *Headache.* 1979;19:204–208.

93. Drummond PD, Lance JW. Thermographic changes in cluster headaches. *Neurology.* 1984;34:1292–1298.

94. Drummond PD, Lance JW. Facial temperature in migraine, tension-vascular and tension headache. *Cephalgia.* 1984;4:149–158.

95. Finney JW, Holt CR, Pearce KB. Thermographic diagnosis of temporomandibular joint disease and associated neuromuscular disorders. In: *Academy of Neuromuscular Thermography Clinical Proceedings.* Dallas: Postgraduate Medicine Custom Communications; 1985:93–95.

96. Kudrow L. A distinctive facial thermographic pattern in cluster headache—The "Chai" sign. *Headache.* 1985;25:33–36.

97. Swerdlow B. Thermographic documentation in a case of post-traumatic dysautonomic cephalgia. *Thermology.* 1985;1:102–105.

98. Swerdlow B, Dieter JN. The persistent migraine cold patch and the fixed facial thermogram. *Thermology.* 1986;2:16–20.

99. Swerdlow B, Dieter JN. The validity of the vascular "cold patch" in the diagnosis of chronic headache. *Headache.* 1986;26:22–26.

100. Rapoport AM, Sheftel FD, Altemus M. Correlations of facial thermographic patterns and headache diagnosis. In: Abernathy M, Uematsu S, eds. *Medical Thermology.* Washington, DC: American Academy of Thermology; 1986:56–61.

101. Uricchio JV. Thermography: The clinical use of thermography in orthopedic practice. In: *Academy of Neuromuscular Thermography Clinical Proceedings.* Dallas: Postgraduate Medicine Custom Communications; 1985:62–64.

102. Uricchio JV. Blinded reading of electronic thermography. In: *Academy of Neuromuscular Thermography Clinical Proceedings.* Dallas: Postgraduate Medicine Custom Communications; 1985:47–53.

103. Adatto KN, Phillips SI, Mandale BL, et al. CT and thermogram: A comparison of 91 patients. *Ortho Trans.* 1985;9:215.

104. Harway RA. A comparison of the results of thermography, computerized tomography scanning, and myelogram evultions in 66 patients with lumbar pain. In: *Academy of Neuromuscular Thermography Clinical Proceedings.* Dallas: Postgraduate Medicine Custom Communications; 1985:73–77.

105. Fischer AA. The present status of neuromuscular thermography. In: *Academy of Neuromuscular Thermography Clinical Proceedings.* Dallas: Postgraduate Medicine Custom Communications; 1985:26–33.

106. Weinstein SA, Wesinstein G. A review of 500 patients with low back complaints: Comparison of five clinically-accepted diagnostic modalities. In: Academy of Neuromuscular Thermography Clinical Proceedings. Dallas: Postgraduate Medicine Custom Communications; 1985:40–43.

107. Weinstein SA, Weinstein G. A clinical comparison of cervical thermography with EMG, CT scanning, myelography, and surgical procedures in 500 patients. In: *Academy of Neuromuscular Thermography Clinical Proceedings.* Dallas: Postgraduate Medicine Custom Communications; 1985:44–46.

108. Hubbard JE. Pain evaluation by electronic infrared thermography: Correlations with symptoms, EMG, myelogram and CT scan. *Thermology.* 1985;1:26–35.

109. Brown RKJ, Bassett LW, Wexler CE, Gold RH. Thermography as a screening modality for nerve fiber irritation in patients with low back pain. In: *Academy of Neuromuscular Thermography Clinical Proceedings.* Orlando, Fla: Modern Medicine Public; 1986:86–88.

110. Green J, Reilly A, Schnitzlein N, Clewell W. Comparison of neurothermography and contrast myelography. *Orthopedics*. 1986;9:1699–1704.

111. Goldberg GS. Infrared imaging and magnetic resonance imaging correlated in 35 cases. *Thermology*. 1986;1:207–211.

112. Hubbard JE. Pain evaluation in 805 studies by infrared imaging. *Thermology*. 1986;1:161–166.

113. Weinstein SA, Weinstein G. Trends in clinical practice induced by standardized electronic thermography: A review of 2000 patients. In: *Academy of Neuromuscular Thermography Clinical Proceedings*. Orlando, Fla: Modern Medicine Public; 1986:58–64.

114. Weinstein SA, Weinstein G. Thermography and other accepted diagnostic modalities: A comparison. *Journal of Osteopathic Medicine*. 1988;33–36.

115. Chafetz N, Wexler CE, Kaiser JA. Neuromuscular thermography of the lumbar spine with CT correlation. *Spine*. 1988;13:922–925.

116. Uematsu S, Long DM. Thermography in chronic pain, In: Uematsu S, ed. *Medical Thermology, Theory and Clinical Applications*. Los Angeles: Brentwood Publishing Co; 1976:52–68.

117. Uematsu S, Hendler N, Hungerford D, Long DM, Ono H. Thermography and electromyography in the differential diagnosis of chronic pain syndromes and reflex sympathetic dystrophy. *Electromyogr Clin Neurophysiol*. 1981;21:165–182.

118. Rosenblum JA. Documentation of thermographic objectivity in pain syndromes. In: *Academy of Neuromuscular Thermography Clinical Proceedings*. Dallas: Postgraduate Medicine Custom Communications; 1985:59–61.

119. Adams WJ, Lloyd JT. Empirical evaluation of the chronic pain diagnosis. In: *Academy of Neuromuscular Thermography Clinical Proceedings*. Dallas: Postgraduate Medicine Custom Communications; 1985:86–89.

120. Shandell KE, Saboda S. Thermographic examinations and the differential diagnosis of psychogenic versus organic factors in patients with pain. In: *Academy of Neuromuscular Thermography Clinical Proceedings*. Dallas: Postgraduate Medicine Custom Communications; 1985:83–85.

121. Maultsby JA, Deaton PC, Tannenbaum SI, Underwood DL, Chabon SJ, Madis C. Electronic thermography: A valuable aid in evaluating and treating symptomatic spinal pathology. In: Abernathy M, Uematsu S, eds. *Medical Thermology*. Washington, DC; American Academy of Thermology; 1986:165–169.

122. Maultsby JA, Underwood DL, Chabon SJ, Meek JB, Routon J, Fletcher D. Comparison of thermographic study with topographical pain drawings and correlations with psychological evaluation. In: Abernathy M, Uematsu S, eds. *Medical Thermology*. Washington, DC: American Academy of Thermology; 1986:210–217.

123. Sherman RA, Barja RH, Bruno GM. Thermographic correlates of chronic pain: Analysis of 125 patients incorporating evaluations by a blind panel. *Arch Phys Med Rehabil*. 1987;66:273–279.

124. *Standards for Neuro-muscular Thermography*. Academy of Neuro-Muscular Thermography; 1989.

125. Technical guidelines, edition 2. *Thermology*. 1986;2:108–112.

126. Hobbins WB. Protocol for autonomic challenge test. Initial, private publ. Thermal Image Analysis, Madison, Wis: 1990;2(1):8–10.

127. *Neuromusculoskeletal Thermographic Protocol*. American Chiropractic College of Thermology; 1988.

128. Policy statement on guidelines for thermography in chiropractic practice, American Chiropractic College of Thermology and ACA Council on Diagnostic Imaging, ratified by ACA House of Delegates, June 13, 1991.

129. *CPT: Physicians' Current Procedural Terminology*. Chicago: American Medical Association; 1989:33.

130. Uematsu S, Jandel WR, Edwin DH, et al. Quantification of thermal asymmetry: Part 2. Application in low back pain and sciatica. *J Neurosurg*. 1988;69:556–561.

11

Standards for Contraindications to Spinal Manipulative Therapy

Meridel I. Gatterman

It is especially important to identify the risk factors that contraindicate a specific health care procedure. Because manipulation is the primary therapeutic procedure used by chiropractic,[1] and because manipulation involves the forceful passive movement of a joint beyond its active limit of motion,[2] chiropractors must identify the risk factors that contraindicate manipulation.

Manipulation is defined as "a passive manoeuvre in which specifically directed manual forces are applied to vertebral and extravertebral articulations of the body with the object of restoring mobility to restricted areas."[3] Successful spinal manipulation involves the application of a mobilizing force to the areas of the spine that are stiff or hypomobile while avoiding areas of hypermobility or instability.[4]

Haldeman classified manipulations as either nonspecific, long-lever manipulations or specific, short-lever, high-velocity, low-amplitude manipulations (ie, the chiropractic adjustment).[5] The long levers include the leg, shoulder, pelvis, and thoracic spine. It is difficult to direct the long-lever manipulation to a particular segment; often, such a mobilization affects the hypermobile vertebral segment rather than the one in which movement is restricted. Therefore, chiropractors most commonly use the more specific short-lever, high-velocity thrust directed specifically to the fixated or blocked vertebral motion segment. Palmer advocated the use of the shorter levers, including the spinous and transverse processes of the vertebrae, to deliver the chiropractic adjustment.[6]

Contraindications to spinal manipulative therapy range from nonindication, where manipulation causes no harm; to lack of a clear indication; to absolute contraindication, where manipulation can be life-threatening. Frequently, manipulation is contraindicated in one area of the spine, yet beneficial in another region.[7,8] Although hypermobility may be a relative contraindication to manipulation in one area of the spine, for example, it may be compensatory to movement restriction in another area where manipulation is the treatment of choice.[6,9] The patient who has suffered a "whiplash" injury frequently exhibits restricted motion in the upper cervical articulations, [9,10] while stretching of the ligaments at the apex of the cervical curve in the midcervical spine has allowed the joints in this area to become hypermobile. Specific short-lever manipulation of the upper cervical joint with restricted motion permits the stretched ligaments in the midcervical region to heal, but manipulation of the sprained midcervical segments is contraindicated. In this case, short-lever manipulation of the restricted joints is the treatment of choice to prevent compensatory hypermobility from continuing,[11] whereas long-lever nonspecific manipulation is contraindicated.

In other clinical situations, forceful manipulation may be precluded, while other, less forceful manual therapies are appropriate.[12] Manual therapy includes manual traction, mobilization, passive stretching, massage, ischemic compression of trigger points, and reflex techniques designed to reduce pain and muscle spasm.[7]

VASCULAR ACCIDENTS

Generally considered the most serious of all complications of spinal manipulative therapy are vascular accidents. An aneurysm involving a major blood vessel, especially the abdominal aorta, is an absolute contraindication to manipulation.[12,13] Compromise of the vertebral arteries that interrupts the blood supply into the basilar area of the brain can result in a number of symptoms and, in the most serious cases, can lead to death[14] (see Chapter 6).

A number of risk factors have been associated with vertebral artery compromise.[7,15-19] Among them are anomalous vertebral arteries; atherosclerosis; abnormal bony structures in opposition to the vertebral arteries by virtue of degenerative changes, such as osteophytic proliferation; and anomalous malformation, such as ponticulus posticus. A cause-and-effect relationship between cervical spine manipulation and stroke has yet to be established, but—because chiropractic manipulation can be a temporal factor to be considered in the relationship—careful screening of patients at risk is necessary (see Chapter 6).

Long-term anticoagulant therapy has also been identified as creating a risk of vascular accidents for patients undergoing spinal manipulative therapy, because intraspinal bleeding as a side-effect of the medication may result in hematoma formation. Dabert, Freeman, and Weis commented that the incidence of hemorrhage complications of spinal adjustments on patients receiving anticoagulation therapy varies from 3.5% to 48%.[20] In 1970, they reported a case of spinal meningeal hematoma with subsequent neuropathy following a chiropractic adjustment in a patient who had been receiving the anticoagulant warfarin (Coumadin).

Stewart-Wynne, in 1976, reported an iliofemoral psoas hematoma with femoral neuropathy in a patient receiving sodium warfarin, following spinal manipulation by an osteopath.[21] Dabert and colleagues identified physical strain, with bleeding precipitated by manipulation as a common factor in vascular accidents following spinal manipulation.[20] They suggested that the combination of the two modalities, namely spinal manipulation and anticoagulant medication, without appropriate interprofessional communication can have disastrous effects. Grieve stated that manual attentions of any vigor and overpressure to full range of movements are unwise in patients on anticoagulants.[22] Although not an absolute contraindication to manipulation, long-term anticoagulant therapy warrants caution when applying forceful spinal manipulative therapy.

Standard 1: Long-term anticoagulant therapy warrants caution when applying forceful spinal manipulative therapy.

TUMORS

Primary bone tumors are unusual in the spine,[23] but neoplastic disease with metastasis to bone can be a source of back pain. Pathological fracture of bone weakened by a primary or secondary tumor is an obvious risk of manipulation in patients with these conditions. Fisk estimated the incidence of primary or secondary bone tumors to be less than 4/100,000 patients; of these, only 1 in 20 occurs in the spine.[24] The vast majority are secondary to primary tumors in the prostrate, breasts, lungs, and thyroid gland. Of the primary malignant tumors, multiple myeloma is most common. Grieve reported that more than 80% of the tumors that produce neurological defects occur at the thoracic cord level.[22]

Benign Tumors

Hemangiomas, the most commonly occurring vertebral tumors, are found in approximately 10% of all spines. They occur with greatest frequency between T-12 and L-4, and two-thirds of the patients with these tumors are women. Most vertebral hemangiomas are noted as incidental findings and are clinically silent. They are not commonly subject to pathological fracture and offer no contraindication to manipulation unless pathological fracture has already occurred.[25,26] In rare cases, neurological referral is appropriate.

Osteoid osteomas commonly have a small nidus surrounded by reactive sclerosis. Although they do not metastasize, they may extend locally, compressing the nerve structures within the canal. Lesions may occur in association with idiopathic scoliosis.[27] Young patients (most often between the ages of 9 and 14) who complain of pain that is worse when they are recumbent should be screened carefully to rule out osteoid osteoma. A bone scan is suggested if the radiographic findings are equivocal. The presence of an osteoid osteoma is not a contraindication to manipulation, but the practitioner should be aware that the patient's pain is most likely caused by the tumor, which warrants further investigation.

Malignant Tumors

Multiple myeloma, while rare, is the most common type of primary malignancy seen in chiropractic offices, as a large percentage of patients with multiple myeloma complain of back pain. It is most common in patients between the ages of 35 and 65,[22] who report poorly localized back pain that is worse when they are lying in bed at night. As the myeloma penetrates and destroys the vertebral bodies, wedging, marked flattening, and compression may appear on radiographs, along with osteopenia. Although gentle manual therapy may offer symptomatic relief, forceful manipulation is contraindicated. Prompt referral to an oncologist or diagnostic specialist is essential. Serum protein electrophoresis and marrow biopsy provide a more definitive diagnosis.

Metastatic Tumors

Spinal metastases are common (36.1%) in patients who are dying of neoplastic disease.[28,29] Next to vertebrae, the most common sites for metastatic disease are the pelvis, proximal long bones, and ribs.[28] Certain cancers have a predilection for metastasis to bone; breast and prostate cancers metastasize to bone most frequently, followed by lung, kidney, and thyroid cancers. Batson demonstrated that the complex vertebral venous system, with its nonvalvular anastomoses, may be the route of dissemination of the tumor emboli.[29]

Like pain produced by primary tumors, the pain associated with metastatic tumors is characteristically of insidious onset, gradually increasing with the passage of time. It is frequently worse at night or at rest. A sudden onset of pain or an acute exacerbation of pain in the back following mild or no trauma may represent a pathological fracture and may be the presenting complaint.

Tumor metastasis may be osteoclastic (bone destructive) or osteoblastic (bone forming); moreover, both of these types of metastasis may occur simultaneously. The osteoclastic (lytic) metastasis frequently leads to vertebral collapse and destruction of the cortex and/or pedicle. The osteoblastic metastasis characteristically occurs when the primary tumor is in the prostate or breast and appears as an area of increased density. Metastatic disease to the spine should be suspected in any patient with a history of malignant disease who has an insidious onset of low back pain. Metastatic disease can become apparent 5 to 10 years after treatment of disease at the primary site.[23]

Careful inspection of each pedicle, transverse process, spinous process, and lamina is necessary to rule out the presence of lesions at these sites. Even with presumably normal spine radiographs, laboratory screening and further diagnostic imaging is warranted if neoplasm is suspected. A bone scan demonstrates increased uptake of technitium in vertebrae with relatively small lesions before they can be visualized on routine spine films.[23]

Chiropractors do not treat neoplastic disease, and forceful manipulation of the spine is contraindicated in these patients. Gentle manual techniques may offer symptomatic relief in patients with malignant disorders of the spine, however. Such palliative care should be rendered concomitantly and in consultation with the physician in charge of treating the malignancy. Complications following manipulation of patients with primary or secondary neoplastic disease have been reported.[30,31] Bone weakened by neoplasm is an absolute contraindication to forceful manipulation. Careful evaluation of each case will indicate prompt referral of patients who may have a bone malignancy.[32]

> *Standard 2:* Bone weakened by neoplasm is an absolute contraindication to forceful manipulation.

INFECTIONS

Bone infections are rare and usually exhibit readily identifiable patterns. The practitioner should be on guard when the patient is both ill and in pain. These patients generally appear to have a systemic illness with febrile symptoms. The infectious agent may be bacterial, tubercular, or mycotic, and the infection may follow spinal surgery, result from a distant focus of infection, or develop idiopathically. A primary site, such as the lungs, urinary tract, or gastrointestinal tract, is typically found with tuberculosis of bone. A staphylococcal furuncle or carbuncle often precedes osteomyelitis. Most chronic infections of bone occur in the young, but they have become rare since the advent of antibiotic drugs.

Tuberculosis of the spine (Pott's disease) accounts for more than half of all bone and joint tuberculosis and is most often seen in early childhood.[33] Laboratory analysis shows an elevated sedimentation rate, and a tuberculin skin test is positive. During the early stage, radiographs may reveal an osteolytic lesion in the anterior part of the vertebral body, with a regional osteoporosis and narrowing of the adjacent intervertebral disk. In the advanced stage, extensive destruction and collapse of the anterior vertebral body, spread to adjacent vertebrae, and a paravertebral abscess may be seen.

Osteomyelitis of the spine is usually hematogenous from a distant primary site. Pain and rigidity from protective muscle spasm are the earliest clinical symptoms.[34] There may be evidence of soft tissue swelling after a few days, mandating laboratory procedures such as a white blood cell count and a determination of the sedimentation rate. After the first week of osteomyelitic infection, there is evidence of bone destruction. The primary risk of spinal manipulation in patients with bone infection, as in those with bone tumors, is pathological fracture. Because of this risk, manipulation of the affected area is absolutely contraindicated.[35] Radiographic examination, coupled with appropriate tests, can detect suspected bone infection and prevent a dangerous delay in treatment.

ARTHRITIDES

The presence of inflammatory joint disease is generally considered an absolute contraindication to manipulation of the affected articulation.[36,37] The most serious complication of manipulation in the presence of the systemic arthritides (eg, ankylosing spondylitis, rheumatoid arthritis, psoriatic arthritis, and Reiter's syndrome) is rupture of the transverse ligament with dislocation of the atlas.[12] Flexion radiographs of the cervical spine will reveal an increase in the atlanto-odontoid interspace. Amounts greater than 5 mm in children or 3 mm in adults are indicative of anterior slippage of the atlas on the axis. Because there is a possibility of total luxation with central cord compression, this slippage is an absolute contraindication to forceful manipulation of this region.[12]

Standard #3: The presence of inflammatory joint disease is a relative contraindication to chiropractic manipulation of the affected articulation.

Standard #4: In systemic arthritides (eg, rheumatoid arthritis), an atlanto-odontoid interspace greater than 5 mm in children or 3 mm in adults as determined by flexion radiograph precludes cervical manipulation.

Ankylosing Spondylitis

Injuries to the vertebral column, spinal cord, and spinal nerves have been reported as complications of chiropractic manipulation of patients with ankylosing spondylitis.[38,39] Schmidley and Koch noted that "the spondylitic spine is especially liable to fracture, particularly when, in addition to being completely ankylosed, it is severely osteoporotic, as it often is in longstanding AS [ankylosing spondylitis]."[39]

Ankylosing spondylitis, which is more common in males than in females, typically occurs in patients between 15 and 35 years of age. The common initial complaint is low back pain of insidious onset following a nontraumatic event. The sacroiliac joints may be involved first. Radiographs may show ill-defined joint margins with reactive sclerosis on both sides of the articulations. The spine may slowly fuse, with accompanying back stiffness, as the disease progresses from caudal to cephalad. Mild anemia and an elevated erythrocyte sedimentation rate are common, but the most helpful laboratory finding is the presence of HLA-B27 antigen, which is found in the serum of more than 80% of patients with ankylosing spondylitis.

Although most authors agree that manipulation is contraindicated during the inflammatory stage of ankylosing spondylitis,[8,12,25,37,40] Stoddard expressed the opinion that manipulation of the spine and exercise to maintain mobility are not contraindicated following the acute phase.[8] Gentle manipulation of the costovertebral joints is beneficial when the disease is quiescent in order to maintain near normal respiratory movement, which improves the general health of the patient. Gentle manipulation and adjunctive soft tissue therapy are not precluded in the quiescent phase; on the contrary, they may have significant palliative effects in many cases, provided that excessive force is avoided.

Rheumatoid Arthritis

A systemic disorder, rheumatoid arthritis is characterized by the destruction of synovial tissue. As the disease progresses, the joint surfaces are destroyed, with the subsequent development of ligamentous laxity and osteoporosis. In the spine, rheumatoid arthritis affects primarily the cervical area. The risk of rupture of the transverse ligament of the atlas precludes manipulation of this region in patients with longstanding rheumatoid arthritis. The cervical spine may be dislocated in these patients, even when they have been totally asymptomatic.[34] Although longstanding rheumatoid arthritis is an absolute contraindication to forceful manipulation, gentle mobilization may relieve pain in these patients.[37]

Psoriatic Arthritis and Reiter's Syndrome

In the spine, psoriatic arthritis is indistinguishable radiographically from Reiter's syndrome. Both are associated with a sacroiliitis similar to that of ankylosing spondylitis; paraspinal ossifications may span vertebral bodies in both conditions. Reiter's syndrome can occur in women and children, but it generally occurs in young men. It is characterized by urethritis, conjunctivitis, and arthritis. Between 20% and 30% of patients with psoriatic arthritis have spinal involvement. The HLA-B27 antigen is found in the serum of 80% of patients with Reiter's syndrome and in 50% of those with spinal involvement in psoriatic arthritis.[41]

Osteoarthritis

Not only does osteoarthritis of the spine result in pathological, degenerative changes in the posterior facet joints, but also it occurs concomitantly with degeneration of the intervertebral disc. The two posterior facet joints and the intervertebral disc comprise a three joint complex with degeneration at any one component affecting the mechanics of the other two. Kirkaldy-Willis has outlined three phases of degenerative change in the lumbar spine, each one blending into the other.[42] The earliest phase, dysfunction, is characterized mainly by abnormal function. This is followed by a phase of instability, during which manipulation has proved beneficial in relieving back pain.[42] Sandoz described an additional stage in which reversible joint restriction occurs following the unstable phase.[43] It appears that, during the second phase when the holding elements of the vertebral motion segment become slack because of the thinning of the intervertebral disc, the patient experiences recurring episodes of joint locking. At this point, manipulation becomes the treatment of choice. The third phase described by Kirkaldy-Willis is restabilization, which occurs with loss of disc substance, fibrosis, and, ultimately, formation of osteophytes around the posterior joints and disc. As one segment of the spine stabilizes, adjacent segments degenerate in the same pathological pattern.

Osteoarthritis of the cervical spine is not an absolute contraindication to manipulation, but Stoddard noted that it is a relative contraindication, depending on the experience of the practitioner.[35] Terrett reported that patients with ischemic symptoms following neck manipulation are at no greater risk when they exhibit accompanying arthritis and noted that otherwise the older group would be at a significantly greater risk than they are.[19]

Maitland recommended gentle mobilization in the treatment of patients with osteoarthritis, followed by more vigorous manipulation in the absence of very painful joints.[37] Stoddard recommended manipulation as a treatment to improve circulation in osteoarthritic spinal joints.[35] Thus, osteoarthritis of the spine is not an absolute contraindication to manipulation, provided that the patient's condition is carefully assessed before the manipulation.

METABOLIC DISORDERS

Forceful manipulation of bone weakened by metabolic disorders is contraindicated because of the risk of pathological fracture.[35,37] The use of soft tissue and mobilizing techniques may prove beneficial to patients with osteoporosis and osteomalacia for whom more forceful procedures are precluded, however. The spine is particularly vulnerable to osteoporotic fracture, and those patients who have a history of long-term steroid therapy and women who have passed menopause are most susceptible. Osteoporosis is the most common metabolic bone disease in adults, and 70% of all fractures in the elderly occur as the result of this disorder. Even minor trauma to the spine, such as the stress caused by a cough or sneeze, may result in the collapse of weakened vertebrae.[23]

More than 30% of bone substance must be lost before there is radiographic evidence of osteoporosis, with the "codfish vertebra," vertebral collapse, and rarification of bone characteristic. The vertical striations and end-plates remain well defined, but the horizontal trabeculae are lost. Laboratory values are typically normal in osteoporosis although there may be a very slight increase in alkaline phosphatase if there has been a recent fracture. Changes in the serum levels of calcium, phosphorus, and alkaline phosphatase occur with osteomalacia. Patients with a history of longstanding steroid therapy, treatment with anticonvulsive medication, malabsorption syndrome, or nutritional deficiencies, as well as the postmenopausal woman, must all be screened carefully for radiographic changes of osteopenia. Forceful manipulation of patients showing evidence of bone thinning is contraindicated.

Standard #5: Forceful manipulation of patients showing evidence of bone thinning is contraindicated in the adjacent joints.

TRAUMA AND HYPERMOBILITY

Although trauma is not an absolute contraindication to spinal manipulation, patients who have suffered traumatic events require careful examination for areas of excessive motion, which may range from mild hypermobility to segmental instability. Grieve defined the hypermobile joint as an overflexible link in a series of articular bodies.[44] According to Muhlemann, hypermobile joints or segments commonly preserve their stability under normal conditions (ie, they are functional for weight bearing and motion) within certain limits.[45] He suggested that hypermobility can evolve into segmental instability. White, Southwick, and Panjabi defined instability as

> the loss of the ability of the spine under physiological loads to maintain relationships between vertebrae in such a way that there is neither damage nor subsequent irritation to the spinal cord or nerve roots and, in addition, there is no development of incapacitating deformities or pain due to structural changes.[46]

White, Southwick, and Panjabi considered a motion segment "unstable" if either all of its anterior or all of its posterior holding elements were destroyed.[46] McGregor and Mior defined clinical instability as the pathological state of motion at an intervertebral level in the cervical spine that results in clinically intolerable symptoms as in cord or root damage, requiring prolonged bracing or surgery. Also involved are abberations in neutral and/or flexion-extension x-rays, such as greater than 3 mm to 5 mm translations and/or greater than 11° difference in vertebral angulation.[47]

Both acute trauma and repetitive microtrauma can lead not only to fracture, but also to excessive segmental mobility. Radiographs must be scrutinized carefully for both fractures and evidence of soft tissue injury.[47,48] Persistent swelling, focal pain, and deteriorating neurological signs all require additional imaging, such as flexion-extension radiographs, bone scan, computed tomography (CT), or magnetic resonance imaging (MRI).

McGregor and Mior reported that radiographs may not reveal underlying instability at first because of technologically inadequate x-rays, inappropriate views, or latent evidence of trauma.[47] In the latter case, reexamination may reveal the classic signs of instability.[49] Herkowitz and Rothman referred to latent evidence of trauma as "subacute instability."[50] The initial absence of observable bony displacement is purported to be due to continued stretching of the holding elements until plastic deformation results; later evidence of instability is also alleged to be the result of spontaneously reduced muscle spasm.[51]

The causes of segmental hypermobility and instability are varied; the mechanical basis appears to be overload by axial compression and torsion.[52] Causes of hypermobility other than trauma include microtrauma due to occupational stress, activities that require excessive flexibility (eg, gymnastics and ballet), hormonal influences (eg, pregnancy and the effects of estrogen medication), compensation for adjacent hypomobile segments (congenital, functional, or surgical), general joint laxness, infections, neoplasms, and metabolic disorders.[9,p170] Repeated forceful and nonspecific manipulation has also been suggested as a cause of hypermobility.[8,53] Nall noted that correction of hypermobility by manipulating only fixed areas produces fewer side-effects.[54] Hypermobile and unstable vertebral motion segments represent an absolute contraindication to forceful nonspecific manipulation.

Standard #6: Hypermobile and unstable vertebral motion segments represent an absolute contraindication to forceful, nonspecific manipulation.

PSYCHOLOGICAL FACTORS

It is important to consider psychological factors in the overall treatment of patients who seek chiropractic care. Failure to differentiate patients with psychogenic complaints from those with organic disorders can result in inappropriate treatment. Furthermore, it can delay appropriate referral. Patients who may need referral include malingerers, hysterics, hypochondriacs, and those with dependent personalities.[9,(p162)]

REGIONAL COMPLICATIONS OF MANIPULATIVE THERAPY

Manipulation is a relatively safe and effective means of relieving painful biomechanical problems of the spine, including the neck. As with all treatments, however, complications can arise. Neurological complications, as well as vascular accidents, have been reported.

Cervical Region

Many of the incidents that have been reported following cervical manipulation involve the use of excessive force or inappropriate maneuvers. Horner's syndrome has been observed following a neck manipulation in which a forceful thrust at the base of the neck may have caused a traction or avulsion injury to the white ramus communicans between the first thoracic nerve and the first thoracic or inferior cervical sympathetic ganglion where it runs in front of the first rib. In this case, the injury was thought to be due to forward movement of the left transverse process following a sharp, downward thrust with both thumbs placed deeply at the base of the neck while the patient was in side posture.[55]

Diaphragmatic paralysis has also followed manipulation of the cervical spine. Although it is possible that the patient's prior neck injury and osteoarthritic vertebral spurring may have predisposed her to the nerve damage, the nerve dysfunction was attributed directly to a vigorous manipulation that was followed immediately by pain radiating along the trapezius ridge and ipsilateral phrenic nerve dysfunction. Because both structures are innervated largely from the fourth cervical trunk, the resultant paralysis of the hemidiaphragm and dyspnea were attributed to the forceful manipulation.[56]

Three cases of myelopathy following cervical spine manipulation have been reported.[57] All three patients noted an increase in cervical pain following manipulation, developed significant sensorimotor deficits within 24 hours, and became tetraparetic. One incident occurred after a sitting manipulation in which the neck was rotated sideways, followed by a sudden forceful forward flexion. The patient's cord lesion was attributed to the ventroflexion and rotational forces. In another case, the patient had prior neurological problems that were thought to result from a small intraspinal subarachnoid hemorrhage, but the neurological deterioration following cervical manipulation was attributed to additional bleeding in the cervical cord that further compromised the patient's neurological function. Pathological fracture of the C-5 vertebral body in an osteoporotic patient with osteophytes at the intervertebral foramina of C5-C6 bilaterally, and a narrow spinal canal at C4-C6, led to tetraplegia 2 hours after cervical manipulation in the third patient.

Cervical disk lesions can cause severe neurological complications in both the upper and lower extremities. Protrusion of the intervertebral disk affects the upper extremities through involvement of the nerve root; symptoms in the lower extremities indicate direct cord involvement. Early recognition of these conditions and immediate referral for neurological decompression is essential to prevent permanent neurological deficits.[9,p66] Techniques requiring excessive extension with rotation are contraindicated in the cervical spine.

Thoracic Spine

Although few cases are reported in the literature, one of the most common complications of manipulation in the thoracic spine is rib fracture and costochondral separation following the excessively forceful application of torque forces while the patient is positioned in side posture. Grieve cautioned that the ribs are particularly vulnerable to injury in patients with osteoporosis or rheumatoid disease.[22] He also cautioned that "the neural canal between T4 and T9 is a critical vascular zone, where the canal is narrowest and the blood supply poorest."

Lumbar Spine

Major complications following manipulation of the lumbar spine can be neurological or vascular, according to the primary tissue that is damaged. Probably the most common serious complication of lumbar manipulation is an increase in neurological symptoms that originally resulted from disk injury.[58] Ladermann concluded that manipulation can exacerbate the symptoms that it is originally intended to relieve.[59]

The most serious neurological complication following manipulation of the lumbar spine is cauda equina syndrome. Some of the cases that have been attributed to manipulative therapy have probably followed the natural course of the discopathy, as cauda equina syndromes generally occur without manipulation. A number of cases of cauda equina syndrome have been associated with spinal manipulation in the literature, however. Ladermann collected 30 cases in which cauda equina syndrome was associated with manipulation in the French, German, and English literature reported between 1900 and 1980.[59] Only 8 of these cases were related to chiropractic treatment. He noted that, had these patients not been manipulated, the outcome would probably have been the same; a menial effort involving an impulsive strain (eg, coughing, sneezing, laughing, or straining at stool) would have replaced the rupturing effect of the manipulation.

In 1982, Malmivaara and Pohjola reported a case of cauda equina syndrome in which the patient was manipulated in side posture.[60] The manipulation reportedly involved thrusting the right thigh forcefully in extension and adduction. In this case, the patient had not had prior low back pain, leg pain, or numbness, but developed these symptoms immediately after the manipulation. Subsequently, he developed bowel incontinence, difficulty with micturition, and impotence. His only low back complaint prior to manipulation had been a prior complaint. Thus, rotary manipulation that involves the application of torsional stress throughout the lumbar spine carries a risk of cauda equina syndrome, even in the absence of prior radicular symptoms, when the neural reflex guards are bypassed either by rapid manipulation or by manipulation under general anesthesia.

Gallinaro and Cartesegna reported a case of cauda equina syndrome, as well as three cases of lumbar disk rupture, associated with spinal manipulation between June and December of 1982.[61] Based on the few reported cases of complications following manipulation and their own experience, they concluded that "chiropraxis may be more dangerous than useful, and the favorable results claimed are more likely to be related to the high rate of spontaneous remission of low back pain than to manipulation itself."[61] Fortunately, this attitude is not uniformly held. There is sufficient evidence of effectiveness to warrant chiropractic treatment not only of back pain, but also of radicular complaints.[60,62-65] There is unanimous agreement, however, that emergency decompressive surgery is required in all patients who show signs of cauda equina syndrome. Prompt referral of these patients, as of any patient showing advancing neurological deficits, is imperative.[66]

> *Standard #7:* Emergency decompressive surgery is required in all patients who show signs of cauda equina syndrome. Prompt referral of these patients, as of any patient showing advancing neurological deficits, is imperative.

A case of meralgia paresthetica has also occurred as a complication of chiropractic therapy.[67] In this case, the application of a trochanteric belt compressed the lateral femoral cutaneous nerve, causing neurological symptoms. A sensory examination should be performed to rule out the existence of this syndrome before any type of encircling belt is prescribed in the pelvic region.

An aneurysm involving a major blood vessel is an absolute contraindication to manipulation.[9,p58] The regional examination of the lumbar spine must include abdominal palpation, because an aortic aneurysm can cause severe back pain and be the presenting complaint of patients in the older age range. Winterstein found 35 abdominal aortic aneurysms on retrospective analysis of 2,000 consecutive x-ray reports.[68] Of these patients, 26 were men, with an average age of 74.19 years, and 9 were women, with an average age of 70.44 years. Radiographs should be carefully screened for signs of aortic aneurysm. Patients with suspected aortic aneurysm should be referred to a vascular surgeon for evaluation and treatment prior to any manipulative therapy.[69]

> *Standard #8:* Aneurysm involving a major blood vessel is an absolute contraindication to manipulation.

PREVENTION OF COMPLICATIONS FROM MANIPULATION

Many incidents and accidents that result from manipulative therapy can be prevented by careful appraisal of the patient's history and examination findings. There is no substitute for asking the mandatory questions and no shortcut for obtaining an adequate history. Information must be sought about co-existing disease and use of medication, including long-term steroid use and anticoagulant therapy. A detailed and meticulous examination, including ancillary procedures such as x-ray studies, laboratory tests, and enhanced imaging when indicated, are all necessary for an accurate diagnosis. The use of appropriate technique is essential. Specific short-lever manipulation with a high-velocity thrust of low amplitude, with the least amount of force effective, lessens the chances of injury. The avoidance of techniques known to be hazardous, for example, excessive rotation in the cervical spine[22] or use of the knee-chest position for patients who are unable to relax in this posture or who have spondylolisthesis and hyperlordosis,[70] is basic. Any attempt to rectify a procedure that produced an adverse reaction by performing by a second manipulation is folly. Finally, treatment should be guided by assessment and reassessment throughout.[22]

> *Standard #9:* The physician must avoid techniques known to be hazardous, such as excessive rotation in the cervical spine or use of the knee-chest position for patients who are unable to relax in this posture or who have spondylolisthesis and hyperlordosis.

"Primum non nocere," as Hippocrates admonished us. First, do no harm.[71]

REFERENCES

1. Vear HJ. Standards of chiropractic practice. *Journal of Manip Physio Thera.* 1985;8:1-33–43

2. Gatterman MI. Indications for spinal manipulation in the treatment of back pain. *ACA J Chiro.* 1982;19(10):51-66.

3. *Dorland's Illustrated Medical Dictionary.* 25th ed. Philadelphia: WB Saunders; 1965:909.

4. Cassidy JD, Potter GE. Motion examination of the lumbar spine. *JMPT.* 1979;2:3.

5. Haldeman S. Spinal manipulative therapy in the management of low back pain. In: Finneson GE, ed. *Low Back Pain.* 2nd ed. Philadelphia: JB Lippincott; 1980:260-280.

6. Palmer DD. *The Science, Art, and Philosophy of Chiropractic.* Portland: Portland Printing House; 1910:101.

7. Gatterman MI. Contraindications and complications of spinal manipulative therapy. *ACA J Chiro.* 1981;15:575-586.

8. Stoddard A. *Manual of Osteopathic Medicine.* 2nd ed. London: Hutchinson; 1983;290-291.

9. Gatterman MI. *Chiropractic Management of Spine Related Disorders.* Baltimore: Williams & Wilkins; 1990.

10. Hviid. Functional radiography of the cervical spine. *Ann Swiss Chiro Assn.* 1965;3:35-65.

11. Mealy K, Brenner H, Fenelon GCC. Early mobilization of acute whiplash injuries. *Br Med J*. 1986;8:656–657.

12. Kleynhans AM. Complications of and contraindications to spinal manipulative therapy. In: Haldeman S, ed. *Modern Developments in the Principles and Practice of Chiropractic*. East Norwalk, Conn: Appleton-Century-Crofts; 1980: 359–384.

13. Kornberge E. Lumbar artery aneurysm with acute aortic occlusion resulting from chiropractic manipulation: A case report. *Surgery*. 1988; 103(1):122–124.

14. Gotlib AC, Thieb H. The vertebral artery syndrome: Part B. Annotated literature review. In: Vernon H, ed. *Upper Cervical Syndrome*. Baltimore: Williams & Wilkins; 1988:207.

15. Houle JOE. Assessing hemodynamics of the vertebrobasilar complex through angiolipsis. *J Can Chiro Assoc*. 1972;16(2):35–36, 44.

16. George PE, Silverstein HT, Wallace H, Marshall M. Identification of the high risk pre-stroke patient. *ACA J Chiro*. 1981;18:S26–S28.

17. Pyo J, Lowman KM. The "ponticulus posticus" of the first cervical vertebra. *Radiology*. 1959;72:850–854.

18. Buna M, Coghlan W, DeGruchy M, Williams D, Zmigwsy O. Ponticles of the atlas: A review and clinical perspective. *J Manip Physiol Therap*. 1984;7:261–266.

19. Terrett A. Vascular accidents from cervical spine manipulation: The mechanisms. *J Aust Chiro Assn*. 1987;17(4):131–144.

20. Dabert O, Freeman DG, Weis AJ: Spinal meningeal hematoma, warfarin therapy and chiropractic adjustment. *JAMA*. 2058, 1970;214:112058.

21. Stewart-Wynne EG. Iatrogenic femoral neuropathy. *Br Med J*. 1976;1:263.

22. Grieve GP. Incidents and accidents of manipulation. In: Grieve GP, ed. *Modern Manual Therapy*. New York: Churchill Livingston; 1986:873–889.

23. Finneson BE. *Low Back Pain*. 2nd ed. Philadelphia: JB Lippincott; 1980:519–532.

24. Fisk JW. *A Practical Guide to Management of the Painful Neck and Back: Diagnosis, Manipulation, Exercise and Prevention*. Springfield, Ill: Charles C Thomas; 1977:6.

25. Manning HJ. Symptomatic hemangioma of the spine. *Radiology*. 195;56:58.

26. Holta O. Hemangioma of the cervical vertebra with fracture and compression myelomalacia. *Acta Radiol*. 1942;23:423.

27. Freiberger RE. Osteoid osteoma of the spine: A cause of backache and scoliosis in children and young adults. *Radiology*. 1960;75:232.

28. Wong D, Formasia VL, Macnab I. Spinal metastasis: The obvious, the occult and the imposters. *Spine*. 1990;15:1–4.

29. Batson OU. The vertebral vein system. *Am J Roentgenol*. 1957;78:195.

30. Livingston CP. Spinal manipulation causing injury: A three year study. *Clin Orthop*. 1971;81:82–86.

31. Austin RT. Pathological vertebral fractures after spinal manipulation. *Br Med J*. 1985;291:1114–1115.

32. Marback N. Complications in a low back case. *ACA J Chiro*. 1980.

33. Salter RB. *Textbook of Disorders and Injuries of the Musculoskeletal System*. Baltimore: Williams & Wilkins; 1970:311.

34. D'Ambrosia. *Musculoskeletal Disorders, Regional Examination and Differential Diagnosis*. 2nd ed. Philadelphia: JB Lippincott; 1977:312.

35. Stoddard A. *Manual of Osteopathic Practice*. London: Hutchinson; 1969:279.

36. Greenman PE. *Principles of Manual Medicine.* Baltimore: Williams & Wilkins; 1989:99.

37. Maitland GD. *Vertebral Manipulation.* 3rd ed. London: Butterworth's; 1973:4.

38. Rinsky LA, Reynolds GG, Jameson RM, Hamilton RD. A cervical spinal cord injury following chiropractic manipulation. *Paraplegia.* 1976;13:223-227.

39. Schmidley JW, Koch T. The non-cerebrovascular complications of chiropractic manipulation. *Neurology.* 1984;34:684-685.

40. Mainge R. *Orthopedic Medicine: A New Approach to Vertebral Manipulations.* Springfield, Ill: Charles C. Thomas; 1972:169, 208.

41. Forrester DD, Brown JC, Nesson JW. *The Radiology of Joint Disease.* 2nd ed. Philadelphia: WB Saunders; 1978:596-597.

42. Kirkaldy-Willis WH. *Managing Low Back Pain.* 2nd ed. New York: Churchill Livingstone; 1988.

43. Sandoz R. The natural history of a spinal degenerative lesion. *Ann Swiss Chiro Assn.* 1989;9:149-192.

44. Greive GP. Lumbar instability. In: Greive GP, ed. *Modern Manual Therapy and the Vertebral Column.* London: Churchill Livingstone; 1986:416-441.

45. Muhlemann D. Hypermobility as a common cause for chronic back pain. *Ann Swiss Chiro Assn.,* in press.

46. White AA, Southwick WO, Panjabi MM. Clinical instability in the lower cervical spine: A review of past and current concepts. *Spine.* 1976;1:15-27.

47. McGregor M, Mior S. Anatomical and functional perspectives of the cervical spine: Part III. The "unstable cervical spine." *J Can Chiro Assoc.* 1990:145-152.

48. Sandoz RW. Technique on interpretation of functional radiography of the lumbar spine. *Ann Swiss Chiro Assn.* 1965;3:66-110.

49. Rifkinson-Mann S, Mormino J, Sachdev VP. Subacute, cervical spine instability. *Surg Neurol.* 1986;413-416.

50. Herkowitz HN, Rothman RH. Subacute instability of the cervical spine. *Spine.* 1985;9:138-357.

51. Evans DK. Anterior cervical subluxation. *J Bone Joint Surg.* 1976;58:318-321.

52. Kirkaldy-Willis WH, Farfan HF. Instability of the lumbar spine. *Clin Orthop.* 1982;165:110-123.

53. Greive GP. Lumbar instability. *Physiotherapy.* 1982;68:2-8.

54. Nall SK. The role of specific manipulation towards alleviating abnormalities in body mechanics and restoration of spinal motion. *J Manip Physiol Therap.* 1982;5:11-15.

55. Grayson MF. Horner's syndrome after manipulation of the neck. *Br Med J.* 1987;295:1382-1383.

56. Hefner JE. Diaphragmatic paralysis following chiropractic manipulation of the cervical spine. *Arch Intern Med.* 1985;145:562-563.

57. Kewalramani LS, Kewalramani DL, Krebs M, Saleem A. Myelopathy following cervical spine manipulation. *Am J Phys Med.* 61:165-175.

58. Bromley W. National Chiropractic Mutual Insurance Company: Stronger than ever. *J Am Chiro Assoc.* 1989;26:52.

59. Ladermann JP. Accidents of spinal manipulation. *Annals Swiss Chiro Assoc.* 1981;7:162-208.

60. Malmivaara A, Pohjola R. Cauda equina syndrome caused by chiropraxis on a patient previously free of lumbar spine symptoms. *Lancet.* 1982;986-987.

61. Gallinaro P, Cartesegna M: Three cases of lumbar disc rupture and one of cauda equina associated with spinal manipulation (chiropraxis) *Lancet.* 1983;411.

62. Quon JA, Cassidy JD, O'Conner SM, Kirkaldy-Willis WH. Lumbar intervertebral disk herniation: Treatment by rotational manipulation. *J Manip Physiol Ther.* 1989;12:220–227.

63. Kuo P, Loh Z. Treatment of lumbar intervertebral disc protrusion by manipulation. *Clin Orthop.* 1987;215:47–55.

64. Mathews JA, Yates DAH. Treatment of sciatica. *Lancet.* 1974;1:352.

65. Cox JM, Aspergen DD. A hypothesis introducing a new calculation for discal reduction: Emphasis on stenotic factors and manipulative treatment. *J Manip Physiol Ther.* 1987;10:287–294.

66. Hooper J. Lowback pain and manipulation: Paraparesis after treatment of low back pain by physical methods. *Med J Aust.* 1973.

67. Terrett AG. Meralgia paresthetica: A complication of chiropractic therapy. *J Australian Chiro Assn.* 1984;14:29–30.

68. Winterstein JF. Abdominal aortic aneurysm. *Roentgenological Briefs.* 1984;11:84.

69. Boline PD, Anderson AV. Abdominal aortic aneurysm. *Am J Chiro Med.* 1989;2:114–115.

70. Plaugher G, Lopes MA. The knee-chest table: Indications and contraindications. *Chiropractic Technique.* 1990.

71. Terrett AG. It is more important to know when not to adjust. *Chiropractic Technique.* 1990;2:1–8.

12

Chiropractic Jurisprudence and Malpractice Considerations

Robert L. Hirtle, Jr.

Chiropractic malpractice cases are extensions of medical malpractice lawsuits, which have been based on the legal theory of tort or negligence. The theory is that persons who have suffered injury through the fault of a professional doctor should recover fair, just, and adequate damages for those injuries. Thus, the tort system or negligence system of tort lawsuits is based on the principle of responsibility. It originated in the common law of England; if a person injured another person as a result of carelessness, the common law held the person who was careless to be responsible for the resulting injuries and losses of the injured person.

THE COURT SYSTEM

The problem that most doctors have with malpractice cases is not with the theory of malpractice, but with the court system. Traditionally, malpractice cases are tried before a jury in an adversarial system, which may be described as civilized combat. On one side of the courtroom is the injured party (ie, the plaintiff) with an attorney, and on the other side of the courtroom is the defendant-doctor with an attorney. Although a judge presides over all malpractice cases, the judge in a jury trial only makes rulings of law; the jury decides the facts.

At the end of the case, the judge delivers a charge or legal instructions to the jury. The judge sets forth those principles of law to which the jury must adhere in reaching its verdict. Most doctors find it disturbing that the jury system allows the jurors to be the sole arbiters of the factual findings in the case. In other words, a lay jury decides whether the doctor has committed malpractice and, if so, awards the damages to the plaintiff as compensation. The very idea of a lay panel making a decision on an issue of malpractice, which frequently involves complicated medical determinations, is abhorrent to most doctors.

In order to make sure that the jury applies appropriate standards of due care, skill, and diligence to the actions of the defendant-doctor, the courts require a plaintiff to present competent medical testimony through an expert witness to establish the standard of due care, skill, and diligence for the jury and further to establish whether the defendant-doctor has breached the standard.

Likewise, the defendant-doctor has the opportunity to present expert testimony to establish the standards of due care, skill, and diligence by which he or she is to be judged and opinion testimony as to whether those standards were breached. The jury members, after hearing expert witness testimony on both sides of an issue, are free to choose which expert they are going to believe. They may also elect to believe part of what one witness says and part of what another witness says, as long as the information is not inconsistent, so the ultimate jury verdict can be based on evidence received from any of the medical experts who testified.

ALTERNATIVE MALPRACTICE RESOLUTION SYSTEMS

There have been alternative systems suggested from time to time to resolve malpractice cases, which would obviate the need for a malpractice case to go before a jury. The most obvious alternative is to have malpractice cases tried before a judge. Without specialized medical training, however, a judge is usually in no better position to assess the actions of a doctor than is any other layperson. The typical training and background of a judge includes no meaningful education in the medical field. A judge may or may not be more learned than are educated persons sitting on the jury and would have the same difficulty in judging the testimony of medical experts that the lay jury would have. A plaintiff may waive the right to a jury trial and have the malpractice case heard by a judge, but such an action is highly unusual. A plaintiff's lawyers generally perceive juries to be more favorably disposed to an injured person's case than a judge sitting without a jury.

Various no-fault type solutions have been proposed. For example, it has been suggested that awards for injury be determined by a workers' compensation type schedule or that general damages for what is called pain and suffering be limited. These legislative restrictions are very difficult to draft without infringing upon the constitutional right to jury trial, however.

Mandatory arbitration has also been suggested as a solution for malpractice disputes. These proceedings are usually more informal and less time-consuming than is a court trial, and the matters are heard generally by either one arbitrator or by a panel of arbitrators. There is a national organization, the American Arbitration Association, that is devoted to the promotion and practice of arbitration. It both supplies panels of arbitrators and arranges for the hearings themselves. Because the arbitration system requires the agreement of both sides, however, it is not generally used.[1]

Beginning in the mid-1970s, some state legislatures enacted malpractice reform acts in an attempt to provide for pre-trial mediation panels. These acts usually require the submission of all malpractice claims to a panel prior to trial. The panels are made up of qualified medical practitioners and attorneys who review the claims in an attempt to weed out frivolous lawsuits and, thus, avoid costly trial expenses.[2] The screening panel legislation has generally been more successful in passing constitutional muster than other types of reform statutes, which have raised the problem of infringement of the right to jury trial.

STANDARDS OF DUE CARE, SKILL, AND DILIGENCE

Chiropractic physicians are bound to use toward their patients reasonable care, skill, and diligence—that is, the care, skill, and diligence that chiropractors in the same line of practice ordinarily have and exercise in like cases.

In the past, the standard of care was limited not only to that exercised by practitioners in the same line of practice, but also to that exercised by practitioners in the same locality. The locality rule has now been set aside, both by legislatures and by courts, in most states. Most courts use a national standard, prompted by the fact that all states now use the national boards for medical examinations.

With the advent of national boards for chiropractic examinations and the establishment of uniform curriculum standards by the Council on Chiropractic Education (CCE), most courts are now switching from the locality standard to a national standard for chiropractic malpractice cases as well. Notwithstanding the national trend, there is still a strong argument that the locality standard should apply in chiropractic cases. The practice of chiropractic is not uniform from state to state, and the scope of practice, therefore, varies from community to community.

The law does not require a chiropractic physician to possess any professional skill and learning other than that ordinarily possessed by chiropractic practitioners. No chiropractic physician guarantees the success of treatment. The fact that the result of treatment was not as favorable as had been hoped for by the patient, the family, or the chiropractor raises no presumption of lack of proper care or skill. The law recognizes that the science of chiropractic has not been so perfected that every treatment or procedure will be successful.

The law also recognizes that there are different schools of medicine, but does not favor one school to the exclusion of others. A chiropractor's care and skill cannot be measured by the treatment that a medical doctor would give, for example, but rather by the principles and practices of chiropractic physicians. The fact that some other method of treatment existed or that some other physician might have used different treatment does not of itself establish negligence or improper treatment. The test is whether the treatment given by the chiropractic physician was a reasonably skillful, careful, and prudent method of treatment or course of conduct.

Causation

Even a jury's verdict that a defendant-doctor was negligent does not necessarily afford a plaintiff a basis for a recovery. There must be satisfactory proof that the negligence was the proximate cause of the injury claimed. In order to be the proximate cause, the negligence must have been a substantial factor in producing the injury. If the injury would have occurred without the defendant-doctor's negligence, then the negligence is not the proximate cause of the injury.

Damages

In a malpractice suit, the damages awarded must be fair, just, and reasonable. Juries are given only very general guidelines for the award of damages: (1) to award medical expenses and lost wages to the plaintiff; (2) to award a sum of money to compensate the plaintiff for his or her injury and, if the injury is permanent, to consider the plaintiff's life expectancy and degree of disability in making the award; and (3) to compensate the plaintiff for any pain and suffering that the injury has caused. These guidelines contain no mathematical formulas.

The only control that the judge has is by way of additur or remittitur (ie, a court-ordered addition or reduction in an award of damages) if the verdict shocks the conscience. A judge who feels that a jury has awarded damages in an amount that is below the reasonable range for the injury suffered can order the award increased. Similarly, a judge who feels that the amount of damages awarded exceeds the reasonable range for the injury can reduce the award. Judges seldom interfere with jury verdicts, however.

The Expert Witness

As mentioned earlier, expert testimony by those having special knowledge about the requirements of proper skill and care is necessary in a malpractice case. Ordinarily, a chiropractic physician is required to testify in a chiropractic malpractice action in order to establish the chiropractic standards of due care, skill, and diligence and to offer an opinion about whether the conduct of the defendant-doctor breached those standards. There are cross-over areas, however, in which experts in more than one field can express opinions. A radiologist, a chiropractor, and an orthopedic surgeon, for example, are all qualified to interpret x-ray films.

As a general rule, chiropractors are competent to testify in a personal injury case as expert or medical witnesses concerning matters within the scope of practice of chiropractic. They are competent to express their opinion as to the causation of the injury; the permanency of the injury, if any; the medical treatment rendered; and the likely course of future medical treatment.[3,4]

CHIROPRACTIC PRACTICE—THE LEGAL VIEW

Patient Histories

The first step in the processing of a new patient should be the taking of a proper patient history. Many good printed forms are available for this purpose. Usually, there is a portion of the form for the patient to complete. After the patient has done so, the chiropractic physician should sit down with the patient and discuss those areas that need clarification and amplification, based on the patient's complaint and initial answers.

Failure to take a patient history is malpractice. Failure to take a patient history appropriate to the complaint is also malpractice. If the history discloses a previous condition that may affect the present diagnosis or treatment, the practitioner should obtain the medical records associated with that condition. Past x-rays should also be sent for and reviewed, if appropriate.

Physical Examination, Testing, and Diagnosis

After taking the patient history, the practitioner should perform a physical examination appropriate to the complaint. The physical findings should be noted in the record, along with the results of any tests performed. Once again, numerous printed forms are available to facilitate the record keeping.

In all states, a chiropractic physician may legally use x-ray for diagnostic purposes. Care should be taken not to expose the patient needlessly to radiation, however. If prior films are available and they are of recent origin, they should be reviewed before additional views are taken. Because of the uniform acceptance of x-ray examination for chiropractic diagnosis, the failure to order x-ray studies when appropriate may result in a breach of the standard of care.

The purpose of a diagnosis is two-fold. First, the chiropractic physician must identify the patient's problem before treating it. This identification is sometimes called a working diagnosis or a differential diagnosis. Even those chiropractic physicians who do not like to use the term *diagnosis* are legally required to perform an evaluation and arrive at an opinion about the patient's problem before undertaking treatment. There is no legal distinction between diagnosis and evaluation, insofar as legal sufficiency under case law.

The second legally required purpose of the physical examination, testing, and diagnosis is to screen out those patients who have conditions for which medication, surgery, or some other treatment beyond the scope of chiropractic practice is necessary. The law mandates referral of such patients to appropriate medical practitioners. Failure to refer a patient when indicated is a breach of the standard of care.

Plan of Treatment

The chiropractic physician is legally required to formulate a plan of treatment and to note it on the patient's chart. The plan of treatment should set forth the proposed therapy, the frequency of the therapy, any modalities to be used in support of the therapy, and an indication of the duration of the therapy before reevaluation.

Although the original plan of treatment is successful in some cases and the patient may reach maximum medical improvement in a timely fashion, a practitioner often must reevaluate the patient's condition and revise the plan of treatment. The record should clearly indicate when the reevaluation is done and should include the results of any tests performed and the doctor's revised diagnosis, if appropriate. A new or revised plan of treatment should be recorded in the patient's chart, once again with an expected length or duration of treatment and an anticipated reevaluation date.

The Chiropractor's Judgment

If the practitioner has complied with the basic legal requirements that have been outlined, the fact that another chiropractor who saw the same patient and performed the same tests might have undertaken a different plan of treatment has no legal significance. As long as the chiropractor's judgment is consistent with his or her training and education, and with the treatment plans used by other chiropractors in similar circumstances, the chiropractor's judgment cannot be legally questioned.

SCOPE OF PRACTICE

State Regulation

Each state has a chiropractic practice act that sets forth a definition of chiropractic and establishes the parameters for the scope of chiropractic practice within that state. Inasmuch as there is great variance in practice statutes from state to state, chiropractic physicians who enter practice in a particular state must acquaint themselves with the scope-of-practice requirements of that legal jurisdiction.

The scope-of-practice statutes generally address two different areas of practice; diagnosis and treatment. The more liberal statutes permit a chiropractor to use any method of diagnosis that is taught in the chiropractic colleges; the more conservative statutes limit methods of diagnosis and may restrict a chiropractor's use of such procedures as blood and urine testing. In the area of treatment, the more liberal statutes permit a chiropractor to use any therapy taught in the chiropractic colleges, including such items as physical therapy and nutritional counseling in support of the chiropractic therapy. The more conservative scope-of-practice statutes may restrict the modes of therapy, may exclude physical therapy or nutritional counseling, or may limit the modalities that may be used in support of chiropractic adjustment.

If a court determines that a chiropractic physician has acted beyond the legal scope of practice, various consequences may result. First, the chiropractor may lose his or her state license. Second, the chiropractor not only may have committed a breach of the standards by practicing beyond the scope of practice, but also may have nullified his or her malpractice insurance coverage. Most malpractice insurance policies cover chiropractic physicians only while they are conducting their activities within the scope of practice as determined by state law.

Established practitioners who attend continuing education seminars on new techniques and treatment must ascertain whether these new techniques are within the scope of practice as determined by state law in their jurisdiction before incorporating such practices into their daily office routine.

Federal Regulation

Ordinarily, the chiropractic physician is not really concerned with federal regulation concerning scope of practice, because it is a matter determined by state law. There are two primary exceptions, however: federal workers' compensation and Medicare. The two are interrelated because the workers' compensation law uses the definition of chiropractic found in the Medicare law.[5] Under the definition of the term *physician* in the Medicare law, a chiropractor is a physician "only with respect to treatment by means of manual manipulation of the spine (to correct a subluxation diagnosed by x-ray to exist) which he is legally authorized to perform by the state or jurisdiction in which such treatment is provided."

The first problem in defining chiropractors as physicians only when they are treating a subluxation demonstrated by x-ray is that chiropractic physicians treat many conditions that do not involve subluxations. The second problem is that the law seems to require an x-ray film to be taken each time that an elderly person seeks treatment at a chiropractor's office. Obviously, there is some question whether each and every patient should be exposed to radiation.

The Medicare definition is clearly not consistent with the day-to-day practice of chiropractors in the United States and is sorely in need of revision. The Medicare law treats all other types of physicians as physicians within the parameters of their state scope-of-practice laws. If Congress amends the Medicare law in the future so that it treats chiropractors the same as other healing arts physicians, chiropractic physicians will no longer have to concern themselves with a restrictive definition of chiropractic in either Medicare or federal workers' compensation cases.

CAUSES OF MALPRACTICE SUITS

Certain categories of malpractice suits can be derived from the medical literature and malpractice insurance statistics.

Failure To Refer

Lawsuits based on the failure to refer generally involve a patient who has a condition that requires treatment by medication or surgery and a chiropractic physician who failed to refer the patient for necessary medical treatment. For example, numerous cases have been reported in the legal literature in which a chiropractor undertook the treatment of a patient who had a cancerous tumor and who subsequently died of the cancer; the doctor was then sued for malpractice for failure to refer. In many of these cases, the cancerous tumor was demonstrated on the x-ray film that the chiropractor took, but the chiropractor either ignored the tumor, failed to recognize the tumor, or persisted with chiropractic treatment in spite of the tumor's presence. When the survival rates of patients with that type of cancer are high following either resection or chemotherapy, juries almost always return a verdict for a plaintiff for failure to refer.

Juries often reach a similar verdict in those cases involving infectious disease in which the chiropractor has either failed to recognize the infection or failed to refer the patient for appropriate treatment of the infection. Once again, where the medical statistics show excellent treatment results with drug therapy or surgery, juries almost always hold a chiropractor guilty of malpractice for failure to refer such patients for treatment.

It should be noted that the chiropractor can provide concurrent treatment, even in a referral case. It is generally accepted that chiropractic treatment may assist the healing process in any disease condition.

Failure To Diagnose

Another large category of malpractice cases involving chiropractic physicians results from the failure to diagnose. In addition to the cancer cases that have been discussed, there are many involving fractures. There are numerous case references in which a chiropractic physician took x-ray films at the initial treatment visit and failed to discover a fracture. In some patients, the fracture became displaced after chiropractic treatment and required surgical reduction. These cases turn on the causation rule; that is, the plaintiff must prove that the chiropractic treatment was the proximate cause of the displacement of the fracture.

The same proximate cause rule applies to the category of cases that involve the treatment of herniated or ruptured disks. Frequently, a patient who underwent chiropractic treatment and later required surgery for a ruptured disk sues the chiropractor for malpractice. Chiropractors frequently treat patients with a herniated or ruptured disk with good results, and a treatment failure does not mean that the chiropractor committed an act of malpractice. The plaintiff must prove that the chiropractic treatment was the cause of the plaintiff's injuries. In this type of case, the legal burden is to prove that the patient's condition at the time of surgery was different from the patient's condition at the time that the chiropractor undertook treatment of the patient.

Stroke Cases

Approximately 107 cases of vascular accidents following spinal manipulative therapy have been documented in the medical literature. Insults to the vertebral artery and the carotid artery have been reported to have resulted from compression of the artery, bisection of the artery, or other trauma producing damage to the arterial wall.[6,7] Since the development of the so-called George test in 1981, most lawsuits involve the question of whether the chiropractor used a screening procedure that consists of one or more steps: (1) case history, (2) bilateral blood pressure readings, (3) neck auscultation, and (4) functional vascular tests. Most juries now consider failure to use the pre-screening tests to be a breach of the standard of care.[8]

Phrenic Nerve Cases

One case of phrenic nerve paralysis following chiropractic adjustment was reported in 1985. Since that time, there have been no reported further incidents of phrenic nerve paralysis. When a patient sues a chiropractic physician for malpractice, claiming that the chiropractic therapy resulted in phrenic nerve paralysis, it is important to know whether the patient's diaphragm was elevated prior to chiropractic therapy. The chiropractor should have copies of prior chest x-ray films and the x-ray films that he or she took on the patient's visit, prior to performing chiropractic therapy. In cases of thoracic complaint, it is also helpful if the chiropractor notes in the clinical findings the presence of an elevated diaphragm on the right, left, or bilateral, if it exists.[9]

Failure To Notify the Patient of an Unfavorable Diagnosis

The issues surrounding a practitioner's failure to inform the patient of an unfavorable diagnosis again arise in cancer type cases. Whether the non-disclosure is negligent or intentional, it creates a situation in which the plaintiff may claim that diagnosis at the time of the chiropractic physician's examination would have enabled him or her to obtain early medical treatment and increased the likelihood of a cure. Many of these cases follow the death of the patient as a result of the condition in question, and the claim for damages is high. The chiropractic physician has a legal duty to diagnose and inform the patient of any condition that is found. A jury never tolerates concealment.

The "Brittle" Patient

Another line of cases deal with the "brittle" patient. Certain patients, such as those who suffer from osteoporosis or those who are aged, may be predisposed to injury in chiropractic treatment. Obviously, the chiropractic physician has a duty to screen these patients and not to perform therapy that would injure them. Of course, when the patient has been properly screened and, through no fault of the chiropractic physician, properly applied therapy results in a bone fracture, the chiropractic physician is not considered at fault.

Use and Nonuse of X-ray

As stated earlier, all states now sanction the use of x-ray by chiropractic physicians. The x-ray has become such a common diagnostic tool that the standard of care frequently requires the chiropractic physician to perform certain standard x-ray tests prior to reaching a diagnosis and undertaking the treatment of the patient. Malpractice claims involving x-ray generally fall into two categories: overexposure to radiation and failure to take x-ray films.

As part of the patient history, the chiropractic physician should inquire about x-ray films that were taken earlier. In the event that the patient has already had the same type of x-ray study that the chiropractic physician needs to reach a diagnosis, the chiropractor has a duty to call for and examine those x-rays before exposing the patient to further radiation. Failure to do so is a breach of the standard of care.

Cases that involve the failure to take x-rays sometimes arise because the patient, before seeking chiropractic treatment, had x-ray films taken by a medical doctor and reported to the chiropractor that the results were normal. In such cases, the x-ray film may indeed be normal; on the other hand, the chiropractic physician may have seen something significant by reviewing the x-ray film. In any event, it is generally considered a breach of the standard of care for a chiropractic physician to fail to review previous x-ray films and to fail to take x-ray films before reaching a diagnosis, if the x-ray film would have had significant value in determining the patient's condition.

STATUTES OF LIMITATION

Every state has a statute of limitations that pertains to medical malpractice suits. These statutes run from 1 to 3 years or more, and their purpose is to set a time period beyond which suit cannot be brought. For instance, if the statute of limitations on a malpractice claim is 2 years and the patient does not bring a lawsuit within 2 years of the time of injury, suit is barred.

By statute and by case law, a statute of limitations may be tolled; that is, the time for the filing of the lawsuit may be extended by various circumstances. The concealment of the injuries so that the patient could not reasonably have discovered it, for example, is a reason for tolling the statute of limitations. In such cases, the statute does not begin to run until the patient reasonably should have discovered the injury. A lawsuit arising from an appliance left in the patient after surgery and not discovered until some later date is the most common example of such a case.

When a practitioner attempts to collect an unpaid bill from a recalcitrant patient, the patient may respond by bringing a counterclaim in malpractice. If the counterclaim is brought within the statute of limitations, the recovery on the counterclaim can be unlimited. For example, if the practitioner sues for a $100 bill, the patient can counterclaim for $1,000,000 in malpractice damages. If the practitioner brings a suit for nonpayment of the bill after the statute of limitations on malpractice has run, the patient can still bring a counterclaim for malpractice. The patient's recovery is limited to an offset, however; the patient can recover for malpractice no more than the practitioner is claiming for nonpayment of the bill. For this reason, most attorneys recommend that practitioners not bring suit to collect unpaid bills—if they suspect that the patient may counterclaim in malpractice—until after the statute of limitations has run.

INFORMED CONSENT

A frequent issue in malpractice cases is whether the patient consented to the specific treatment received. The patient is deemed not to be able to consent to a procedure without first receiving adequate information about the procedure. There are three basic prerequisites for informed consent: (1) the patient must have the capacity to reason and make judgments; (2) the decision must be made voluntarily and without coercion; and (3) the patient must have a clear understanding of the risks and benefits of the proposed treatment, alternatives, or nontreatment, along with a full understanding of the nature of the disease and the prognosis.

A practitioner is not required to disclose all possibilities that are reasonably foreseeable, such as the consequences of deviations from the applicable standard of treatment, but occur so infrequently as to be remote. It is generally felt that the risk of injury from chiropractic treatment is so remote that chiropractic physicians need not use informed consent forms. On the other hand, it is certainly prudent for the chiropractic physician to use informed consent forms when there are documented case histories of injury following the chiropractic adjustment to be performed. The use of informed consent procedures eliminates one of the causes of negligence or malpractice that is commonly used by plaintiff's attorneys in bringing a malpractice suit.

Although expert testimony is required in a malpractice case to establish what a reasonable practitioner should disclose to a patient, the degree of risk involved is a question of fact that the jury will decide, based on the expert testimony received. Malpractice cases resulting from lack of informed consent normally arise after treatment is concluded, and the results of treatment did not meet the patient's expectations. The plaintiff must establish a causal relationship between the alleged lack of consent and the resulting injury, but the risk is already manifested at the time the claim is made. Thus, it is difficult for the practitioner to defend against a claim when an informed consent procedure has not been used.

MALPRACTICE INSURANCE

According to a recent study, 8% of the practicing physicians in the United States will become defendants in a medical malpractice action.   Clearly, it behooves the chiropractic physician to obtain and maintain adequate malpractice insurance coverage. Several private insurance companies write malpractice coverage for chiropractors. In addition, there is the National Chiropractic Mutual Insurance Company, which is the largest carrier in the field and is controlled by chiropractic physicians.

A malpractice insurance policy provides the practitioner with two important benefits. First, the insurance provides the practitioner with a competent legal defense in the event of a malpractice claim. The cost of litigation is high, and the benefit of having that cost borne by the insurance company is important. Second, any recovery obtained against the practitioner for malpractice within the scope of practice will be covered by the insurance policy up to the limits of the policy.

Statistically, more than 50% of the physicians who are sued for medical malpractice win their cases with a defendant's verdict. The average jury verdict in malpractice cases against chiropractic physicians in 1988 was substantially below $100,000. At the same time, however, there are several malpractice verdicts each year in which awards to plaintiffs exceed $1,000,000; there are numerous awards in the $300,000 to $800,000 range. Thus, low limits of coverage may be adequate for the average chiropractic verdict, but the chiropractic physician would be wise to have the maximum limits available for a case involving death or disabling injury.

If the chiropractic physician is uninsured a plaintiff may request property attachments or other security at the time a suit is instituted. In the absence of insurance coverage, most courts will grant such a request for security. Property attachments granted as prejudgment remedies may tie up the practitioner's real estate or other assets for the duration of the litigation, which may be for years. In the event of a plaintiff's verdict, the attachment may be converted to a judgment lien, which is retroactive to the date of the original attachment. Failure to pay the verdict may result in foreclosure of the judgment lien, resulting in a public auction of the property. Appropriate insurance coverage avoids all these consequences. Obviously, the chiropractic physician who practices today without adequate insurance is foolhardy.

REFERENCES

1. Medical malpractice arbitration: Time for a model. Act. 33 Rutgers L. Rev. 454 (1981).

2. Recent medical malpractice legislation: a first checkup. 50 Tulane L. Rev. 655 (1976).

3. 52 American Law Review 2d, 1384.

4. *Miller v. Drowin,* 183 Conn. 189 (1981).

5. 42 USC § 1395x(r).

6. Terrett A. Vascular accidents from cervical spine manipulations: The mechanisms. *ACA Journ of Chiropr.* 1988;25(5):59.

7. Terrett A. Vascular accidents from cervical spine manipulation: Report on 107 cases. *ACA Journ of Chiropr.* 1988;25(4):63.

8. George PE, Silverstein HI, Wallace H, Marshall M. Identification of the high risk pre-stroke patient. *ACA Journ of Chiropr.* 1981;18(3):S26–8.

9. Hefner J. Diaphragmatic paralysis following chiropractic manipulation of the cervical spine. *Arch Intern Med.* 1985;145(3):562–564.

13

Standards of Practice in Third-Party Relationships

Charles A. Simpson and Richard H. Tilden

> *The doctor's responsibility is not primarily to*
> *a colleague*
> *an attorney*
> *an insurer*
> *It isn't even to the patient.*
> *It is to the TRUTH, even when politically or economically inconvenient to the doctor.*

The primary focus of standards of practice for chiropractic physicians is the doctor-patient relationship. Physician behavior and activity with respect to the patient is the principal concern. In today's climate of medical care delivery, however, the doctor-patient relationship and the physician's activities in this relationship are no longer the only areas of concern in developing standards of practice. Many third-party interests intersect with the doctor-patient relationship, and established standards may be applied to these third-party relationships.

THIRD PARTIES

Purchasers of health care services, patients' attorneys, various administrative agencies, and employers share concerns about the interactions between a doctor and a patient. The emergence of managed care organizations (MCOs) creates another third party with a legitimate interest in the primary doctor-patient relationship. Relationships between physicians and third-party payers can be critical in that a breakdown in such relationships can compromise the outcome of health care services as effectively as can inadequate diagnosis or treatment. It is incumbent on practitioners to understand the necessary requirements of third-party payers, if the highest standard of chiropractic practice is to be realized. Purchasers of health care services have a right to examine a physician's interaction with a patient to determine eligibility for benefits, as well as the reasonableness and necessity of diagnostic and treatment procedures.

Patients may also be claimants in a compensation system (eg, workers' compensation, personal injury, social security). A patient in litigation involving health care is generally represented by legal counsel. These advocates are dependent on the treating or examining physician for expert medical testimony in making the case for their client. A physician who is able to perform adequately in this arena renders a service to the patient that can be as valuable as are the services rendered through the physician's clinical expertise and technical skill.

In a similar fashion, various administrative agencies, such as workers' compensation agencies, the Social Security Administration, and welfare and state employment services, depend on information from treating physicians in making administrative determinations. Physician awareness of the particular demands of each of these agencies facilitates communication and can further promote effective health care.

Employers rely on efficient health care providers to assist their employees in recovering from illness and injury. In addition, they often rely on the medical judgment of an employee's doctor in determining the workload that is appropriate for that employee, the need for physical restrictions on work activities, and the need for temporary total disability. Employers can benefit from the special knowledge of chiropractic physicians concerning the biomechanical aspects of ergonomic design in the workplace. Expertise in these areas enhances a physician's ability to serve patients.

The advent of MCOs has expanded the circle of interested third parties. Like third-party payers, MCOs are interested in physician behavior in treating patients, but with an added focus on utilization review and quality of care. When a chiropractic physician agrees to participate in an MCO, there is an incumbent responsibility to provide the MCO with the data relevant to clinical encounters. Understanding this necessity and performing accordingly become nearly as important as knowing how to develop a successful doctor-patient relationship, formulate an accurate diagnosis, and provide appropriate treatment.

PHYSICIAN RESPONSIBILITIES COMMON TO ALL THIRD PARTIES

Interaction with third-party payers emphasizes the importance of certain physician activities and behaviors. Although each class of interested third parties may have its own particular interests, some physician behaviors are necessary for all these groups.

Clinical Documentation

Practitioners must provide clinical documentation of diagnosis and the plan of treatment to the interested third party under appropriate circumstances. The elements of the history, the diagnosis, the treatment offered, and the clinical outcome must be consistent. In providing this documentation, the chiropractic physician is called upon to advocate the patient's need for care. It is imperative for the effective physician to be able to communicate with the interested parties regarding this need.

Complete documentation of the clinical interaction is the key element in third-party relationships. The medical chart documents a patient's condition through a record of past and present medical history, symptoms, examination findings, diagnosis, treatment, and outcome. Chiropractic care cannot be described as appropriate unless it has been documented. From a legal point of view, if it has not been written down, it has not happened.

Third-party payers, attorneys, administrative agencies, and MCO utilization committees depend primarily on the written records provided by the treating physician. The ability to generate and maintain adequate clinical notes is crucial if the appropriate standard of care is to be achieved. Haldeman proposed a system of clinical record keeping that originated in the problem-oriented medical record developed by Weed.[1,2] Although this format for record keeping has not received universal acceptance, it is widely recognized as an acceptable standard by which clinical records may be judged. State statutes and rules governing chiropractic practice routinely refer to clinical record keeping. For example, the Oregon Administrative Rules state: "It will be considered fraud not to keep complete detailed and correct records and case histories of the services (diagnostic and therapeutic procedures employed) rendered to each patient."[3] Most state chiropractic laws have similar provisions.

Standard:
The practitioner must provide for appropriate sharing of information within the confines of patient confidentiality.

Chart Notes

Properly developed clinical chart notes provide timely documentation of a patient's condition, some indication of that condition's course, the type and extent of treatment rendered, and an assessment of the likely outcome of treatment. These notes should include clinical examination findings, both at initial evaluations and at subsequent reevaluations. Treatment notes also should record objective findings at every visit. Dates of treatments and an interim history of exacerbations or new injuries must be clearly recorded.

The clinical findings, both objective and subjective, should provide reasonable indications for the treatment offered.

The medical history, in conjunction with the examination findings, should support the diagnosis through a logical chain of clinical reasoning. A statement of the diagnosis should be in the medical record. The problem-oriented clinical record offers a scheme for updating the diagnosis by maintaining a "problem list." As a particular condition is brought to resolution, the "problem" is eliminated from the list. New and emerging problems can be added to the list at any time when supported by clinical and historical data entered into the record. Haldeman and Weed opposed keeping separate files for multiple injuries,[1,2] as the medical record is for the benefit of the patient and must provide continuity.

The treatment modalities employed, the frequency of treatment, and the time span over which treatment is to proceed should be specified in the medical record. This course of treatment and the time frame should be consistent with the pathological features known to be associated with the diagnosis and displayed by that particular patient. If, during the course of treatment, new information emerges or other signs and symptoms appear, the treatment plan can be altered to reflect the new contingencies. In addition, failure of the patient to progress with the original treatment plan dictates different treatment approaches, consultation, referral to another specialty, or discharge from treatment. Continued treatment in the absence of documented improvement is rarely justifiable.

Standard:
Treatment must be efficient and effective.

Patient Advocacy

With this rational approach, the attending practitioner can reasonably justify the patient's need for treatment. Failing to comply with these guidelines in one of the areas of history, examination, diagnosis, or treatment plan lessens the credibility of the treating practitioner and detracts from the effectiveness of his or her advocacy for the patient. Patient advocacy is inappropriate when treatment is rendered on the basis of subjective complaints only and without supportive objective findings of improvement.

Standard:
Objectivity lends credence to advocacy.

Clinical Communication

In addition to creating documents that capture all aspects of the clinical encounter, the attending practitioner should be able to communicate relevant information both orally and in writing. Whether informally by telephone or in a sworn statement, such as a deposition or court testimony, the practitioner's ability to communicate orally about clinical issues can be of paramount importance in representing the patient. Written narratives, brief reports, and updated reports are all routinely called for by interested third parties. The ability to generate chiropractic reports that are meaningful to nonchiropractic professionals is an important service to the patient.

Standard:
   Maintaining objectivity and a commitment to rational analysis is incumbent upon the treating chiropractor.

UNIQUE NEEDS OF THIRD PARTIES

Although third parties have many needs in common, other needs are unique to a particular party. Payers' interests are quite different from those of the patient's employer. These, in turn, are distinct from the needs and interests of other third parties, such as attorneys and others.

Payers

In managing claims for health benefits, payers have unique needs. Communication with payers of all types consists primarily of billings for services rendered. Each type of payer may have particular requirements for additional documentation, depending largely on the benefit design (eg, workers' compensation, personal injury, health and welfare).

Beginning in the 1960s, the health care industry began standardizing procedures. Increasingly, government and private health care insurance programs have come to rely on formalized descriptions and identifications for health care procedures in the private office, hospital, or other medical setting. The most widely used form of procedural coding, *Current Procedural Terminology* (CPT), has been adapted to the chiropractic profession and its unique service.[4]

Inherent in this formalized approach to billing is a tension between the intent of the system and a tendency to maximize return on services rendered. At root, the intent of the CPT codes or similar systems is to provide terminology for procedures and services common to all fields of medical practice. Certain management practices in the health care professions encourage "laundry list" approaches to billing, however, effectively "gaming" the system. For example, a routine visit to a chiropractor's office can be "unbundled" to include an office call, a manipulation, a manipulation to a second and third area, massage, trigger point therapy, and one or more physical therapy modalities. Each procedure has its own code, and each has an available fee.

Ethical and legal guidelines in this area are sketchy, but so-called "unbundling" of fees is a misuse of CPT codes and distorts relationships between payers and service providers. The practitioner clearly has the right to be compensated for services rendered. Presenting the bill for service in a format designed to produce maximum revenue can compromise the efficient delivery of health care, however. Decisions relative to the amount and necessity of treatment are the proving ground of an individual physician's clinical honesty, as the legal climate in the antitrust area has constrained the ability of physicians to determine fees as a group.

Some health care delivery systems such as workers' compensation, are unaffected by antitrust, and relative value schedules that effectively set fees are in place. It remains for individual practitioners to make ethically driven decisions in the development of billings.

The emergence of for-profit MCOs is a market-driven attempt to control medical costs. As managed health care systems replace the usual fee-for-service style of medical care at an increasing rate, the physician's ability to determine the level of his or her fee schedule will diminish. The manner and combination in which the services are delivered will be similarly constrained in a managed health care environment.

Ideally, fees should reflect the degree of knowledge and skill required to perform the procedure or service, as well as the time needed for the treatment. Fees for treatment rendered should be consistent across all sources of payment. Statutes and rules in many states frequently specify this point. For example, the Oregon Administrative Rules state, "Insurance carriers, including workers' compensation carriers, shall not be expected to pay a fee greater than an individual physician normally charges patients who are paying their own bills."[5]

Fees are often reduced by contractual agreements (eg, with MCOs), by rule (eg, in most workers' compensation systems), or by other arrangements. The responsibility for the difference between the billed charges and the reimbursed fee may also be determined by contractual agreement or by rule, or it may be negotiated directly with the consumer. The health care provider must be sensitive to the reimbursement environment of each patient. The terms of contracts and the rules of compensation systems differ widely. Open lines of communication among providers, consumers, and payers can serve to clarify questions and solve problems. Insurance relations committees of physicians' trade groups, provider committees in health maintenance organizations (HMOs), and utilization review committees of MCOs all facilitate this communication.

Workers' Compensation Systems

Few other primary care providers have as much to offer injured workers as does a chiropractor. Although many injuries require treatment that is outside the scope of chiropractic practice, a high percentage of on-the-job injuries are of a musculoskeletal nature. The conservative chiropractic approach has a great deal to offer workers who have suffered strains, sprains, and cumulative trauma disorders. A chiropractor's special expertise in conditions of the spine can provide an efficient and effective solution to the most common clinical problem in industrial medicine—back injuries.

Health care providers' participation in workers' compensation systems carries certain responsibilities. Workers' compensation insurance is different from other forms of health insurance. It is intended primarily to protect injured workers from losses due to injuries on the job. Compensation for lost wages (ie, temporary disability), lost physical capacity (ie, permanent disability), or death is a primary function of all systems. An equally necessary, but secondary, function is payment for medical expenses that arise in connection with an on-the-job injury. The physician's role in determining the necessity of treatment and in evaluating the degree of impairment is pivotal in the success of workers' compensation systems.

The reporting requirements of most workers' compensation systems are unique and often arbitrary. Patients who are seeking workers' compensation are often in a dilemma that affects the doctor-patient relationship and sometimes affects the response to treatment. When compensation is paid on the basis of length of disability or degree of permanent impairment of physical function, there may be strong financial incentives for a patient not to get well. The effects of compensation on recovery are well recognized and controversial. Moreover, the ethical issues that surface in the workers' compensation arena are unique in chiropractic practice. In the usual doctor-patient relationship, the doctor's primary responsibilities flow to the best interests of the patient. Primary responsibilities in a worker's compensation case, however, flow both to the patient's interest and to the employer. What is best for the patient may not be best for the employer. Managing this conflict requires practical knowledge of problem solving involving ethical issues.

By and large, physicians control access to medical treatment in a workers' compensation system. They also provide the medical evidence that forms the basis of compensation for temporary or permanent disability. Managing this complex role appropriately is a challenge to all health care professionals and reflects directly on the credibility and respect given to a profession. Physicians who expect to deliver and be paid for services rendered to injured workers must understand practical matters, such as documentation and reporting requirements, and must use appropriate forms and terminology. Although an accurate and complete diagnosis is as important in workers' compensation systems as in other insurance settings, determination of causation becomes critical for workers' compensation.

The chiropractic physician must be able to differentiate job-related conditions from non–job-related injuries, preexisting problems, and congenital or degenerative conditions. Treatment rendered for the latter conditions is not usually compensable in workers' compensation systems. Impairment that arises from them may also not be compensable.

An understanding of the key terms commonly used in workers' compensation systems is a basic necessity (see Glossary). Individual systems often have particular usage, as well as peculiar and unique terminology. These are defined in the administrative rules of the various states and provinces and may vary significantly. Knowing the meaning of these terms and the correct way to use them facilitates communication in the system. Obviously, it is the responsibility of the participating physician to be informed about the prevailing workers' compensation system. In some systems, there are special educational requirements and programs for participating physicians.

Personal Injury Insurance

Patients frequently seek chiropractic care as a result of injury caused by motor vehicle accidents. The chiropractic physician who chooses to treat patients covered by motor vehicle accident insurance bears certain responsibilities that are peculiar to this third-party environment.

Like workers' compensation systems, personal injury protection laws are often quite specific about reporting requirements, time constraints, dollar limits, and other regulations. The treating chiropractor must be conversant with the laws, rules, and procedures of his or her locality. Patients often rely on their doctor for basic information regarding laws and rules, as well as for medical help. Referral to appropriate legal counsel is also a responsibility that frequently falls to the treating doctor; in this matter, a full measure of objectivity and financial disinterest is essential.

Objectivity is also the byword in representing the medical aspects of a patient's motor vehicle accident claim. As in workers' compensation, the more objective the treating physician, the greater the weight of his or her medical opinion. Inappropriate advocacy by a treating physician compromises that physician's credibility and limits the influence of the medical opinions offered.

As with all clinical encounters, the medical record creates a permanent documentation of the injured patient's condition, the treatment offered, and the outcome. Although the primary function of the medical records is to facilitate appropriate case management, they also may become key elements in a legal proceeding.

> Medical records not only should be complete and legible, but also should clearly indicate subjective and objective findings, diagnosis, treatment, and outcome.

Medical records are an exception to the hearsay rule. They are regarded as reliable, because they were prepared at the time of the events that were recorded. If the events are not captured in writing, for legal purposes, they did not occur.

> Chiropractic physicians who elect to treat patients injured in motor vehicle accidents shall accept the responsibility of offering testimony in legal proceedings.

Treating physicians are often required to submit written reports or to give oral testimony in hearings, trials, or arbitration proceedings. Accurate clinical records are the factual underpinnings of reports and testimony. The skill necessary to translate clinical data into language that is understood by the layman, whether attorney, judge, or jury, is critical.

The most common role for the chiropractic expert in a legal proceeding is in support of his or her own patient, but chiropractors are increasingly used as defense expert witnesses as well. In general, a chiropractor who acts as a defense witness should demonstrate the same thoroughness and clinical objectivity that he or she would demonstrate as the plaintiff's doctor. The relationship of the defense expert to the patient is, of course, quite different. Many of the standards governing the usual doctor-patient relationship also apply, however.

The defense expert may see the patient in an independent medical examination. In this setting, no actual doctor-patient relationship is created in that no treatment or advice is given to the patient. All recommendations made by the independent examiner should be offered for consideration to the patient's chiropractor.

The defense medical expert usually examines the patient. Great care and sensitivity are necessary in this role. The patient frequently perceives the relationship to be adversarial, which can compromise the history and examination. A friendly, nonthreatening, and objective approach to a patient examined on behalf of the defense is usually rewarded with candid and compliant behavior on the part of the patient.

Health Benefits Insurance

Payers of health benefits have a contractual relationship with their enrollees to pay for medical services. Most contracts specify that payment will be made only for reasonable and medically necessary services. The chiropractic physician who renders service to a patient with health insurance must understand the concepts of reasonable and necessary. Furthermore, certain policies may have particular exceptions, exclusions, or limits on diagnoses or treatments that are allowed by any particular health care provider.

The reasonable test is most often applied to the dollar amount billed for the service provided. Reasonable charges for service can be derived from customary charges or from usual charges. The customary charge can be determined from a survey of the fees that a physician has charged his or her patients for a particular service; the range or charges in such a survey indicates the median charge, which is considered the "customary" charge of that particular physician for that particular service. Usual (or prevailing) charges are those that similar providers in a given area most frequently charge for a particular service. The area is often defined in geographical and/or socioeconomic terms. When they are considered for payment, a chiropractor's billed charges are often compared with customary and usual fees to determine the reasonableness of the bill. The chiropractic physician must be aware of the limits implicit in the concepts of usual, customary, and reasonable fees if he or she expects satisfactory compensation for services provided. Failure to recognize these constraints penalizes the patient who may otherwise assume that the insurance carrier will pay for the services delivered.

The test of medical necessity may also be applied to a chiropractor's bills when they are considered for payment. Medically necessary services are those within the standards of good chiropractic practice in the chiropractic community. Necessary services are appropriate for the evaluation of symptoms, diagnosis, and treatment of the patient's condition. Necessity also requires that the level of service provided (ie, brief, intermediate, or comprehensive) be appropriate for the condition. Finally, medically necessary services are not primarily for the convenience of the patient, the physician, or another health care provider, but depend on the medical condition and the requirements for diagnosis and treatment.

Chiropractors who choose to treat insured patients must understand these concepts of reasonable and necessary. Failure to consider these concepts in billing for services can cause unnecessary aggravation and financial hardship for the patient. In addition, the credibility and reputation of the chiropractor is at stake. Bills that are at wide variance from the usual and customary charges or appear to include fees for procedures of questionable medical necessity reflect poorly on the individual practitioner and the chiropractic profession as a whole.

Fee-for-service and prepaid health insurance plans frequently require copayments as part of the contract with the enrollee. Co-payments may restrain the unnecessary use of medical services, but such out-of-pocket expenses may also prevent a patient from obtaining necessary or even critical health care. Many chiropractic physicians forgive co-payments for patients who cannot afford them, as the forgiveness of co-payments makes the difference between receiving and not receiving needed care.

Lachs and his colleagues pointed out that, from the payer's perspective, forgiving co-payments represents an unacceptable tinkering with the contractual and actuarial relationships that underlie health insurance systems.[6] If, for example, a 20% co-payment is required, forgiving co-payments amounts to a 20% discount on services from which only the patient benefits. Were the discount shared equally, the insurance company would be responsible for 80% of the discounted fee, and the patient would be responsible for the remainder. Furthermore, forgiving co-payments can lead to the delivery of unnecessary services, increasing the inefficiency of the health care system. The legal standards in this area have yet to be defined.

Health insurance policies may have a wide range of special provisions. For example, health insurance policies often contain special provisions related to diagnosis. For example, medical conditions that existed before the patient's enrollment are frequently exempted from the benefit. A patient with an old back problem may not have coverage for treatment directed to this problem. In addition, most health benefits policies do not cover problems that result from work activity or motor vehicle accidents. Health benefits carriers sometimes provide special coverage for acute accidental injuries, however. Co-payments are often waived if a medical condition results from an accident rather than a constitutional or degenerative condition. Moreover, maintenance and preventive care are often outside the scope of health benefits policies; these services become the patient's own responsibility.

Chiropractors routinely complain about "health" insurance being in actuality "illness" insurance. Philosophically, chiropractors adhere to a preventive approach to treatment. Unfortunately, the clinical data necessary to support this point of view are not available at present. Although there is a great deal of anecdotal evidence to support preventive chiropractic treatment, most health benefits insurance carriers refuse to pay for treatment rendered on a preventive or maintenance basis.

Medicaid

State-administered health care plans for the poor may include provisions for chiropractic services. Chiropractors who choose to accept Medicaid patients must accept the requirements and limitations inherent in most Medicaid programs, however. Administrators of these programs are constantly hamstrung by inadequate funding. Each state agency handles the problem differently, but the usual result for the provider of medical services is a significantly reduced fee and, sometimes, no reimbursement at all.

Medicaid programs may include provisions that may restrict the use of diagnostic and therapeutic procedures. Keeping aware of these restrictions and using resources appropriately, both inside and outside of the Medicaid programs, are perhaps the best services that a chiropractor can perform for those less fortunate.

The fundamental tenet in chiropractic ethics is to act always for the greatest good of the patient. Practical experience suggests that success in a doctor-patient relationship depends in large measure on the expectations to pay for and to receive compensation for services. If no fee is asked and no payment expected, the value of the service declines to zero. On the other hand, to refuse to render effective treatment to a suffering patient whose circumstances do not allow payment for those services is also unacceptable. Therefore, although doctors of chiropractic are entitled to receive reasonable compensation for their professional services, common sense and longstanding professional sensibilities direct the chiropractic physician to offer treatment irrespective of the patient's ability to pay and the doctor's expectation of compensation.

The legal profession has developed the standard of *probono* service. It is expected that 10% of legal work will be done without expectation of compensation. It may be incumbent on all of the learned professions to give away at least a portion of their services for the good of all.

Medicare

The inclusion of chiropractic in the provision of health care to Medicare recipients was a political breakthrough for the profession. Medicare patients have benefited from chiropractic treatment for many years. Physician participation in the Medicare program has become increasingly constrained during this time, however, because of various attempts to keep Medicare costs in line with the available resources. Among the administrative attempts to control costs are caps on fees, screens, limits on allowable diagnoses and treatments, and the emergence of diagnosis-related groups (DRGs) and resource-based value schedules (RBVS).

Chiropractors who choose to accept Medicare patients must be willing to adapt to the special requirements of the program. Learning the vagaries of Medicare reimbursement and staying abreast of the ever-changing Medicare rules and procedures requires constant attention and considerable patience.

Attorneys

Litigation is a routine feature of chiropractic practice. Many states have joint bar-chiropractic liaison committees that attempt to oversee attorney-chiropractor relations. The very existence of these joint committees testifies to the importance of this interprofessional dialogue. Standards developed by these liaison committees for attorney-chiropractor relationships are enforced by mutual cooperation and rarely have the power of law.

> A primary obligation of the chiropractic physician to the patient and the patient's attorney is to provide a comprehensible interpretation of the patient's condition.

The chiropractor's professional knowledge and understanding are well suited to medical-legal situations involving conditions of and injuries to the musculoskeletal system, particularly the spine. Chiropractors specialize in the diagnosis and treatment of musculoskeletal injuries that often defy precise pathological definition, but nonetheless may cause significant disability. Assisting a patient and his or her attorney toward an appropriate and just compensation is a valuable service.

An awareness of basic legal protocol is fundamental for the chiropractic physician who is to be a witness in medical-legal matters. One important aspect of this protocol is the attorney-chiropractor conference. The chiropractor's obligation is to explain in lay language basic information about chiropractic and about musculoskeletal physiology, injury, and repair. This explanation should include chiropractic terminology and concepts, the relationship of the injury to the patient's condition, the measure of impairment, and the extent of the resultant disability.

> An objective appraisal of the medical facts, combined with a coherent interpretation of the clinical history, is a solid basis for any medical-legal case. The chain of clinical reasoning must follow logically through the patient's history, examination findings, treatment plan, and outcome.

The diagnostic and therapeutic procedures that were provided should lie within the mainstream of chiropractic practice. The testimony will be closely scrutinized by other chiropractors and by medical physicians, who may review the facts and opinions. To the extent that the procedures employed are validated by these other observers, the credibility of the chiropractic physician's testimony will be enhanced.

Employers

The ethical demands of occupational medical practice deserve special mention. The obligations of a chiropractor who chooses to treat an injured worker flow in many directions and sometimes appear to be diametrically opposed. Not only is the chiropractic physician expected to act in the patient's best interests and advocate appropriately for the patient's need for treatment, but also the chiropractor must address the needs of the employer and the worker's compensation system. The two sets of responsibilities create tension and ambiguity in the delivery of medical care to an injured worker. Confronting and managing this ethical dilemma effectively is an integral part of treating injured workers.

As attending practitioners in many workers' compensation systems, chiropractors are called upon to document permanent physical impairment and ability to work. In order to be effective in this arena, a treating chiropractor must be able to document the objective physical examination findings and understand their relationship to a determination of physical impairment. Administrators, claims adjudicators, referees, attorneys, and other physicians routinely review disability determinations made by chiropractors. To the extent that the treating chiropractor's observations and statements remain solidly grounded in objective facts and are well reasoned clinically, the opinions as to impairment and disability ratings will be credible.

The treatment of injured workers requires the recognition of important factors that go beyond physical injury and physiological response. Hadler urged the acceptance of the concept of the "predicament" of the injured worker,[7] which places the patient with the injury and need for treatment against a background of associated social, economic, and psychological factors. The literature on the effect of compensation on injury and recovery is not univocal, however, the negative effect of compensation has been demonstrated. The successful treatment of workers' compensation patients requires a thorough and practical understanding of the psychosocial and economic dimensions of the patient's problem. The inability to discriminate psychosocial and economic problems from purely physical and physiological problems leads to the inefficient delivery of health care services, prolonged disability, and the risk of fostering unnecessary chronic pain behavior.

Social Security Administration

The chiropractic physician's role in Social Security disability determination is limited. Although chiropractors do not usually participate directly in disability evaluation, they may be called on to supply routine medical evidence, such as examination findings, x-ray films and laboratory reports, and treatment chart notes. Responding to requests from the Social Security Administration for information about an applicant is an obligation to be fulfilled on behalf of the patient. Social Security does not provide reimbursement for this service.

Patients are often not aware of the most basic elements of the Social Security disability system. Therefore, a practitioner's a fundamental knowledge of Social Security benefits and eligibility requirements can be quite helpful to patients in making their decision to apply for benefits. The Social Security Administration has published a handbook for physicians, *Disability Evaluation under Social Security,*[8] that contains evaluation criteria and listings of the impairments that form the medical basis for disability. The chiropractic physician must understand the basics of "impairment" and "disability" in the Social Security disability system in order to advise patients appropriately.

Managed Care Organizations

The economics of health care is in the midst of a revolution. The traditional supply-and-demand economics of fee-for-service medical care has largely given way to alternative forms of financing because of upward-spiraling health care costs; increasingly expensive medical technology; and changes in public expectations and perceptions about health, well-being and doctors. The public policy debate over health care is no longer framed in terms of how much society wants or needs, but how much society can afford.

In this climate of rising costs and dwindling resources, various systems of health care delivery have been developed in an effort to provide adequate care for an affordable and predictable cost. A variety of prepaid health insurance plans now offer managed health care delivery, and health care providers of all kinds are seeing their patients enroll in managed care systems. There is little practical choice for health care providers but to participate in these systems as well.

Chiropractic participation in managed care is in its infancy at present, and standards in this area of practice are yet to be developed. To be an effective participant in MCOs, however, the chiropractic profession must meet the particular needs of these systems. Doing so may require fundamental changes in the professional outlook that has characterized the profession during its first century of existence.

Chiropractors have frequently claimed to be cost-effective, especially in the treatment of spine-related problems. If the chiropractic profession can demonstrate that chiropractic care can resolve certain health problems more economically than the medical alternative can, MCOs will direct patients with those conditions toward chiropractors. The challenge to chiropractic is to develop the data that confirm its cost-effectiveness and then to demonstrate this efficiency in performance in a managed care setting.

Participation in MCOs will present a series of challenges and opportunities for the chiropractic profession and for individual chiropractic physicians. Basic requirements of MCO inclusion are procedures for credentialing, peer review, utilization review, and quality assurance. Certain of these processes are familiar ground to chiropractors. Others may require a measure of professional introspection and growth.

Credentialing Process

Credentialing is the process by which a prospective provider applies to and is screened by the MCO. The provider generally must pay a fee, after which the MCO screens the provider according to various criteria. Of primary interest are practice patterns, fee structures, and other indicators of performance by the chiropractic physician. In this manner, the MCO can assure its client payers in advance of some measure of predictable performance by the providers in the MCO. The credentialing procedure requires that the physician-applicant be willing and able to open his or her practice to intense scrutiny.

Practitioner/Utilization Review

The essential feature of all MCOs is the review and improvement of physician performance. The practice patterns of panel physicians can be compared with those of other members of the panel and with external standards. Physicians whose patterns of practice appear to fall outside the norms can become the subject of further scrutiny. In a corrective action model, this information is reported back to the physician or the panel. More detailed information about the problematic pattern of practice may explain the reasons for the deviation from the norm or may establish a basis for further education of the provider.

A utilization review focuses on the appropriateness, efficiency, and economy of health care services and resources by means of concurrent and/or retrospective review of data on provider performance. Consideration is given to the level and duration of care, units of service, and use of ancillary services. Additional factors include evidence that the diagnosis is supported by the medical records. Is there a causal relationship sufficient to establish third-party responsibility? Is appropriate use made of ancillary services and of diagnostic and treatment referrals? Professional review during claim analysis ensures consistency between the clinical factors of history, findings, diagnosis, and treatment plan. This further level of concurrent review is critical if utilization review is to be successful.

Medical records are routinely reviewed for clinical consistency of history, diagnosis, and treatment. The focus is on appropriate use of diagnostic procedures, level, intensity and frequency of treatment, and cost per unit of service. This process is common in medical practice, especially in the hospital setting. Traditionally, chiropractors have not been subject to this type of review; however, it will be increasingly common in chiropractic in the immediate future.

Quality Assurance

A less direct method of evaluation, quality assurance focuses on measured treatment outcomes and the means by which care is dispensed. Its goal is to ensure organizational excellence and the best possible ambulatory care. Krantz and Hendrickson defined quality of care as "the degree to which care is provided in an appropriate manner, within an appropriate time frame."[9] Vear considered quality to be "concerned with outcomes which can be verified by the direct measurement of the improved health of the individual or the population served."[10]

The Institute of Medicine defined quality health care as that which is "effective in bettering the health status and satisfaction of a population, within the resources that society and individuals have chosen to spend for that care."[11] Palmer described five "dimensions" of quality.

> The dimensions encountered . . . are:
> - *Effectiveness.* The power of a particular procedure or treatment to improve health status.
> - *Efficiency.* The delivery of a maximum number of comparable units of health care for a given unit of health resources used.
> - *Accessibility.* The ease with which health care can be reached in the face of financial, organizational, cultural, and emotional barriers.
> - *Acceptability.* The degree to which health care satisfies patients.
> - *Provider Competence.* The core, because it is concerned with the provider's ability to use the best available knowledge and judgment to produce the health and satisfaction of consumers. Provider competence can refer to an individual's technical and interpersonal skills . . . [or] to a health care delivery system and the way in which it functions as a whole.[12]

In the health care marketplace, then, these dimensions of quality "speak directly to the delivery of health care that *works*, that is cost effective, that is delivered by appropriate providers, that extends to all who need it when they need it, and that satisfies the full set of the customer's requirements."[13]

All aspects of practice and the entire range of services of all provider and ancillary personnel are subject to quality assurance. The initial focus of investigation can be provider-specific or an entire group practice. A baseline review of current performance, the medical literature, and other sources will establish the generally accepted standards. A reasonable threshold is set, and information pertaining to the performance of the panel is collected. Outcome measurements are used to evaluate the results of care, patient satisfaction, and payer satisfaction. If necessary, a plan is developed for corrective action; this involves education and feedback. Periodic restudy is necessary to see if practice patterns have improved. The process continues to evolve as the factors used to ensure improvement and increased sophistication of the reevaluation process are modified.

As managed care concepts come to dominate health care delivery, "price" will diminish as a driving force in the market. In its place, "quality" will be the commodity most highly valued. In a cost-cutting environment with an increasing concern over quality, any organization that can demonstrate high-quality care will have a decided competitive advantage.

REFERENCES

1. Haldeman S. Important record keeping in evaluation of chiropractic results. *ACA Journal of Chiropractic.* 1975; 9:108–114

2. Weed LL. Medical records that guide and teach. *N Engl J Med.* 1986; 278:593–600, 652–657.

3. Or. Admin. R., chap 8, div. 15, § 005 (1987).

4. Llewellyn JK. *CA-ICD-9-CM.* Corvallis, Or: Chiropractic Publishing Service, 1983.

5. Or. Admin. R., chap 8, div. 15, § 000(2) (1987).

6. Lachs MS, Sindelar JL, Horwitz RI. The forgiveness of coinsurance. *N Engl J Med.* 1990; 322(22): 1599–1602.

7. Hadler NM. *Clinical Concepts in Regional Musculoskeletal Illness.* Orlando, Fl.: Grune & Stratton; 1987.

8. US Department of Health, Education and Welfare. *Disability Evaluation under Social Security; A Handbook for Physicians.* Washington, D.C.: HEW Pub. No. (SSA) 79-10089, 1979.

9. Krantz KC, Hendrickson RM. *Chiropractic and the HMO-PPO Challenge.* Washington, D.C.: International Chiropractors Association; 1988.

10. Vear HJ. Standards of chiropractic practice. *Journal of Manipulative and Physiological Therapeutics.* 1985; 8(1):33–43.

11. Institute of Medicine. *Advancing the Quality of Health Care: Key Issues and Fundamental Principles.* Washington, DC: National Academy of Sciences; 1974.

12. Palmer RH: *Ambulatory Health Care Evaluation: Principles and Practice.* Chicago: American Hospital Association; 1983:15.

13. Benson DS, Townes PG. *Excellence in Ambulatory Care.* San Francisco: Jossey-Bass; 1990:56.

Appendix A _____
Attributes of Chiropractic Practice Guidelines

The following attributes of practice guidelines provide guidance for the development of new guidelines as well as the evaluation of existing ones.

ATTRIBUTE 1

Chiropractic standards and guidelines should be developed by or in conjunction with chiropractic organizations.

Organizations and individuals participating in the development of chiropractic standards and guidelines should be characterized by the following:

- scientific and clinical expertise in the content areas of the guidelines;
- broad-based representation of doctors and chiropractic likely to be affected by the guidelines; and
- process capabilities for facilitating panels, providing evidence and viewpoints to panels and reviewing draft guidelines.

Relevant chiropractic organizations should have the opportunity to review and comment on practice guidelines during their development.

ATTRIBUTE 2

Reliable methodologies that integrate relevant research and appropriate clinical expertise should be used to develop chiropractic standards and guidelines.

Documentation—the procedures followed in developing guidelines, the participants involved, the evidence used, the assumptions and rationale accepted, and the analytic methods employed must be documented meticulously and described.

Documentation of review of relevant literature and other appropriate research should be available:

- description of the process for reviewing the clinical and scientific literature and appropriate research is noted or available on request, and
- description of the evidence reviewed is included or available upon request.

Expert clinical judgment and review should be provided, including use of appropriate consensus methods, the methodology of which is evidenced by:

- description of clinical review process and credentials of consensus facilitator is documented and available upon request; and
- special chiropractic procedure interests, specialty affiliations and other credentials of groups or individuals providing clinical expertise and review is documented and available upon request.

Findings from the review of relevant research findings and clinical judgment, including substantive minority reports should be incorporated into practice standards and guidelines and evidenced by:

- statements regarding the basis (e.g., scientific literature, clinical judgment) for the practice standards or guidelines are noted or available upon request.

ATTRIBUTE 3

Practice standards and guidelines should be as comprehensive and specific as possible.

Validity—Practice guidelines are valid if, when followed, they lead to better health outcomes. A prospective assessment of validity will consider the substance and quality of the evidence cited, the means used to evaluate the evidence, and the relationship between the evidence and recommendations.

Reliability/Reproducibility—Practice guidelines are reproducible and reliable if (1) given the same evidence and methods for guideline development, another set of experts produces essentially the same statements, and (2) given the same clinical circumstances, the guidelines are interpreted and applied consistently by practitioners (or other appropriate health care providers).

Clinical Applicability—Practice guidelines should be as inclusive of appropriately defined patient populations as evidence and expert judgment permit, and they should explicitly state the population(s) to which they apply.

Clinical Flexibility—Practice guidelines must identify the specifically known or generally expected exceptions to what is recommended.

Clarity—Practice guidelines must use unambiguous language, define terms clearly, and use a logical and easy-to-follow mode of presentation.

Guidelines should consist of statements noting indications for appropriate management in specific clinical situations.

Guidelines should be designed to assist clinicians by providing a framework for the evaluation and treatment of the more common patient problems confronting the chiropractor. They are not intended to replace either the clinician's clinical judgment or to establish a protocol for all patients with a particular condition. It should be understood that some patients will not fit the clinical conditions contemplated by such guidelines and that a guideline will rarely establish the only appropriate approach to the problem.

ATTRIBUTE 4

Practice standards and guidelines should be based on current information.

Scheduled Review—Practice guidelines must include statements about when they should be reviewed to determine whether revisions are warranted, given new clinical and research evidence or professional consensus (or lack of it).

There should be provisions for periodic reviews and revisions, when appropriate, of the practice guidelines as evidenced by:

- date of publication, or completion, is specified, and
- initial writing, review, or revision has occurred within the last three years.

ATTRIBUTE 5

Practice standards and guidelines should be widely disseminated.

There should be plans for wide distribution of the guidelines to the chiropractic practice community, evidenced by:

- source where guidelines will be available are noted and published, and
- mechanism by which guidelines will be distributed are identified.

Organizations of health care practitioners, health care consumers, peer reviewers, accrediting bodies, chiropractic academic centers, chiropractic educators, researchers, payers, and other appropriate groups will be encouraged to disseminate the guidelines to their members and constituents.

Successful implementation will depend on many factors in addition to the quality and credibility of the guidelines and their design process. Among those factors are: (1) the funding for dissemination and other implementation activities; (2) the incentives and supports for the guidelines to be used by practitioners, health plans, and others; (3) the accessibility, scope, accuracy, and timeliness of a variety of organizational information systems; and (4) the ability of multiple parties to plan and execute the various steps needed to implement guidelines.

Source: Reprinted with permission from *Attributes of Chiropractic Practice Guidelines* by Consortium for Chiropractic Research, March 1991.

Appendix B

General and Managed Care Glossary

Acute Care
Care for people whose illnesses or health problems are of a fairly serious nature, lasting over a fairly short period of time. General hospitals are usually classified as acute care facilities.

Acute Condition
A condition that has "lasted less than three months and which has involved either medical (chiropractic) attention or restricted activity," according to the National Center for Health Statistics.

ACS Contract
A contract between an insurance company and a self-funded plan where the insurance company performs administrative services only and does not assume any risk. Services usually include claims processing, but may include other services such as actuarial analysis and utilization review.

Actuarial Assumptions
The assumptions that an actuary uses in calculating the expected costs and revenues of the plan. Examples are utilization rates, age and sex mix of enrollees, and cost for medical services.

Algorithm
A logical progression of questions that should be asked of any procedure under evaluation. Throughout this scheme, various elements of the scientific method are incorporated. The analysis focuses on such principal issues as the identification of parameters, relation to known information, and published research.

Alternative Delivery System (ADS)
Usually HMOs and PPOs as alternatives to the traditional fee-for-service method of financing and delivery of health care services.

Anecdotal/Empirical
Depending on experience and observation. This includes categories and classifications of procedures, technologies, or equipment that have not received the benefit of the experimental method.

Appropriate
Having a reasonable chance to affect the patient's health positively in a cost-effective manner. Appropriate care neither undertreats nor overtreats the patient.

Aspect of Care
A significant quality-related component of a health care program. It is one of many such components that flow from a "scope of services" inventory conducted by the organization. When taken with other aspects of care, it provides a functional evaluation of organizational performance.

Assessment
The process of comparing performance against selected criteria and standards. Basically it equates to the monitoring and evaluation phase of the overall two-phase quality assurance process.

Audit
A structured system to generate data continuously for quality assurance monitoring and evaluation activity. It obtains information from a larger sample, generally through asking specific questions.

Benefit Package
The group of medical, hospital, and other health care services that an HMO or PPO provides to an enrollee in exchange for a premium fee.

Capitation
Method of payment for health services in which an HMO, medical group, doctor, or hospital is prepaid a fixed amount for each person served. The amount of money paid covers services provided, regardless of the actual number, nature, or value of those services and is usually expressed in units per member per month.

Case Law
Law established by judicial decisions.

CHAMPUS
Civilian Health and Medical Program of the Uniformed Services.

Chiropractic
A discipline of the scientific healing arts concerned with pathogenesis, diagnostics, therapeutics, pain syndromes, and neurophysiological effects related to the statics and dynamics of the locomotor system, especially of the spine and pelvis.

Chiropractic Physician
A health care professional licensed to treat human ailments without the use of drugs, medicine, and operative surgery; a primary health care provider and portal of entry to the health care delivery system.

Closed Panel
A managed health care plan that contracts with physicians on an exclusive basis for services, not allowing members to see physicians outside of the limited exclusive panel of providers for routine care.

CMP (Competitive Medical Plan)
A federal designation that allows a health plan to obtain eligibility to receive a Medicare risk contract without having to obtain qualification as an HMO. Requirements for eligibility are somewhat less restrictive than are those for an HMO.

Co-insurance
A provision in a member's (or covered insured) coverage that limits the amount of coverage by the plan to a certain percentage, commonly 80%. Any additional costs are paid by the member out-of-pocket.

Complainant
One who applies to the court for legal redress.

Comprehensive
Inclusive and of broad scope.

Concurrent
Validity designs that provide strategies for judging the extent to which an observation measures what it is intended to measure. This research paradigm involves the assumption that some previously developed measurement method is valid.

Concurrent Utilization Review
The process of monitoring the diagnosis and ensuing care decisions of a plan member while such care is being administered for the purpose of determining or confirming the appropriateness of the care. The objective is to provide optimum quality of care, while avoiding overutilization.

Consensus Development Program
A public evaluation of scientific information concerning biomedical technologies and arrival at consensus statements that will not only be useful to health care providers and the public at large, but also will serve as contributions to scientific thinking about the technologies in question.

Consent
A voluntary act by which one person agrees to allow someone else to do something. For medical liability purposes, consent should be in writing with an explanation of the procedures to be performed (*see* Informed Consent).

Consumer
One who may receive or is receiving health services. Although all people at times consume health care services, a consumer as the term is used in health legislation and programs is usually someone who is never a provider (ie, is not associated in any direct or indirect way with the provision of health services).

Co-payment
Fees or charges over and above the periodic fixed premium levied on plan-provided services on a per unit basis, as agreed upon in the plan contract. For example, some plans assess members an additional amount for each office visit or each prescription filled under the plan.

Cost Containment
Various methods used to control health care costs.

Cost-Effectiveness
The descriptive term used to contrast and compare types or schedules of care producing similar outcomes in terms of cost comparison. If a less expensive routine of care is proved to bring about a satisfactory outcome (ie, the same outcome as a more expensive routine of care), the less expensive routine is said to be "cost-effective."

CPT-4
Current Procedural Terminology, 4th edition. A set of five-digit codes that apply to medical services delivered. Frequently used for billing by professionals.

Criteria
Measurable characteristics of a health care service; predetermined elements against which the necessity, appropriateness, or quality of health care services may be compared. Often used synonymously with guidelines (*see* Standards).

Data
Information (either objective or subjective). Data provide the necessary means to compare actual performance with a standard of perceived quality.

Data Source
A place to find information needed to evaluate performance relative to established organizational standards for indicators of quality.

Deductible
That portion of a subscriber's (or member's) health care expenses that must be paid out-of-pocket before any insurance coverage applies. Deductibles are not allowed in federally qualified HMOs and are often not allowed under state HMO regulations, although co-payment requirements can achieve exactly the same result. They are common in insurance plans and PPOs.

Deposition
A sworn statement made out of court, which may be admitted into evidence if it is impossible for a witness to attend in person.

Diagnosis
The art and science of determining the nature and cause of a disease and differentiating among diseases or illnesses.

Disease
Literally, "without ease," a failure of the adaptive mechanisms of an organism to counteract adequately, normally, or appropriately the stimuli and

stresses to which it is subject, resulting in a disturbance in the function or structure of some part of the organism.

Disease is multifactorial and may be prevented or treated by changing any of the factors. Disease is very elusive and difficult to define, being largely socially defined. Thus criminality and drug dependence presently tend to be seen as diseases, whereas they were previously considered to be moral or legal problems (*see* Health).

Effectiveness

The degree to which diagnostic, preventive, therapeutic, or other actions achieve the intended results. Effectiveness requires a consideration of the cost of outcomes to be measured. It does not require consideration of the cost of the actions, although one way of comparing the effectiveness of actions with the same or similar intended results is to compare the ratios of their effectiveness to their costs.

Efficiency

The relationship between the quantity of inputs or resources used in the production of medical services and the quantity of outputs produced; the ability to produce the desired effect with a minimum of effort, expense, or waste.

Epistemology

The branch of philosophy dealing with the study of the nature of knowledge, its origin, foundations, limits, and validity.

EPO (Exclusive Provider Organization)

A form of CMP that is similar to an HMO. It uses primary care physicians as gatekeepers, often capitates providers, has a limited provider panel, and uses an authorization system; EPOs are generally regulated under insurance statutes rather than HMO regulations, however. Many states do not allow them, on the ground that EPOs are really HMOs.

(ERISA Employee Retirement Income Security Act)

A federal law that allows self-funded plans to avoid paying premium taxes or complying with state-mandated benefits, even when insurance companies and managed care plans must do so. Another provision requires that plans and insurance companies provide an explanation of benefits (EOB) statement to a member or covered insured in the event of a denial of a claim, explaining the reason that a claim was denied and informing the individual of his or her rights of appeal.

Evaluation

Comparison of actual performance with preestablished criteria and standards. This comparison may be based on actual data or on subjective judgment.

Experimental/Investigational

Not yet proved safe. This includes categories and classifications of procedures, technologies, or equipment not in widespread use within or among individual branches of health care disciplines, but nevertheless of such a nature, based on testing and clinical trial, that there is no organized scientific opposition to their use in health care. Although not orthodox, such items are removed from empiricism or quackery.

Expert Witness

An individual with sufficient expertise to establish the standard of due care, skill, and diligence for the jury and, further, to establish whether the standard has been breached.

Explicit

Objective and predetermined, as opposed to "implicit."

Fault

See Theory of Fault

Fee-for-Service

A method of charging whereby a physician or other practitioner bills for each encounter or service rendered. This is the usual method of billing by the majority of US physicians.

Gatekeeper

The primary care physician who, according to the rules and provisions of the plan contract, exercises responsibility for and control of the utilization of services of a given enrollee. The concept of "gatekeeper physician" is the cornerstone of HMO/prepaid plan efforts to deliver care at the optimum level and to avoid both underutilization and overutilization.

Health

"A state of complete physical, mental and social well-being and not merely the absence of disease or infirmity," according to the World Health Organization. Experts recognize, however, that health has many dimensions (eg, anatomical, physiological, and mental) and is largely culturally defined. The relative importance of various disabilities varies, depending on the cultural milieu and the role of the affected individual in that culture. Most attempts at measurement have taken a negative approach in that the degree of ill health has been assessed through morbidity and mortality rates. In general, the detection of changes in health status is easier than the definition and measurement of the absolute level of health.

Health Care System

The network of personal health care services, consisting of persons who give services, facilities and resources that support these services, financing mechanisms, the legal framework, and the communications and relationships that link one part of the system to another.

HCFA (Health Care Financing Administration)
The federal agency that oversees all aspects of health care financing for Medicare and also oversees the Office of Prepaid Health Care.

HMO (Health Maintenance Organization)
Prepaid organization that provides for health care in return for a preset amount of money on a per member per month basis. This is a group of physicians and other health care professionals who are organized to provide a wide range of services. There are four general types of HMO arrangements:
Group Model—an HMO with an exclusive contract with group practice physicians to provide health care to enrollees.
Staff Model—usually a clinic type facility in which the physicians work exclusively for the HMO.
Independent Practice Association—an HMO often organized by a group of physicians in a community. IPA physicians provide medical services in their own offices to prepaid plan subscribers *and* to traditional fee-for-service patients.
Network Model—a hybrid HMO that blends or combines elements of IPAs, group and staff models.

ICD-9-CM
International Classification of Diseases, 9th Revision, Clinical Modification. The classification of disease by diagnosis, codified into four-digit numbers. It is frequently used for billing purposes by hospitals.

Implicit
Subjective: based in opinion or judgment (often by "experts"), as opposed to "explicit."

Indemnity Insurance
Traditional medical insurance in which the insurance carrier reimburses individual persons or their providers for services *after* the service has been rendered.

Indicator of Quality
An important subset of an aspect of care that is actively monitored to determine how well the organization is doing with respect to a related aspect of care. Each indicator is important as part of an overall quality assurance program. Each should have its own standard, and each has the potential to affect the health of the patient in some fashion.

Individual Practice Association (IPA)
An organization of physicians who contract with an HMO to provide services to HMO members. The HMO pays the IPA; the IPA, in turn, compensates its member physicians, usually on a fee-for-service basis. IPA physicians work in their own offices, serving both HMO members and their own patients. There are several variations of the IPA model. In one, the individual physicians are reimbursed on a capitation rather than fee-for-service basis. In

another, (Network IPA) the HMO contracts with individual physicians, as well as with groups of physicians. In still another, the IPA is responsible for management and enrollment, as well as for delivering health care services.

Informed Consent

Consent, preferably in writing, obtained from a patient for a specific medical, surgical, or research procedure after the proposed procedure and risks involved have been fully explained in nontechnical terms and are understood by the patient. If the patient is a minor or is incapable of understanding or communicating, such consent may be obtained from a close adult relative, legal guardian, or the person with authority to grant consent.

Joint Commission on Accreditation of Healthcare Organizations

A private, nonprofit organization whose purpose is to encourage the attainment of uniformly high standards of institutional medical care.

Liability

An obligation that one has incurred or might incur through any act or failure to act.

Maintenance Services

A regimen designed to provide for the patient's continued well-being or to maintain the optimum state of health while minimizing reoccurrence of the clinical problem.

Malpractice

Professional misconduct, improper discharge of professional duties, or failure to meet the standard of care of a professional, resulting in harm to another.

Managed Care Organization (MCO)

A comprehensive, planned, and coordinated program of health care with emphasis on preventive care. Managed care is usually associated with HMO programs.

Manipulation (ACA definition)

Therapeutic application of manual force. Spinal manipulative therapy broadly defined includes all procedures in which the hands are used to mobilize, adjust, manipulate, apply traction, massage, stimulate, or otherwise influence the spine and paraspinal tissues with the aim of influencing the patient's health.

Manipulation (Gatterman)

A passive maneuver in which specifically directed manual forces are applied to vertebral and extravertebral articulations of the body with the object of restoring mobility to restricted areas.

Medical Necessity

Generally recognized reasons for treatment. When physicians accept patients for health care, the doctors automatically acknowledge that the patients' conditions will be recognized ones and that the examinations, tests and treatments used will be based on scientific studies and principles that are generally accepted by the profession at large as being necessary and appropriate to diagnose and treat patients with the particular conditions presented. Third-party contracts usually call for a direct relationship between covered services and medical necessity.

Medical Record

A record kept for each patient containing sufficient information to identify the patient, to justify the diagnosis and treatment, and to document results accurately. The content of the record is confidential.

Medically Stationary

The point in the care of a patient when no further improvement can be expected. This point is based upon the clinical evaluation of the patient.

Medicare (Title XVIII)

A nationwide health insurance program for people aged 65 and over, for persons eligible for Social Security disability payments for more than 2 years, and for certain workers and their dependents who need kidney transplantation or dialysis.

Meta-Analysis

The systematic evaluation and combination of results from separate studies of a particular subject. Such an analysis can be useful when individual studies disagree in their findings or are too small to yield conclusive answers.

Mixed Model

A managed care plan that mixes two or more types of delivery systems, traditionally an HMO that has both closed panel and open panel delivery systems.

Negligence

Carelessness, failure to act as an ordinary prudent person, or action contrary to that of a reasonable person.

Open Panel

A managed care plan that contracts (either directly or indirectly) with private physicians to deliver health care in their own offices. Examples are a direct contract HMO and an IPA.

Orthodox/Mainstream

Based on the scientific method. This includes all categories and classifications of procedures, technologies, or equipment in widespread use within or among individual branches of the health disciplines.

Outcome Measures

A measure of the quality of health care in which the standard of judgment is the attainment of a specified end result or outcome. The outcome of care is measured with such parameters as improved health, lowered mortality and morbidity, and improvement in abnormal states (eg, elevated blood pressure).

Overutilization
Treatments and/or tests performed in health care that are performed unnecessarily without therapeutic or diagnostic benefit.

Palliative Care
Relief of the symptoms of exacerbations with no net improvement in the patient's stationary condition.

Patient Satisfaction
The degree of confidence and gratification accompanying the delivery of health care services. Patient satisfaction relates strongly to perceptions on the part of the patient that his or her wishes are being carried out, that quality care is being delivered, and that patient sensitivities are being respected. These perceptions are based on subjective patient feelings and they may or may not deal with issues of technical appropriateness of care or outcomes.

PCP (Primary Care Physician)
Generally, an internist, pediatrician, family physician, general practitioner, and occasionally an obstetrician/gynecologist.

Peer Review
Generally, the evaluation by practicing physicians or other professionals of the effectiveness and efficiency of services ordered or performed by other practicing physicians or other members of the profession whose work is being reviewed (peers).

Performance Audit
A "peer review" audit of the performance of an organization's providers, based on the medical record. It generally collects information that only a member of the provider staff is competent to evaluate.

Perjury
The willful giving of false testimony under oath.

Plaintiff
The party to a civil suit who brings the suit seeking damages or other legal relief.

Point-of-Service Plan
A plan in which members do not have to decide how to receive services until they need them. For example, members of a simple PPO may receive coverage at a greater level if they use preferred providers than if they choose not to do so. These plans provide a dramatic difference in benefits (eg, 100% coverage vs 60% coverage), depending on whether the member chooses to use the plan providers and comply with the authorization system or go outside the plan for services.

Practice Guidelines
Standardized specifications for care developed by a formal process that incorporates the best scientific evidence of effectiveness with expert opinion.

Predictive Validity
Research that seeks to determine how well a measurement tool can forecast future performance or clinical outcome.

Preferred Provider Organization (PPO)
A health care plan that can be sponsored by business, labor, third-party payers, consumers, or providers. It offers a set of services to groups of individuals or provides incentives for groups of individuals to use selected providers. These services are provided on a contractual or predetermined basis.

Preventive Care
Treatment procedures considered necessary to prevent the development of clinical problems.

Primary Care
Basic or general health care that emphasizes the point at which the patient first seeks assistance from the health care system; care of the less complex and more common illnesses. The primary care provider usually assumes ongoing responsibility for the patient in both health maintenance and therapy of illness.

Privileged Communication (Confidential)
Any statement or communication made in confidence or trust to a person recognized by law as responsible for holding such communication in trust.

Problem Resolution
The second phase of the two-phase quality assurance process. When the first phase (monitoring and evaluation) identifies a problem (or opportunity to improve), this phase ensures that the identified problem is solved (or the opportunity to improve is taken advantage of).

Procedure Audit
An audit of the medical record to assess how well procedures are performed and documented by provider and support staff. It is often designed to be performed by clerical personnel.

Prophylaxis
Treatment designed to reduce or eradicate disease by removing or altering the responsible etiologic factors.

Prospective Review
Method of review that requires that each nonemergent hospital admission be authorized for necessity prior to admittance. The primary objective is to avoid unnecessary hospitalization for conditions that could be handled on a more cost-effective outpatient basis. Selected outpatient procedures in a clinical setting may also be reviewed in this way.

Protocol
The foundation for an explicit peer review process. The protocol defines a reasonable expectation of care. Protocols frequently, although not always,

include diagnostic and treatment criteria, as well as documentation criteria. The criteria in the protocol should be predetermined, clinically valid, and developed by the professional staff who will be participating in the peer review process.

Provider
A supplier of health care services (eg, hospital, physician, laboratory, or nursing home).

Proximate Cause
In negligence cases, a careless act that caused injury.

Quality Assurance
Activities and programs intended to ensure high-quality care in a defined health care setting or program. The programs must include educational or other components intended to remedy identified deficiencies in quality, as well as the components necessary to identify the deficiencies, such as peer review or utilization review components, and assess the program's own effectiveness. A program that identifies deficiencies in quality and responds only with negative sanctions, such as denial of reimbursement, is not usually considered a quality assurance program, although the latter may contain such sanctions.

Quality Care
The degree to which health care services for individuals and populations increase the likelihood of desired health outcomes and are consistent with current professional knowledge.

Reasonable and Customary Charge
A usual charge for medical service or treatment in the geographical area in which the treatment is rendered.

Rehabilitation Care
Procedures necessary for re-education or functional restoration of a disabled body system or part.

Retrospective Utilization Review
The examination of patient records and case histories after a care episode has been concluded to determine the appropriateness of the type and amount of care provided. Such procedures serve to identify a physician or physicians who are prone to overutilizing certain services.

Scope of Services Review
The process by which an organization essentially defines itself and its services (of all types). The resulting "inventory" of services facilitates selection of specific aspects of care to be monitored and evaluated.

Secondary Care
Services provided by specialists, who generally do not have first contact with patients (eg, neurologists). However, there has been a trend toward a self-

referral by patients to secondary care providers rather than through primary care providers.

Self-Insured or Self-Funded Plan

A healthcare plan in which the risk for medical cost is assumed by the company rather than the insurance company or managed care plan. Under ERISA, self-funded plans are exempt from certain requirements, such as premium taxes and mandatory benefits. Self-funded plans often contract with insurance companies or third-party administrators to administer the benefits.

Sensitivity

The proportion of correct positive results in a group of patients who actually have the disease in question. Highly sensitive tests are used to exclude or *rule out* disease.

SOAP

A method of recording information in a patient's record based on a problem-oriented clinical approach. It stands for Subjective, Objective, Assessment, and Prognosis.

Specificity

The proportion of correct negative results in a comparison group who do not have the target disease or condition. Highly specific tests are used to confirm or *rule in* the presence of disease.

Standard

An agreed upon level of excellence, established by an authority, custom, or general consent.

Standard, Consensual

Published statements about appropriate and preferred strategies of interaction with patients. Standards provide guidelines by which individual doctors may govern themselves and by which others may judge their professional behavior. Some standards specify purpose and ethics in professional life and are generally stable principles independent of research findings. Others, especially standards related to clinical technique, should depend upon rigorous clinical research as a source of authority.

Standard of Care

1. Those acts performed or omitted that an ordinary prudent person would have performed or omitted. It is a measure against which a defendant's conduct is compared.
2. Statements describing specific diagnostic or therapeutic maneuvers that should or should not be performed in certain clinical circumstances.

Standards of Practice

The patient's Bill of Rights, whereby all patients benefit from appropriate clinical evaluation of their complaint, including but not limited to case history; physical examination; clinical, x-ray, and laboratory tests; diagnosis; referral; and/or consultation. In chiropractic practice, this refers to those clinical standards taught in and through colleges accredited by the Council on Chiropractic Education.

Statute of Limitations

A legal limit on the time allowed for filing suit in civil matters, usually measured from the time of the wrong or from the time that a reasonable person would have discovered the wrong.

Stop-Loss

A form of re-insurance that provides protection for medical expenses above a certain limit, generally on a year-by-year basis. This may apply to an entire health care plan or to any single component.

Subpoena

A court order requiring one to appear in court to give testimony.

Subrogation

The contractual right of a health care plan to recover payments made to a member for health care costs after that member has received such payment for damages in a legal action.

Subscriber

Enrollee in an HMO or other health care plan.

Suit

A court proceeding in which one person seeks damages or other legal remedies from another.

Support Staff

Those staff members in an ambulatory care organization whose job is to support the provider staff in some manner in the care of patients. Among them are medical assistants, receptionists, cashiers, laboratory technicians, and x-ray technicians. Nurses and therapists may be classified as either provider staff or support staff, depending on their role in a particular organization.

Theory of Fault

The theory that persons who have suffered injury through the fault of a professional doctor should recover fair, just, and adequate damages for those injuries.

Therapeutic

Able to return the patient to a preclinical status or establishing a stationary status.

Third-Party Payer

Any organization, public or private, that pays or insures individuals and their families for health or medical expenses. The individual generally pays a premium for such coverage in all private and some public programs. Payments made on behalf of the covered person are called "third-party payments."

Threshold
A term developed by the Joint Commission on Accreditation of Healthcare Organizations to describe prospectively how close an organization must come to meeting a criterion before in-depth, second-level evaluation must be initiated.

Tort
The principle of responsibility. If a person is careless, and as a result of that carelessness, injures another person, the common law held the person who was careless to be responsible for the resulting injuries and losses of the injured person.

TPA (Third-Party Administrator)
A firm that performs administrative functions (eg, claims processing or membership) for a self-funded plan or a start-up managed care plan.

Treatment
The management and care of a patient for the purpose of combating disease or disorder; the application of medical-surgical knowledge and skill based upon a diagnosis.

Triple Option
The offering of an HMO, a PPO, and a traditional insurance plan by one carrier.

Two-phase Process
The sum of the two major components of the generic concept of quality assurance: (1) monitoring and evaluation, and (2) problem resolution.

UCR (Usual, Customary, and Reasonable Reimbursement)
A method of profiling prevailing fees in an area and reimbursing providers based on that profile. One common technology is to average all fees and choose the 90th percentile. This approach may be used concurrently with a fee schedule when the fee schedule is set relatively high.

Unbundling
The reduction of a multistep procedure to its components for the purpose of assigning multiple billing codes, thereby increasing charges.

Underutilization
The provision by a plan of less than an appropriate or adequate amount of proper care.

Underwriting
Bearing the risk for something (ie, a policy is underwritten by an insurance company); analyzing a group to determine rates or to determine if the group should be offered coverage at all.

Usual Charges
See UCR.

Utilization
The extent to which a given group uses specific services during a specific period of time.

Index

About the Editor

Herbert J. Vear, DC, LLD, is a professor in Chiropractic Sciences. He is Dean Emeritus at the Canadian Memorial Chiropractic College and President Emeritus from the Western States Chiropractic College. He authored *An Introduction to Chiropractic Science,* and he has pioneered concerns for consensus definitions and descriptions for chiropractic practice, scope of practice, standards of practice, and standards of care. Currently, he is retired, with an active interest in a number of chiropractic professional organizations.

About the Contributors

Robert Anderson, DC, MD, PhD, is a professor of Anthropology at Mills College, Oakland, California, and a Research Associate in Anthropology, at the University of California, Berkeley. He is a professor with the Life Chiropractic College, San Lorenzo, California, and a Fellow of the North American Spine Society. He was Research Director at Life Chiropractic College from 1978 to 1983.

Robert Boal, PhD, has been a faculty member of Western States Chiropractic College since 1976, and he is the Chair of the Basic Science Division at WSCC. He received his doctorate in biochemistry from Boston University.

Meridel I. Gatterman, MA, DC, is an associate professor at the Canadian Memorial Chiropractic College, where she is director of the Division of Chiropractic Sciences. She has served as a test committee member with the National Board of Chiropractic Examiners, and she is the author of the *Chiropractic Management of Spinal Related Disorders,* a textbook published by Williams & Wilkins in 1990. Dr. Gatterman is also a qualified chiropractic orthopedist and is certified as an Independent Medical Examiner in Oregon.

Richard G. Gillette, MS, PhD earned his doctorate with research on how the spinal cord processes noxious input from lumbar and paraspinal structures. He is with the Oregon Health Sciences University and the R.S. Dow Neurological Sciences Institute of Good Samaritan Hospital and Medical Center, Portland. He is an Assistant Professor of Neurophysiology and Associate Director of Research at Western States Chiropractic College.

Daniel T. Hansen, DC, is in private practice in Olympia, Washington. He serves as a technical advisor to the Back Pain Assessment Team of the National Center for Health Services Research and Technology Assessment and numerous health care and risk management groups. He is editorial advisor to *Chiropractic Technique* and *D.C. Tracts,* and associate editor of *Clinical Chiropractic Reports.* His contributions to chiropractic include editing an interim standards of care document for the State of Washington and serving as facilitator for the first two Chiropractic Consensus Conferences.

Donald Henderson, DC, is in private practice in Toronto, Ontario. He is chairman of the Canadian Chiropractic Association's Standards of Practice Committee. He was on the faculty of the Canadian Memorial Chiropractic College, where he was associate clinic director and associate professor of Clinical Sciences. He is chairman of the Chiropractic Advisory Committee of the Healing Arts Radiological Protection Commission, Ministry of Health, Ontario, a quality assurance administration. Currently he is the secretary-treasurer of the Canadian Chiropractic Association and a consultant to the Worker's Compensation Board of Ontario.

Robert L. Hirtle, Jr., JD, has served as a Judge Advocate in the US Navy, and as a Lieutenant Commander in the US Naval Reserves. He is in practice with the law firm of Rogin, Nassau, Caplan, Lassman & Hirtle in Hartford, Connecticut. He is prominent among attorneys specializing in malpractice cases and has been active with the chiropractic profession. He is a charter member, the past president, and now secretary-treasurer of the National Association of Chiropractic Attorneys. He remains a respected consultant to the chiropractic profession on matters of litigation.

Mark Kaminski, MS, is an assistant professor of Basic Science at Western States Chiropractic College. He teaches cell biology, histology, and genetics. Beyond his vigorous teaching responsibilities, Dr. Kaminski continues to pursue the study of his interests in health care evaluation and delayed onset post-exercise muscle soreness. He has served for a number of years as a consultant to the National Board of Chiropractic Examiners, and he currently serves as chairman of the Physiology Test-Assembly Committee.

Joseph C. Keating, Jr., PhD, is assistant editor of *Chiropractic Technique;* vice president of the National Institute of Chiropractic Research; an associate professor at the Palmer College of Chiropractic/West, Sunnyvale, California; and a member of the board of directors of the Association for the History of Chiropractic and the Stockton Foundation for Chiropractic research. He earned his doctorate in clinical psychology at the State University of New York, Albany. He has contributed numerous original papers and articles to the chiropractic literature.

William C. Meeker, DC, MPH, is dean of research, Palmer College of Chiropractic/West and president of the Consortium for Chiropractic Research. He serves on the editorial board of the *Journal of Manipulative and Physiological Therapeutics, Clinical Chiropractic Reports,* and *Chiropractic Technique.* He has consulted with the National Institutes of Health, the Rand Corporation, Corporate Health Policies Group, and the Veterans Administration on matters related to the chiropractic profession. Dr. Meeker has also been active in the American Public Health Association, serving as secretary and program director of the Chiropractic Forum.

David Peterson, DC, is currently an associate professor and chairman of the Division of Chiropractic Sciences at Western States Chiropractic College. He is an active member of the ACA, Council on Technique, Advisory Panel, chairing their terminology subcommittee, and also serves on the editorial review board of the *Journal of Manipulative and Physiological Therapeutics* and *Chiropractic Technique.*

Cynthia Peterson, RN, DC, is currently radiology lecturer at Anglo-European College of Chiropractic, Bournemouth, England. A former chair of the Department of Radiology, Western States Chiropractic College, in Portland, Oregon, she delivered postgraduate lectures for the Oregon Association of Naturopathic Physicians, Oregon X-ray Council, Western States Chiropractic College, and the Swiss Chiropractic Association.

Charles Alfred Simpson, DC, is a diplomate of the American Board of Chiropractic Orthopedists. He is on the staff of Western Medical Consultants in Portland, Oregon and is a consulting Independent Medical Evaluator from his office in Cornelius, Oregon. He has been very active in continuing education programs in Oregon to advance standards of practice and quality of care. He has served on the executive committee of the Chiropractic Society of Oregon for several years.

Richard Henry Tilden, DC, is a reviewer with the Utilization and Standards of Practice Board, Department of Labor and Industries, State of Washington, and chairman, Utilization and Review Committee of ChiroNet, a managed care organization. He is also on the board of directors for the Northwest Chiropractic Network, a Preferred Provider Organization, and chair of the Ethics and Standards of Practice Committee of the Chiropractic Society of Oregon. He has been active with numerous chiropractic organizations throughout the US. He maintains a particular interest in standards of practice, quality assurance, and utilization review processes in chiropractic.

Susan L. Vlasuk, DC, achieved diplomate status in radiology from the American Chiropractic Board of Radiology and is board-certified via examination by the American Chiropractic Board of Thermography. After conducting a general practice for 12 years, she has, for the past 8 years, limited her practice to diagnostic imaging and now operates an outpatient laboratory, providing consulting, thermographic, and radiologic services at the referral of treating doctors. Dr. Vlasuk chaired the American Chiropractic Association House of Delegates Study Committee on Thermology and was the charter president of the American Chiropractic College of Thermology, from 1986 to 1989.

Walter I. Wardwell, PhD, has written numerous papers on chiropractors and their sociological status within the health care movement. He is a sociology authority on the chiropractic profession and continues to study the profession in retirement. Dr. Wardwell is Professor Emeritus from the University of Connecticut, where he served from 1949 to 1984. He is a director of the Association for Chiropractic History.

Printed in Great Britain
by Amazon.co.uk, Ltd.,
Marston Gate.